Lifestyle Psychiatry

Lifestyle Psychiatry

Edited by

Douglas L. Noordsy, M.D.

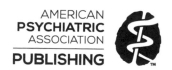

AMERICAN
PSYCHIATRIC
ASSOCIATION
PUBLISHING

Copyright © 2019 American Psychiatric Association Publishing

ALL RIGHTS RESERVED

First Edition

Manufactured in the United States of America on acid-free paper
23 22 21 20 19   5 4 3 2 1

American Psychiatric Association Publishing
800 Maine Avenue SW
Suite 900
Washington, DC 20024-2812
www.appi.org

Library of Congress Cataloging-in-Publication Data

Names: Noordsy, Douglas L., 1959– editor. | American Psychiatric Association Publishing, issuing body.
Title: Lifestyle psychiatry / edited by Douglas L. Noordsy.
Description: First edition. | Washington, D.C. : American Psychiatric Association Publishing, [2019] | Includes bibliographical references and index.
Identifiers: LCCN 2018061024 (print) | LCCN 2018061670 (ebook) | ISBN 9781615372522 (ebook) | ISBN 9781615371662 (pbk. : alk. paper)
Subjects: | MESH: Mental Disorders—therapy | Physical Therapy Modalities | Diet Therapy | Life Classification: LCC RC454 (ebook) | LCC RC454 (print) | NLM WM 400 | DDC 616.89—dc23Style | Health Behavior
LC record available at https://lccn.loc.gov/2018061024

British Library Cataloguing in Publication Data
A CIP record is available from the British Library.

Contents

PART I
THE BASIS OF LIFESTYLE PSYCHIATRY

PART II
EXERCISE IN THE PREVENTION AND MANAGEMENT OF SPECIFIC PSYCHIATRIC DISORDERS

PART III
HEALTHY BODY, HEALTHY MIND

PART IV
INSPIRING HEALTHY LIVING

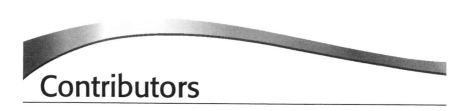

Contributors

Donna Ames, M.D.
Professor in Residence, David Geffen School of Medicine at UCLA, Los Angeles, California

Stephen J. Bartels, M.D., M.S.
Director, The Mongan Institute, and James J. and Jean H. Mongan Chair in Health Policy and Community Health, Department of Medicine, Massachusetts General Hospital, Harvard Medical School, Boston, Massachusetts

Fiona Barwick, Ph.D.
Clinical Assistant Professor, Stanford Sleep Medicine Center, Department of Psychiatry and Behavioral Sciences, Stanford University School of Medicine, Redwood City, California

Kacy Bonnet, M.D.
Staff Psychiatrist, Counseling and Psychological Services, University of California Santa Cruz, Santa Cruz, California

Jonathan Burgess, M.D.
Master of Public Health degree candidate, Columbia University Mailman School of Public Health, New York, New York

Rebekah Carney, Ph.D.
Research Associate, Youth Mental Health Research Unit, Greater Manchester Mental Health NHS Foundation Trust, Manchester, UK; Research Associate, Faculty of Biology, Medicine and Health, University of Manchester, Manchester, UK

Robert O. Cotes, M.D.
Medical Director, Inpatient Psychiatry at Grady Memorial Hospital; Director, PSTAR Clinic at Grady Memorial Hospital; Associate Residency Training Director, Department of Psychiatry and Behavioral Sciences, Emory University School of Medicine, Atlanta, Georgia

Laura Dunn, M.D.
Professor of Psychiatry and Behavioral Sciences and Director, Geriatric Psychiatry Fellowship Training Program, Department of Psychiatry and Behavioral Sciences, Stanford University, Stanford, California

Kayla Fair, Dr.P.H., R.N., M.P.H.
Postdoctoral Researcher, Department of Psychiatry, UT Southwestern Medical Center, Dallas, Texas

J. Kaci Fairchild, Ph.D.
Co-associate Director, Sierra Pacific Mental Illness Research Education Clinical Center (MIRECC) and Clinical Geropsychologist, VA Palo Alto Health Care System, Palo Alto, California; Clinical Assistant Professor, Stanford School of Medicine, Stanford, California

Erica Frank, M.D., M.P.H.
Professor and Canada Research Chair in Preventive Medicine and Population Health, University of British Columbia, Vancouver, British Columbia, Canada; Founder and President, www.NextGenU.org, Clear Lake, Washington; Principal Investigator, Healthy Doc=Healthy Patient, Nanoose Bay, British Columbia, Canada

Joseph Firth, Ph.D.
Senior Research Fellow, NICM Health Research Institute, Western Sydney University, Westmead, New South Wales, Australia; Honorary Research Fellow, Division of Psychology and Mental Health, University of Manchester, Manchester, UK; Honorary Research Fellow, Centre for Youth Mental Health, University of Melbourne, Melbourne, Victoria, Australia

Matthew J. Friedman, M.D., Ph.D.
Senior Advisor, National Center for PTSD, Veterans Administration Medical and Regional Office Center, White River Junction, Vermont; Professor of Psychiatry and Vice Chair for Research, Department of Psychiatry, Geisel School of Medicine, Dartmouth College, Hanover, New Hampshire

Michelle Guo, B.A.
Medical student, Department of Psychiatry, Perelman School of Medicine at the University of Pennsylvania, Philadelphia, Pennsylvania

Antonio Hardan, M.D.
Professor, Department of Psychiatry and Behavioral Sciences, Stanford University Medical Center, Stanford, California

Debora Holmes, M.E.S.
Chief Editor, NextGenU.org, Clear Lake, Washington

Keith Humphreys, Ph.D.
Esther Ting Memorial Professor, Department of Psychiatry and Behavioral Sciences, Stanford University, and Senior Research Career Scientist, Veterans Affairs Health Services Research and Development Service, Palo Alto, California

Masha Krasnoff, B.A.
Graduate student, UCLA, Los Angeles, California

Scott Kutscher, M.D.
Clinical Assistant Professor, Stanford Sleep Medicine Center, Department of Psychiatry and Behavioral Sciences, Stanford University School of Medicine, Redwood City, California

Anna Lembke, M.D.
Associate Professor of Psychiatry and Behavioral Sciences, Stanford School of Medicine, Stanford, California

Bethany Lerman, B.A.
Research Assistant, Sunnybrook Health Sciences Centre, Toronto, Ontario, Canada

Emeran A. Mayer, M.D.
Director, G. Oppenheimer Center for Neurobiology of Stress and Resilience, and Co-director, CURE: Digestive Diseases Research Center, Vatche and Tamar Manoukian Division of Digestive Diseases, David Geffen School of Medicine at UCLA, Los Angeles, California

Christie Mead, M.S.
PGSP-Stanford Psy.D. Consortium, Palo Alto University, Palo Alto, California

Douglas L. Noordsy, M.D.
Clinical Professor of Psychiatry and Behavioral Sciences, Stanford University School of Medicine, Stanford, California; Professor of Psychiatry, Geisel School of Medicine at Dartmouth, Hanover, New Hampshire

Amer Raheemullah, M.D.
Clinical Instructor, Psychiatry and Behavioral Sciences, Stanford School of Medicine, Stanford, California

Neil A. Rector, Ph.D.
Psychologist, Senior Scientist, and Director of Research, Thompson Anxiety Disorders Centre, Sunnybrook Health Sciences Centre; Professor, Departments of Psychiatry and Psychological Clinical Science, University of Toronto, Toronto, Ontario, Canada

Margaret A. Richter, M.D.
Associate Scientist, Sunnybrook Health Sciences Centre; Associate Professor, Department of Psychiatry, University of Toronto, Toronto, Ontario, Canada

Hyo Jin Ryu, B.S.
Research Associate, G. Oppenheimer Center for Neurobiology of Stress and Resilience, Vatche and Tamar Manoukian Division of Digestive Diseases, David Geffen School of Medicine at UCLA, Los Angeles, California

Tyler Sasser, Ph.D.
Acting Assistant Professor, Department of Psychiatry and Behavioral Sciences, University of Washington School of Medicine, Seattle, Washington

Erin Schoenfelder, Ph.D.
Assistant Professor, Department of Psychiatry and Behavioral Sciences, University of Washington School of Medicine, Seattle, Washington

Anup Sharma, M.D., Ph.D.
Research Fellow, Department of Psychiatry, Perelman School of Medicine at the University of Pennsylvania, Philadelphia, Pennsylvania

Alexander Sones, M.D.
Resident Physician, UCLA Semel Institute for Neuroscience, Los Angeles, California

David Spiegel, M.D.
Jack, Samuel and Lulu Willson Professor in Medicine, Department of Psychiatry and Behavioral Sciences, Stanford University, Stanford, California

Mark A. Stein, Ph.D., ABPP
Professor, Department of Psychiatry and Behavioral Sciences, and Adjunct Professor, Department of Pediatrics, University of Washington School of Medicine, Seattle, Washington

Shuichi Suetani, B.Sc., M.B., Ch.B., FRANCZCP
Psychiatrist, Metro South Mental Health and Addiction Services, Brisbane; Adjunct Research Fellow, Queensland Centre for Mental Health Research, The Park Centre for Mental Health, Wacol; Adjunct Research Fellow, Queensland Brain Institute, University of Queensland, St. Lucia, Queensland, Australia

Michael E. Thase, M.D.
Professor, Department of Psychiatry, Perelman School of Medicine at the University of Pennsylvania and the Corporal Michael J. Crescenz VAMC, Philadelphia, Pennsylvania

Madhukar H. Trivedi, M.D.
Professor of Psychiatry, Betty Jo Hay Distinguished Chair in Mental Health, Department of Psychiatry, and Director, Center for Depression Research and Clinical Care, UT Southwestern Medical Center, Dallas, Texas

Davy Vancampfort, Ph.D.
Lecturer, Department of Rehabilitation Sciences, KU Leuven–University of Leuven, Leuven; Research Fellow, UPC KU Leuven–University of Leuven University Psychiatric Centre, Kortenberg, Belgium

Janani Venugopalakrishnan, M.D., M.P.H.
Clinical Assistant Professor, Department of Psychiatry and Behavioral Sciences, Stanford University, Stanford, California

Marcus Vicari, B.S.
M.D. candidate, Perelman School of Medicine, University of Pennsylvania, Philadelphia, Pennsylvania

Martha C. Ward, M.D.
Director, Emory Psychiatry Residency Outpatient Psychotherapy Training Program, and Assistant Course Director, Essentials of Patient Care, Department of Psychiatry and Behavioral Sciences, Department of Medicine, Emory University School of Medicine, Atlanta, Georgia

Lynn Yudofsky, M.D.
Clinical Instructor, Department of Psychiatry and Behavioral Sciences, Stanford University, Stanford, California

DISCLOSURE OF INTERESTS

The following contributors to this book have indicated a financial interest in or other affiliation with a commercial supporter, a manufacturer of a commercial product, a provider of a commercial service, a nongovernmental organization, and/or a government agency, as listed below:

Robert O. Cotes, M.D.   *Advisory board*: Alkermes. *Speakers bureau*: Otsuka. *Speakers bureau*: Otsuka. *Research funding*: Alkermes, Lundbeck, Otsuke.

Douglas L. Noordsy, M.D.   *Research grant funding*: Janssen.

Emeran A. Mayer, M.D.   *Scientific advisory boards*: Axial Biotherapeutics, Amare, Danone, Pharmavite, Prolacta, Viome, Whole Biome. *Consultant*: General Mills, Host Therabiotics, Kelloggs, Kevita, Nestlé.

Michael E. Thase, M.D.   *Advisory/consultant*: Acadia, Alkermes, Allergan (Forest, Naurex), AstraZeneca, Cerecor, Eli Lilly, Fabre-Kramer Pharmaceuticals, Inc., Gerson Lehrman Group, Guidepoint Global, Johnson & Johnson (Janssen, Ortho-McNeil), Lundbeck, MedAvante, Inc., Merck, Moksha8, Nestlé (PamLab), Novartis, Otsuka, Pfizer, Shire, Sunovion, Takeda. *Grant support*: Agency for Healthcare Research and Quality, Alkermes, AssureRx, Avanir, Forest Pharmaceuticals, Janssen, Intracellular, National Institute of Mental Health, Otsuka Pharmaceuticals, Takeda. *Royalties*: American Psychiatric Foundation, Guilford Publications, Herald House, W.W. Norton & Company, Inc. *Spouse's employment*: Peloton Advantage, which does business with Pfizer and AstraZeneca.

The following contributors have indicated that they have no financial interests or other affiliations that represent or could appear to represent a competing interest with the contributions to this book:

Donna Ames, M.D.; Fiona Barwick, Ph.D.; Jonathan Burgess, M.D.; J. Kaci Fairchild, Ph.D.; Michelle Guo, B.A.; Debora Holmes, M.E.S.; Keith Humphreys, Ph.D.; Masha Krasnoff, B.A.; Scott Kutscher, M.D.; Hyo Jin Ryu, B.S.; Tyler Sasser, Ph.D.; Anup Sharma, M.D., Ph.D.; Alexander Sones, M.D.; David Spiegel, M.D.; Shuichi Suetani, B.Sc., M.B., Ch.B., FRANCZCP; Janani Venugopalakrishnan, M.D., M.P.H.; Marcus Vicari, B.S.; Lynn Yudofsky, M.D.

Foreword

Beth Frates, M.D.

Lifestyle prescriptions are powerful medicine. Hippocrates wrote about many of the basic principles of lifestyle medicine centuries ago. Some of these include "Let food be thy medicine and medicine be thy food"; "Walking is man's best medicine"; and "If we could give every individual the right amount of nourishment and exercise, not too little and not too much, we would have found the safest way to health." Thousands of years later, we have research data to support the use of the exercise prescription, nutrition prescription, and the coach approach to counseling patients about adopting and sustaining healthy habits.

My journey in lifestyle medicine started when I was 18 years old and my father had a massive myocardial infarction and subsequent cerebral artery infarct, leaving him paralyzed on the left side. Prior to his heart attack and stroke, my father ate fast food, did not exercise, slept 5 hours or less, worked 80 hours a week, did not socialize much or have close connections with loved ones, and was experiencing chronic stress. My father made a complete recovery (except for some fine motor movement in his left hand), and he made a complete lifestyle change. I have been a firm believer in the powers of lifestyle prescriptions because my father lived the best 27 years of his life after his devastating health setback.

With the help of some of the forefathers in lifestyle medicine, including Nathan Pritikin and Dean Ornish, my father was able to learn about the medicinal benefits of nutrition, exercise, and social connection. In the 1980s, only a few physicians were using lifestyle medicine principles to help patients recover from and prevent disease. Dr. Dean Ornish was doing groundbreaking research at the time, and 30 years later his efforts have resulted in an evidence-based lifestyle program that is covered by insurance. Many other individuals have done groundbreaking work and research that have allowed this new medical subspecialty to exist. Today, resources include the American College of Lifestyle Medicine (www.lifestylemedicine.org), the American Board of Lifestyle Medicine (https://ablm.co), and a certification examination to become a board-certified lifestyle medicine physician or board-certified lifestyle medicine specialist. The field has come a long way.

At the time of my father's stroke, I was in college, and his health setback as well as his recovery inspired me to become premed at Harvard College. My research and focus on exercise, nutrition, and stress started in the mid-1980s. I wrote my thesis about the impact of mental stress on the functioning of the heart. In medical school at Stanford University, I performed research on the impact of different diets on the endothelial cells in the arteries, specifically looking at diets rich in nitric oxide. After medical school, I did an internship in medicine at Massachusetts General Hospital and then completed my residency in the Department of Physical Medicine and Rehabilitation at Spaulding Rehabilitation Hospital. I went on to focus on stroke and completed research on lifestyle medicine topics. One important study I participated in while a resident was on exercise habits, personal habits, and counseling habits of physicians (Abramson et al. 2000). My colleagues and I found that physicians who exercise also counsel on exercise—specifically, physicians who did strength training counseled on strength training, whereas physicians who did aerobic exercise counseled on aerobic exercise. If physicians did both, they counseled on both. If physicians did neither, they counseled on neither. This study has been replicated many different times by others since our original publication in 1999 (see Chapter 18, "Physician Lifestyle and Health-Promoting Behavior").

After residency, I focused on stroke and coauthored a book about preventing a second stroke with some colleagues at Spaulding, Dr. Joel Stein and Dr. Julie Silver (Stein et al. 2006). For that book, I researched diet, nutrition, and stress and read as many studies as possible so that I could make recommendations that were evidence based. The book was published in 2006, and at that time, I started lecturing on the powers of exercise, diet, and stress management. Dr. Edward Phillips, director of the Institute of Lifestyle Medicine (ILM) at Harvard, explained to me that what I was doing was *lifestyle medicine*, a term I had never heard of before. My efforts to get patients to eat a healthy diet, exercise regularly, and manage their stress were all consistent with the work of Dean Ornish and other forefathers in the field of lifestyle medicine. I became the director of medical student education at the ILM, where I served as codirector for continuing medical education courses on exercise and basic lifestyle medicine principles; 2018 marks the tenth year of these courses. In addition, I started the first lifestyle medicine interest group (LMIG) at Harvard, and this LMIG is now an official interest group at Harvard. As faculty advisor, I give some presentations on lifestyle medicine topics and help guide the group with their activities. The idea of LMIGs has been replicated at many different schools now. Stanford was one of the first medical schools to implement them.

With the increasing numbers of patients diagnosed with obesity and diabetes in the United States and worldwide, there is growing interest in lifestyle medicine principles to help prevent, treat, and reverse these conditions. Cardiac disease remains the number one killer (Nichols 2017), and it is well known that exercise, diet, and stress management can help patients avoid and recover from a cardiac event (Mokdad et al. 2004). However, it is not just diseases of the body that are influenced by lifestyle; depression and anxiety are also alleviated by healthy habits such as exercise, healthy diet, stress management, sound sleep, and high-quality social connections. The field of lifestyle psychiatry is rapidly emerging. There are psychiatrists who have set up two treadmills in their offices, side by side. Instead of a patient sitting on a couch for therapy, the patient and the therapist walk during the sessions. Research tells us that exercise helps decrease the state of anxiety and increase "out of the box" thinking and can increase feelings of well-being, all of which can be helpful in a therapy session (Anxiety and Depression Association of America 2018; Wong 2014).

Prescribing exercise is not the same as prescribing antibiotics or antidepressants. There are similarities, in that dose and frequency are determined, but the main difference is that the patient has some say in the prescription details when it comes to a lifestyle medicine prescription. For many practicing physicians in cardiology, physiatry, internal medicine, endocrinology, and other specialties, collaborating with the patient and working together to co-create goals is foreign. Many physicians are used to writing a prescription and dictating the care. Psychiatrists and therapists are much more in tune with the supportive counseling and motivational interviewing techniques that a clinician needs to use to counsel a patient on lifestyle change. As Hippocrates said, "It's far more important to know what person the disease has than what disease the person has." Getting to know patients and meeting them where they are with respect to their interest in making changes is key in lifestyle medicine counseling. This is the area that many physicians find most challenging. Counseling patients to adopt healthy habits is more like a dance than a wrestling match. It is not about convincing the patient to exercise more; rather, it is about giving the patient the space to convince himself or herself that exercise is essential and to determine how it can become a daily or weekly routine. Knowing how to counsel our patients on lifestyle changes is just as important as knowing the guidelines for exercise, diet, or sleep.

It has been thousands of years since Hippocrates first shared some of the major principles of lifestyle medicine, and now these principles are becoming part of mainstream medicine. Dr. James Rippe edited the first major medical textbook in lifestyle medicine in 1999 (Rippe 1999), and the third edition of that textbook is due out in 2019. The textbook is thousands of pages long. To know and practice lifestyle medicine is to keep up with the times and provide the best evidence-based counseling and prescriptions. The book you are reading gives you the information, tools, and tips you need to successfully incorporate lifestyle medicine into your own practice. It might even motivate you to adopt these healthy behaviors yourself if you have not already done so.

Beth Frates, M.D.
Assistant Professor of Physical Medicine and Rehabilitation
Harvard Medical School
Boston, Massachusetts

REFERENCES

Abramson S, Stein J, Schaufele M, et al: Personal exercise habits and counseling practices of primary care physicians: a national survey. Clin J Sport Med 10(1):40–48, 2000 10695849

Mokdad AH, Marks JS, Stroup DF, Gerberding JL: Actual causes of death in the United States, 2000. JAMA 291(10):1238–1245, 2004 15010446

Anxiety and Depression Association of America: Exercise for Stress and Anxiety. Silver Spring, MD, Anxiety and Depression Association of America, 2018. Available at: https://adaa.org/living-with-anxiety/managing-anxiety/exercise-stress-and-anxiety. Accessed January 9, 2019.

Nichols H: The top 10 leading causes of death in the United States. Medical News Today, updated February 23, 2017. Available at: www.medicalnewstoday.com/articles/282929.php. Accessed January 9, 2019.

Rippe JM: Lifestyle Medicine. London, Blackwell Science, 1999

Stein J, Silver J, Frates EP: Life After Stroke: The Guide to Recovering Your Health and Preventing Another Stroke. Baltimore, MD, Johns Hopkins University Press, 2006

Wong M: Stanford study finds walking improves creativity. Stanford News, April 24, 2014. Available at: https://news.stanford.edu/2014/04/24/walking-vs-sitting-042414. Accessed: January 9, 2019.

Preface

My journey in lifestyle psychiatry started with a need for breaks from long hours of studying in medical school. Washington University's medical campus is located on the edge of Forest Park, so I started running along the park's trails. I had enjoyed sports throughout my childhood, but running had always seemed a necessary evil, part of getting in shape for basketball season. Now running transformed into a soothing experience of calm contemplation and connection to the trees, sunshine, and sky outside my room. My excursions gradually lengthened until I could comfortably complete an 8-mile loop around the park. I sustained myself through internship with runs up Goose Pond Road in Canaan, New Hampshire, then entered a fun run around Canaan Lake in the town's Old Home Days celebration. A few years later, I crossed the finish line of the Boston Marathon. I also completed Dartmouth-Hitchcock's annual century ride and have taken up yoga, sculling, kayaking, and cross-country skiing.

As I experienced the value of exercise, diet, and mind-body practice for self-care, I began to raise the topic with my patients. During my community mental health care for young adults with co-occurring substance abuse and severe mental illness, I used physical activity as a backdrop for building therapeutic alliance and reconnecting my patients to their prior passions and the rewards of exercise. Some time later, while supporting a young man with schizophrenia through stages of expanding exercise and recovery, I agreed to run his first marathon with him, only to find myself gasping to keep up with his pace. He greeted me at the finish line, having crossed 30 minutes prior. The success of these efforts led me to study the literature on lifestyle interventions in psychiatry, discuss it in my teaching and writing, and direct my research toward making a contribution. Coming to Stanford University created the opportunity for me to place lifestyle and sports psychiatry at the center of my career.

This book is dedicated to the many patients who have taught me about the transformative power of living well. I am also indebted to the many chapter authors for their elegant contributions. This book could not have happened without the intellectual stimulation and support of many fine colleagues. I am particularly grateful to Laura Roberts for her vision in encouraging me to pursue lifestyle psychiatry and in asking me to lead the sports psychiatry program at Stanford. Laura conceptualized this book and gave me the opportunity to write it and publish it with American Psychiatric Association Publishing. She also introduced the concept of *the new psychiatry*.

I am grateful to Mickey Trockel and Lynn Yudofsky for their partnership in developing lifestyle psychiatry at Stanford. Francesco Dandekar, Lisa Post, and Kelli Moran-Miller have been invaluable partners in developing the sports psychiatry program at Stanford. Jake Ballon has been a generous and stimulating collaborator in developing the INSPIRE clinic research program on physical exercise for people with psychosis. Kaci Fairchild, Marily Oppezzo, and Jeff Christle were instrumental in developing BrainEx, Stanford's research collaborative on physical exercise and the brain.

Finally, and most importantly, I am grateful to my dear wife, Mary, and my loving family for tolerating my absence during excursions in the natural world, for sharing big brunches on my return, and for patiently tolerating the many hours dedicated to this volume. My beautiful children, Charlotte and Jack, spent their early years on excursions to mountaintops, blackberry patches, and secluded ponds. Our faithful canine companions, Bridey and Zinnia, became my dedicated adventure partners until they could go no more. I also thank my parents for introducing me to the beauty of the natural world and for modeling a lifetime of cultivating living well.

Douglas L. Noordsy
Palo Alto, California
Silver Bay, New York

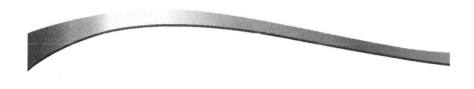

PART I

The Basis of Lifestyle Psychiatry

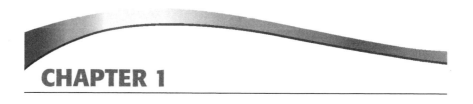

CHAPTER 1

Introduction to Lifestyle Psychiatry

Douglas L. Noordsy, M.D.

KEY POINTS

- Lifestyle psychiatry is a component of lifestyle medicine that focuses on management of psychiatric disorders through an integrated, holistic approach to health.
- The term *lifestyle* in medical care refers to physical activity, diet and nutrition, adequate sleep, and stress management.
- Lifestyle psychiatry goes beyond the biopsychosocial model to include specific recommendations for exercise, diet, sleep, and mindfulness practice for helping people manage their psychiatric disorders.
- Lifestyle interventions may complement medication and psychotherapy by impacting such domains as cognitive impairment, amotivation, and self-efficacy.
- Lifestyle interventions have been demonstrated to exert neurobiological and epigenetic effects; physical exercise is the most potent intervention known for stimulating synaptic plasticity.
- Lifestyle psychiatry offers the opportunity to address life balance and immersion in nature.

This book is designed to open the world of lifestyle psychiatry to primary care and mental health practitioners and their patients. Incorporating lifestyle interventions can make psychiatric practice more gratifying and more effective. We review the burgeoning body of evidence demonstrating the efficacy of physical exercise, diet, mind-body practices, and restorative sleep for preventing and managing psychiatric disorders—in other words, achieving health and wellness. This evidence includes studies in which lifestyle practices are the primary intervention as well as studies that combine lifestyle practices with traditional treatments such as psychopharmacology or psychotherapy. The evidence supporting the efficacy of lifestyle interventions in psychiatry is now so robust that clinicians can feel confident recommending them as evidence-based practices. In fact, public awareness has grown to the point that many patients ask about lifestyle interventions as a component of their care. As providers, our role is to help guide patients in separating evidence-based recommendations from unhelpful or untested ideas.

Lifestyle psychiatry is part of a larger lifestyle medicine movement. Lifestyle medicine was founded on the principle that traditional interventions such as medications and surgery are powerful tools for treatment but have limited efficacy in addressing modifiable risk factors of chronic disease, including poor nutrition, physical inactivity, and chronic stress (Bortz 1984). Lifestyle medicine seeks to reduce disease burden and improve health by addressing the modifiable contributors to chronic illness. It reframes chronic illness syndromes as *lifestyle deficiency syndromes*, which may be more etiologically accurate and can lead to curative interventions. For example, if a person's hypertension is substantially based in overweight, inactivity, stress, and overuse of alcohol, medication will only palliate and will not cure the hypertension. Patients often feel trapped by an endless cycle of trips to the pharmacy, copays, and life-limiting side effects and struggle to balance the pressure to be a good patient with a desire to have more fundamental autonomy in governing their health status. The promise of medicine often devolves into a muddy compromise of using partially effective medications with substantial side-effect burden in order to try to stave off long-term risks while avoiding talking about the powerful agents of daily life health practices.

Practitioners who are frustrated with the limits of prescribing medications that only partially correct blood sugar or blood pressure and result in nausea, fatigue, or sexual dysfunction may be rejuvenated by helping their patients achieve better health and feel better through exercise, diet, and stress management when they adopt lifestyle medicine approaches. However, it may be uncomfortable for providers—and patients—to discuss lifestyle interventions. Providers lack formal education regarding lifestyle interventions, and patients live in an environment of pervasive cultural influences that work against implementing lifestyle recommendations. Lifestyle medicine recognizes that these issues must be addressed in order for patients to receive optimum medical care.

Lifestyle psychiatry is becoming a subspecialty of lifestyle medicine that focuses on the role of diet, physical activity, stress, and sleep in contributing to the onset and maintenance of psychiatric disorders. Lifestyle interventions may have particular relevance in psychiatry because the complicated interplay between mind and brain has limited our capacity to move beyond syndromic diagnosis, and psychosocial factors have been shown to contribute to all psychiatric disorders. Like lifestyle medicine, lifestyle psychiatry is most effective for the prevention and management of chronic illness and has less support in acute illness. Lifestyle medicine's focus on health and wellness brings us back to our roots as healers and, importantly, engages patients in assuming responsibility for their well-being. In this era of questioning the value and risks of psychotropic medications and interventional procedures, providers and patients can find common ground in identifying the value and limits of pharmacological, psychotherapeutic, and lifestyle interventions and developing a plan for how to optimally apply them to meet the patient's goals.

WHAT IS MEDICINE?

According to *Merriam-Webster*, *medicine* can be defined as "the science and art dealing with the maintenance of health and the prevention, alleviation, or cure of disease." Over the 75 years since the introduction of penicillin to treat infections, practitioners and patients have been lured by the exciting possibility that medication and other procedures could cure disease and return people to health. The dramatic rise in placebo response rates over every decade since the 1960s (Weimer et al. 2015) is a testament to public belief in the power of pills. Medicine has become equated with medication. Although the acute illness/cure model remains the archetype of modern medicine, the nonacute management of health and chronic disease may have a more powerful effect on a patient's life course and outcomes.

Although most practitioners would agree that lifestyle factors contribute to their patients' disorders, many feel unprepared to address lifestyle in their care of patients. As practitioners trained in modern medicine, we are indoctrinated in the belief that the realm of medicine is properly those things over which practitioners have exclusive authority. This is what our training focuses on. Medical training is required to order medical tests, procedures, and prescriptions, but anyone can provide advice and make decisions about how often to play tennis and what to eat.

As we enter the age of precision medicine, in which treatment is customized to individual etiology, physicians must think beyond traditional approaches of providing what we are comfortable with or good at and focus on how we can tailor best practices to address the precise causes of each patient's specific disease (Berman 2018). The precision medicine approach requires attention to lifestyle factors as key contributors to disease as well as barriers to full recovery. By contrast, no specific etiological basis has been established for a DSM-5 psychiatric disorder (American Psychiatric Association 2013; Kapur et al. 2012). We will improve the specificity, effectiveness, and cost of our health care system only if we address patients holistically and make treatment recommendations that include the full range of contributors to patients' distress. This is what patients and family members expect of their health care providers and increasingly what society expects of our health care systems.

WHAT IS LIFESTYLE?

The inception of a field is an important point for defining terminology. Lifestyle psychiatry is distinct from classical biopsychosocial psychiatry. The term *lifestyle* has multiple uses and carries connotations that we do not typically associate with the practice of medicine, psychiatry, or psychology. Lifestyle may be used to refer to where one lives or the form of transportation one takes to work. The concept of lifestyle is often used to sell material goods. This leaves the term tainted and imprecise. In conceptualizing this book, I gave extensive thought to alternatives to lifestyle as a defining term.

Wellness is perhaps the best alternative to lifestyle for defining a field that focuses on using health-related behaviors to optimize health. Although the term wellness psychiatry has appeal, it is similarly imprecise because it does not focus attention on life choices and behaviors. Using the term wellness also misses the opportunity to align with the established field of lifestyle medicine at a time when integration of psychiatry and primary care is central to quality care. Therefore, this book uses the term *lifestyle psychiatry* in alignment with the practice of our colleagues in general medicine.

WHAT IS A SYNDROME AND WHAT IS A TREATMENT?

As in lifestyle medicine, there is an underlying philosophical question of whether to view lifestyle interventions as treatments or to view healthy lifestyle as the normal state and exercise deficiency or stress response, for example, as a syndrome. As you read through the chapters of this book, be thoughtful about how you conceptualize illness and treatment. If you find compelling links between lifestyle behaviors and the initiation or perpetuation of the disorders you treat, this may shape the nature of your discussions with patients about how to understand their disorder and where to position lifestyle interventions in the treatment armamentarium. This approach may also help patients to view adopting positive health behaviors as an opportunity to achieve life balance rather than as a constraint, which is more likely to result in collateral and sustained healthy lifestyle changes over time.

HOW DO LIFESTYLE INTERVENTIONS EXERT THEIR EFFECTS?

In Chapter 2 ("Physical Exercise and the Brain"), we focus on the neuroscience of exercise and its impact on brain function and brain health. In the chapters of Parts II and III, we reveal the depth of the science of exercise, mind-body practices, diet, and sleep on specific psychiatric categories. Across these chapters we see patterns, including stimulation of neurotrophic factors that leads to increases in synaptogenesis and regional brain volumes. We also note that sustained lifestyle habits are associated with epigenetic changes that may be passed through generations (Denham 2018).

In Part IV we explore the impact of lifestyle behaviors on self-image and therapeutic alliance. Engaging patients in examining the role of their choices in their distress can feel challenging at first, but it allows a partnership of observation and empowerment to emerge in the treatment relationship. Lifestyle psychiatry is recovery oriented and can create powerful opportunities for patients to develop self-efficacy, which may magnify gains in other domains. Such practices as meditation and exercise may directly trigger brain reward pathways, providing useful alternatives to destructive and addictive reward triggers. Lifestyle practices may also have synergistic power. For example, many mind-body practices incorporate meditation, and sustained exercise is associated with a calm, contemplative mental state. Helping people to find reliable methods within their control to alter their distress can be empowering and build confidence.

It is somewhat remarkable how broadly lifestyle interventions affect mental health and wellness. This suggests the presence of both generalized and specific effects on brain health, which expands the toolkit of psychiatric providers beyond managing neurotransmitter levels. As you review the chapters in this book, allow yourself to be amazed by the breadth of impact a simple intervention such as physical activity can have on mental health and consider the mechanisms that may underlie such generalization. Consider also how patterns of unhealthy lifestyle behavior can interact with and magnify each other during disease onset and perpetuation.

POTENTIAL FOR PREVENTION OF ONSET OF PSYCHIATRIC DISORDERS

Emerging evidence is identifying that, in addition to helping patients manage existing psychiatric disorders, healthy lifestyle behaviors have value for reducing rates of onset of psychiatric disorders (Johnson et al. 2017). Recent evidence of rising rates of psychiatric disorders and suicide, especially among transitional-age youth and young adults, raises concern about the generational consequences of unhealthful lifestyle behaviors as well as the impact of immersion in rapidly disseminating Internet technologies on lifestyle and wellness (Substance Abuse and Mental Health Services Administration 2018). Lifestyle psychiatry has importance for population health as well as individual health and may inform best practices for societal interventions to support the wellness of generations to come.

AN EVOLUTIONARY PERSPECTIVE

As you explore the evidence in this volume detailing the impact of lifestyle behaviors on mental health and well-being, consider why these relationships may exist. What advantages for human survival were created by the association of physical exercise with synaptic proliferation, brain health, and learning? Why might some dietary elements be associated with mental health and others with depression? Why might adequate sleep optimize cognitive and motor function? Why might letting go of our amazing ability to think and plan in order to focus for short periods on the present moment be associated with mental well-being? Although these questions may be largely unanswerable, considering their implications can help place this body of evidence into context and provide useful analogies for working with patients.

BENEFITS OF LIFESTYLE PSYCHIATRY FOR THE PRACTITIONER

In Chapter 18, "Physician Lifestyle and Health-Promoting Behavior," we review evidence on the impact of practitioners' health behaviors on their engagement in lifestyle medicine. There is also potential for the practice of lifestyle medicine to motivate the provider. As we immerse ourselves in the evidence supporting lifestyle practices on health outcomes, it is common to become increasingly interested in trying out various lifestyle steps in our own lives. Reminders of the benefits of eating certain foods or practicing mindfulness may lead to sampling those behaviors. The more we try, the more likely these behaviors may evolve into sustained patterns that have synergies in our own lives and ripple effects for our patients. New evidence emerges all the time and may inspire the attentive psychiatrist or psychologist to continue to fine-tune his or her personal health behaviors.

POTENTIAL RISKS

It is important to acknowledge that there are risks of overdoing in lifestyle practice as in other types of interventions and behaviors. People can become so restrictive in their diet or so excessive in their exercise or meditation practices as to do harm (see case example in Chapter 8, "Exercise and Addiction"). People can become obsessively focused on lifestyle to the point that they are constrained in their interests or daily function. As you assess and monitor health behaviors, keep the possibility of overdoing in mind and be prepared for the need to address balance.

The authors of this volume seek to support the efforts of psychiatrists and mental health and primary care professionals to deliver lifestyle-informed psychiatry well by collating the evidence to support its areas of efficacy as well as effective approaches to delivery. We also aim to provide evidence and wise practices that may inform novel approaches to health care delivery. Finally, we hope to stimulate much-needed conversation about how to maximize the value of health care through incorporating thoughtful, sophisticated approaches to optimizing wellness. After all, health and wellness are about all of us, and we have a responsibility to ensure a society and a health care system that provide our sons, daughters, brothers, sisters, parents, and friends with guidance and care that can support each individual in achieving optimal wellness.

DISCUSSION QUESTIONS

1. Why is lifestyle medicine such a popular concept in modern society?
2. How does lifestyle psychiatry fit the precision medicine model?
3. How can lifestyle psychiatry support a shared decision-making approach and build self-efficacy?
4. Do you think of lifestyle interventions as treatments or as a return to an evolutionarily normative state? How do you present these interventions to your patients?
5. Why is adopting a healthy lifestyle associated with greater efficacy at delivering lifestyle medicine?

RECOMMENDED READINGS

Bortz WM, Stickrod R: The Roadmap to 100: The Breakthrough Science of Living a Long and Healthy Life. St. Martin's Press, New York, 2010
Lam CW, Riba M (eds): Physical Exercise Interventions for Mental Health. Cambridge, UK, Cambridge University Press, 2016

REFERENCES

American Psychiatric Association: Diagnostic and Statistical Manual of Mental Disorders, 5th Edition. Arlington, VA, American Psychiatric Association, 2013
Berman JJ: Precision Medicine and the Reinvention of Human Disease. London, Academic Press, 2018
Bortz WM: The disuse syndrome. West J Med 141(5):691–694, 1984 6516349
Denham J: Exercise and epigenetic inheritance of disease risk. Acta Physiol (Oxf) 222(1):1–20, 2018 28371392

Johnson R, Robertson W, Towey M, et al: Changes over time in mental well-being, fruit and vegetable consumption and physical activity in a community-based lifestyle intervention: a before and after study. Public Health 146:118–125, 2017 28404463

Kapur S, Phillips AG, Insel TR: Why has it taken so long for biological psychiatry to develop clinical tests and what to do about it? Mol Psychiatry 17(12):1174–1179, 2012 22869033

Substance Abuse and Mental Health Services Administration: Key Substance Use and Mental Health Indicators in the United States: Results From the 2017 National Survey on Drug Use and Health (HHS Publ No SMA 18-5068, NSDUH Series H-53). Rockville, MD, Center for Behavioral Health Statistics and Quality, Substance Abuse and Mental Health Services Administration, 2018. Available at: www.samhsa.gov/data. Accessed January 9, 2019.

Weimer K, Colloca L, Enck P: Placebo effects in psychiatry: mediators and moderators. Lancet Psychiatry 2(3):246–257, 2015 25815249

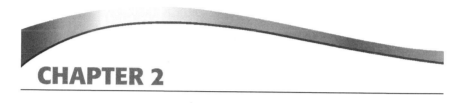

CHAPTER 2

Physical Exercise and the Brain

Joseph Firth, Ph.D.

Rebekah Carney, Ph.D.

KEY POINTS

- The link between physical fitness and cognitive abilities appears to stem from common factors driving functional increases in both of these throughout the course of our evolution as a species.
- There is now compelling evidence from clinical trials that aerobic exercise can significantly improve brain function in both psychiatric samples and the general population.
- The evidence for resistance training affecting the brain is currently nascent but highly promising as an additional approach for improving cognition via exercise interventions.

HEALTHY BODY, HEALTHY MIND: THE HISTORY OF EXERCISE AND THE BRAIN

The concept of physical exercise being inexplicably linked to the healthy mind predates modern medicine itself. The great philosopher Socrates (470–399 B.C.) often spoke of the overarching benefits of physical activity, saying, "Surely a person of sense would submit to anything, like exercise, so as to obtain a well-functioning mind and a pleasant, happy life" (www.hiddendominion.com/socrates-quotes-on-physical-fitness). The Buddha (563–483 B.C.) also saw the cognitive importance of physical fitness, famously saying, "To keep the body in good health is a duty; otherwise we shall not be able to keep our mind strong and clear" (Lu and Ahmed 2010, p. 378). Contemporary great thinkers have further speculated on this mind-body connection, with perhaps the most specific quote coming from President John F. Kennedy: "Physical fitness is not only the key to a healthy body; it is also the basis of dynamic and creative intellectual activity" (Kotecki 2011, p. 210).

Medical science has extensively investigated and quantified whether and how physical exercise may improve brain health. Even before the turn of the twentieth century, 200 studies examining the influence of physical fitness on cognitive performance (Etnier et al. 1997) had been published, with the overall evidence collectively showing a positive and statistically significant relationship between the two. Subsequent research aimed to determine if this relationship persisted across the lifespan. For instance, a meta-analysis by Sibley and Etnier (2003) across 44 studies conducted in children showed the existence of significant associations between physical activity and cognition from an early age. Sofi et al. (2011) analyzed data from 33,000 older adults to demonstrate that individuals who engaged in regular physical activity were less likely to experience aging-related cognitive decline than were sedentary persons.

However, although these large-scale observations demonstrate a clear link between exercise and brain health, the pertinent question still remains: can individuals improve the structure, connectivity, or functional capacities of their brain through engaging in certain types of physical activity? The potential benefits of exercise for brain health are particularly relevant for individuals with psychiatric disorders because both mood disorders and psychotic disorders are associated with impairments in cognition. These impairments are observed across multiple cognitive domains, including processing speed, memory, and reasoning, and often persist despite psychiatric treatment (Bora et al. 2013; Goldberg et al. 2007). Furthermore, cognitive deficits are highly predictive of the long-term functional disability often observed in people with psychiatric disorders (Evans et al. 2014; Green et al. 2000). Given that much of the personal and economic burden of these conditions can be attributed to poor social and occupational functioning, an intervention that could successfully improve cognitive health among individuals with psychiatric disorders would have substantial value from both a patient and a public health perspective.

In this chapter, we present the findings of key epidemiological and clinical studies examining the impact of physical exercise on brain health. Throughout the chapter, we focus specifically on studies of people with psychiatric disorders, particularly schizophrenia, major depression, and bipolar disorder. We consider whether different types of exercise, including aerobic and strength-training activities, can provide effective treatments for the neurocognitive dysfunction associated with these psychiatric conditions. Furthermore, through examination of human and animal studies, we present the neurobiological mechanisms through which these lifestyle-based interventions confer their cognitive benefits.

SURVIVAL OF THE FITTEST: NEUROPROTECTIVE EFFECTS OF AEROBIC EXERCISE

Effects of Aerobic Exercise on Brain Structure

Aerobic exercise can exert many physiological changes, one of which is the propensity to alter brain structure. Magnetic resonance imaging (MRI) studies have enabled us to gain an in-depth understanding of the structure of the human brain. This has allowed us to investigate the effects of behaviors such as physical activity. Although research to date is mixed, there is growing evidence to suggest that physical activity and aerobic fitness can affect the structure of the brain. Imaging research has found that aerobic activity is associated with the following:

- Increased gray matter volume in frontal, occipital, entorhinal, and hippocampal regions and a reduced risk of cognitive impairment (Erickson et al. 2014)
- Changes in the structure and connectivity of white matter regions and increased overall white matter volume (Sexton et al. 2016; Voss et al. 2013)
- Structural changes to the basal ganglia, an area implicated in cognition and overall functioning (Niemann et al. 2014)

Typically, structured exercise interventions involve encouraging people to increase their physical activity levels to a minimum amount, such as 90 minutes of moderate to vigorous activity per week over a given time period (e.g., 12 weeks). Comparing structural MRI scans before and after an exercise intervention can identify structural changes that may occur as a result of increasing aerobic activity.

Hippocampus and Exercise

The hippocampus is believed to be particularly responsive to the effects of physical activity (Cotman et al. 2007). It is a structure found deep within the limbic system that is responsible for memory, emotion regulation, and motivation. The function of the hippocampus is largely related to consolidating information from short-term to long-term memory. Extensive animal studies suggest a link between aerobic exercise and hippocampal size and function. For example, voluntary exercise in rodents is associated with cell growth in the hippocampus (van Praag et al. 2005).

This effect is also observed in human brains. Randomized controlled trials of exercise have shown increases in hippocampal volume over a relatively short period of time (Erickson et al. 2011; Pajonk et al. 2010). A meta-analysis by Firth et al. (2018b) synthesized existing research to determine the impact of physical activity interventions on hippocampal volume in healthy and clinical populations. Fourteen individual trials were included, containing a total of 737 participants who received various interventions such as stationary cycling interventions and treadmill running. For a summary of these 14 trials and the studies by Erickson et al. and Pajonk et al., see Table 2–1.

TABLE 2–1. Studies on the effects of exercise on hippocampal volume

Study	Sample	Description of intervention	Key findings
Burzynska et al. (2017)	124 older adults (31% male)	6-month outdoor walking program (40 minutes 3×/week) at 50%–60% of max HR and progressing to 60%–75% max HR compared with stretching and toning	White matter decreased in both conditions across all major brain regions
Erickson et al. (2011)	120 older adults (33% male)	12-month walking program (40 minutes 3×/week) at 50%–60% HR reserve and progressing to 60%–75% HR reserve compared with stretching and toning	Exercise training increased HCV and improved memory; there were nonsignificant increases in thalamus
Jonasson et al. (2016)	58 older adults (48% male)	6-month jogging and cycling program (30–60 minutes 3×/week) at 40%–80% estimated max HR compared with stretching and toning	No group differences were noted in cortical thickness, but HCV was positively associated with aerobic fitness over time
Krogh et al. (2014)	79 people with MDD (33% male)	3-month stationary cycling (45 minutes 3×/week) at 80% max HR compared with stretching	Exercise did not increase HCV
Lin et al. (2015)	30 females with first-episode psychosis	3-month aerobic training on treadmill and bicycle (45–60 minutes 3×/week) at 50%–60% VO_2 max compared with treatment as usual	Aerobic exercise resulted in small increases in HCV

TABLE 2–1. Studies on the effects of exercise on hippocampal volume *(continued)*

Study	Sample	Description of intervention	Key findings
Maass et al. (2015)	32 older adults (45% male)	3-month treadmill running (30 minutes 3×/week) at 65%–85% HR reserve compared with stretching and muscle relaxation	Exercise increased overall GMV, and improved fitness was associated with increased HCV
Malchow et al. (2016)	39 people with schizophrenia (68% male)	3-month stationary cycling (30 minutes 3×/week) at individualized intensity depending on blood lactate concentration of 2 mmol/L compared with table-top football	Exercise increased volume in left superior, middle, and inferior anterior temporal gyri but did not affect HCV
Morris et al. (2017)	68 older adults with probable Alzheimer's disease (49% male)	24 weeks of supervised aerobic exercise to achieve 150 minutes/week at 60%–75% HR reserve compared with stretching and toning	Exercise did not affect total GMV, but fitness was associated with improved memory and bilateral HCV
Niemann et al. (2014)	30 older adults (35% male)	12-month Nordic walking (45 minutes 3×/week) above aerobic threshold and below anaerobic threshold	Exercise increased volume of the basal ganglia and was associated with improved executive function
Pajonk et al. (2010)	16 males with schizophrenia	3-month stationary cycling (30 minutes 3×/week) at individualized intensity depending on blood lactate concentration of 1.5–2 mmol/L compared with tabletop football	HCV increased in response to exercise and was correlated with improved aerobic fitness

TABLE 2–1. Studies on the effects of exercise on hippocampal volume *(continued)*

Study	Sample	Description of intervention	Key findings
Rosano et al. (2016)	26 older adults (30% male)	24-month moderate-intensity walking (40 minutes, 2×/week) and other activities compared with health education	Exercise increased left HCV
Scheewe et al. (2013)	30 people with schizophrenia (78% male)	6-month stationary cycling (60 minutes 2×/week) increasing from 45% to 75% HR reserve compared with OT	Exercise did not affect global brain and hippocampal volume or cortical thickness
Ten Brinke et al. (2015)	21 older females with MCI	6-month outdoor walking program (60 minutes 2×/week) at 40% HR reserve and progressing to 70%–80% compared with balance and tone training	Aerobic training significantly increased right and left HCV
Thomas et al. (2016)	54 young adults (44% male)	6-week stationary cycling (30 minutes 5×/week) at 55%–85% HR max compared with a waitlist control	Exercise increased anterior HCV but returned to baseline within 6 weeks of not exercising

Note.   GMV=gray matter volume; HCV=hippocampal volume; HR=heart rate; MCI=mild cognitive impairment; MDD=major depressive disorder; OT=occupational therapy ; VO_2=oxygen volume.
Source   Firth et al. 2018b.

Overall, a significant effect of aerobic exercise was observed on left hippocampal volumes ($P=0.003$). In several studies comparing the effects of exercise across hemispheres, the left hemisphere was consistently more sensitive to exercise-induced improvements than was the right (Firth et al. 2018b). This suggests that increasing people's aerobic activity can result in significant structural changes. Although the hippocampus is known to have high levels of structural plasticity, the reasons why exercise exerts such an effect are unclear.

Clinical Populations

Aging population. The propensity for exercise to induce structural changes in clinical populations is of clinical importance. For example, the hippocampus suffers a substantial decrease in gray matter in the aging population, which is associated with pervasive cognitive decline. However, aerobic exercise has the potential to induce positive effects on left hippocampal volume in older adults in particular (Firth et al. 2018b). This is related to retention of hippocampal volume rather than increased neuronal mass per se; however, it does indicate that exercise could exert a neuroprotective effect in later life. Any intervention that has the potential to benefit cognitive functioning in the aging population is worth further investigation and may have significant public health implications.

Schizophrenia. The neurobiological benefits of exercise have also been identified in people with schizophrenia. Two studies found that 12 weeks of aerobic exercise undertaken three times per week significantly increased hippocampal volume compared with control conditions (Pajonk et al. 2010; Lin et al. 2015). For example, Pajonk et al. (2010) randomly assigned men with schizophrenia to either a cycling program or table football for 12 weeks. Following exercise training, hippocampal volume significantly increased in both patients (12%) and healthy subjects (16%), with no change in nonexercise groups.

However, results are often inconsistent; subsequent studies that also used 12 weeks of aerobic exercise did not identify changes in hippocampal volume (Malchow et al. 2016; Rosenbaum et al. 2015). In a recent study, 20 people with schizophrenia were randomly assigned to 3 months of endurance training or a control group (table football). Despite finding no difference in hippocampal volume, participants showed increases in the various regions of the temporal gyri (Malchow et al. 2016).

It is also unclear whether these findings extend to other conditions. Studies including people with depression, mild cognitive impairment, and Alzheimer's disease have all had inconsistent results (Firth et al. 2018b). Therefore, further research is required to explore the neurobiological effect of exercise in clinical populations and across other regions of the brain.

White Matter Pathways and Exercise

White matter refers to the neural fibers, or axons, that connect neurons within the gray matter of the brain. The majority of research has focused on structural changes to gray matter in relation to exercise, and the white matter pathways have been largely underresearched. However, the question remains as to whether aerobic exercise can affect white matter pathways and structural connectivity in the human brain. A recent review sought to clarify this question and identified 29 studies assessing overall white matter volume, lesions in the brain, and individual white matter microstructure across a range of populations (Sexton et al. 2016). Sexton and colleagues found that higher levels of physical activity and fitness were associated with increased global white matter volume and smaller volume of white matter lesions, which often occur during the aging process. Although encouraging, the current studies do pose some limitations, such as small sample sizes and methodological issues, including lack of blinding and inconsistent results. Nonetheless, these preliminary findings are worthy of further exploration.

Effect of Aerobic Exercise on Cognitive Functioning

As well as resulting in structural changes, aerobic exercise has the potential to improve overall cognitive functioning. The majority of previous research showing the cognitive benefits of exercise has been conducted in elderly adults (Cotman et al. 2007). However, studies in healthy adult samples have shown that aerobic exercise can increase attention, processing speed, memory, and executive function (Smith et al 2010) In young people, increasing exercise levels is associated with better academic performance (Monti et al. 2012).

Improving Cognition With Exercise in People With Psychiatric Disorders

The clinical utility of exercise is becoming more apparent in clinical populations who have cognitive deficits and decline. Conditions such as schizophrenia are associated with pervasive deficits in cognitive functioning. Poor working memory, attentional deficits, and difficulties with executive functioning all have a significant impact on overall functioning and quality of life. The positive impact exercise can have on brain health has resulted in growing research assessing the clinical utility of exercise interventions to ameliorate cognitive deficits in clinical populations.

Remaining with the example of schizophrenia, the cognitive benefits of exercise have been reported in several reviews (Firth et al. 2017a; Vakhrusheva et al. 2016; Vancampfort et al. 2014). Indeed, a recent meta-analysis of 10 randomized controlled trials of a total of 385 patients found that aerobic exercise significantly improved overall cognition in people with schizophrenia (Firth et al. 2017a). Particularly large effects were found in the domains of working memory and attention, both of which are necessary for general day-to-day functioning and are predictive of functional recovery after a first episode of schizophrenia. Pajonk et al. (2010)

and Lin et al. (2015) found that structural changes to hippocampal volume corresponded to significant increases in short-term memory. Additionally, just 12 weeks of exercise was associated with significant increases in left anterior lobe volume and improved short-term memory in people with schizophrenia (Malchow et al. 2016).

Social cognition is another domain that can be improved by exercise. Two recent studies in early psychosis observed significant improvements in socio-occupational functioning following participation in an aerobic exercise intervention (Firth et al. 2018a; Nuechterlein et al. 2016). Indeed, the recent meta-analysis by Firth et al. (2017a) identified particularly strong improvements in social functioning. This is important because sociocognitive impairments persevere even in the absence of symptoms and are more predictive of real-world functioning than are other domains of cognition (Fett et al. 2011). Therefore, exercise may have profound real-world benefits for a person's functioning by maximizing the transfer of cognitive improvements to daily life. Additionally, a recent review concluded that just 30 minutes of exercise improved executive functioning in children with attention-deficit/hyperactivity disorder (ADHD), suggesting that exercise can have a clinically meaningful impact from an early age (Grassmann et al. 2017).

However, despite relatively strong evidence with ADHD and psychotic disorders, similar effects are yet to be extended to people with bipolar disorder or depression. A recent meta-analysis of eight randomized controlled trials of exercise for depression identified exercise-induced improvements in visual learning and memory (Brondino et al. 2017); however, no effect was observed on overall cognition. This is not to say there is no effect; low levels of adherence and high attrition rates were observed across these studies that may potentially have masked the true effects of exercise.

How Much Is Enough?

The use of aerobic exercise interventions to improve cognitive functioning and mental and physical health in clinical populations is of particular importance. Despite promising findings, it remains unclear how much exercise is enough to have a clinically significant effect. There is evidence to suggest that greater amounts of exercise and adherence to interventions result in larger improvements in both cognition and symptoms in people with schizophrenia (Firth et al. 2017a; Kimhy et al. 2016). Additionally, the type and intensity of exercise may have an impact on neurobiological changes. A recent study showed that high-intensity interval training had similar benefits for cardiovascular fitness as long-term endurance training (Martins et al. 2016), and this may also be the case for cognitive functioning. Nevertheless, we do know that people with psychiatric disorders typically engage in less physical activity than the general population (Vancampfort et al. 2017) and experience more barriers to living an active lifestyle (Firth et al. 2016). Therefore, future research should seek to clarify the best methods of implementation of exercise interventions to result in clinical benefits.

It may be that rather than specific doses and intensity, cardiovascular fitness is a more viable target for interventions. As discussed earlier, improvements in fitness coincide with neurobiological changes. Exercise-induced fitness improvements are positively associated with greater neurocognitive improvements in both clinical and nonclinical populations (Erickson et al. 2011; Firth et al. 2017a). Therefore, considering the wider benefits of exercise interventions on mental health, metabolic health, and physical health, prescribing exercise to improve fitness may be of particular clinical utility. Focusing on improving fitness rather than specifically looking at neurobiological changes in neural microstructure is a feasible target for an intervention.

Limitations of Current Research

There are some limitations to the evidence discussed.

- A majority of research to date is cross-sectional; therefore, causality cannot be established.
- Many aerobic exercise trials are not randomized and contain small numbers of participants.
- Evidence for the impact of exercise on specific brain areas is mixed, and there are many contradictory findings across studies.
- Most research has focused on the hippocampus despite emerging findings in other brain regions and white matter tracts.

Neurobiological Mechanisms of Aerobic Exercise and Cognition

Supramolecular Processes

There is growing evidence from behavioral and imaging studies that aerobic exercise can exert structural and cognitive changes to the human brain. Nevertheless, the question still remains as to how exercise can have such a profound effect on brain health. There are three main supramolecular processes that occur as a result of exercise: neurogenesis, angiogenesis, and synaptogenesis.

Neurogenesis refers to the creation of new neurons from neural stem cells across the brain. Both human and animal studies have shown that the rate of neurogenesis within the brain is readily upregulated in response to aerobic exercise, particularly in the hippocampus (Cotman et al. 2007; van Praag 2008). Indeed, neurogenesis has been identified as perhaps the primary neural process through which exercise increases brain volume.

Angiogenesis is a further process that occurs as a result of exercise. This relates to a growth in blood vessels and capillaries to specific regions of the brain. Evidence for this comes from increased dentate gyrus cerebral blood volume in rodents following aerobic exercise (van Praag et al. 2005). Human studies have also shown that dentate gyrus cerebral blood volume was significantly associated with increased oxygen uptake after aerobic exercise in healthy and clinical populations (Malchow et al. 2016; Pereira et al. 2007). The cognitive benefits of exercise may be mediated by increased angiogenesis because capacity for aerobic exercise coincides with increased blood flow in the hippocampus (Pereira et al. 2007) and increased cortical capillary blood supply (Colcombe et al. 2006).

Finally, *synaptogenesis* refers to the process of building new synapses, thus enhancing connectivity between brain regions. Aerobic exercise has been shown to increase the number of synaptic connections in the brain, thus creating enhanced neural pathways (Colcombe et al. 2006). Furthermore, the increased connectivity arising from exercise-induced synaptogenesis has also been linked to improved cognitive performance (Colcombe et al. 2006).

What Stimulates These Brain Adaptations?

The precise neurobiological mechanisms underlying the increases in neurogenesis, angiogenesis, and synaptogenesis that result from exercise are not fully established. Nonetheless, there are several possibilities:

- Increased neurotrophic factors such as brain-derived neurotrophic factor (BDNF)
- Increased cardiorespiratory fitness resulting in neurological changes
- Indirect mechanisms that mediate neurological changes in both brain structure and function

The strongest evidence suggests that changes are mediated by increased trophic factors such as an increase in insulin-like growth factor 1 and BDNF. BDNF is the most abundant growth factor in the brain and is upregulated during aerobic exercise, resulting in increased neurogenesis (Szuhany et al. 2015). Evidence from both human and animal studies suggests that an increase in BDNF may explain the significant neurogenesis observed following aerobic exercise (Szuhany et al. 2015).

As well as stimulating neurogenesis, increased BNDF reduces neuroinflammation, thus improving neuronal signaling (Cotman et al. 2007); increases the volume of white matter structures; and improves structural and functional connectivity by stimulating formation of synapses (Svatkova et al. 2015; Voss et al. 2013). It is also associated with cognitive enhancement in both healthy and clinical populations. For example, Kimhy et al. (2015) found that increased BDNF predicted 14.6% of cognitive improvements resulting from an exercise intervention. However, more research is required before determining whether this is the main neurobiological mechanism responsible for changes to brain health. A recent review suggested that the neurological benefits of exercise in humans cannot be attributed solely to increases in BDNF because many studies did not show significant changes in BDNF despite improved cognition (Firth et al. 2017b).

Another possible mechanism of action is through aerobic exercise increasing cardiorespiratory fitness. There is evidence to suggest that improving cardiorespiratory fitness can confer significant changes to brain structure, including overall brain volume and increased hippocampal volume (Erickson et al. 2014; Svatkova et al. 2015). For example, changes in hippocampal volume were correlated with improved aerobic fitness as measured by change in maximum oxygen consumption (Pajonk et al. 2010). Indeed, physiological changes such as increased cardiovascular fitness, weight loss, and improved metabolic health are all linked to increased cognitive performance. This is perhaps due to metabolic benefits of exercise improving glucose regulation, which in turn supports optimal function of the hippocampus (Convit et al. 2003). Improved fitness is also associated with decreased levels of inflammation and greater white matter integrity (Svatkova et al. 2015).

It is also possible that the positive effects on cognition occur indirectly, and there is, in fact, a third factor that could account for changes in brain structure (through neurogenesis, angiogenesis, and synaptogenesis) and real-world functioning. For example, exercise improves mental health and well-being, quality of life, and social functioning as well as having clear benefits to physical health and fitness. All of these factors are associated with neurological functioning and improved cognition. Yet it could also be that the mechanisms of action vary across populations. For instance, in older populations, rather than increasing brain volume, exercise prevents the decline in gray matter volume that is usually observed with age. This contrasts with the cell growth that occurs in younger, healthier individuals. Therefore, exercise has the potential to exert a different neuroprotective effect across populations. Individual differences in the type of exercise as well as the population could also drive different neurological processes. For instance, strength training may act through entirely different neurobiological mechanisms to improve cognitive health. Future studies should compare different exercise programs and assess clinical, cognitive, and neurological outcomes to gain further insight into the cognitive benefits of exercise.

RESISTANCE TO CHANGE: IS STRENGTH TRAINING THE NEW EXERCISE FOR BRAIN POWER?

Resistance training refers to forms of physical activity that involve moving the limbs and/or core against resistance provided by weighted objects (e.g., barbells, dumbbells), elasticated bands, your own body weight, or machines. Resistance training is typically undertaken to improve muscular strength and endurance along with stimulating muscular hypertrophy for both metabolic and aesthetic benefit.

Over the past several decades, the popularity of resistance training across society has increased enormously, accompanied by a concomitant increase in the number of books and research articles dedicated to this topic (Smith and Bruce-Low 2004). This popularity is somewhat spurred by the growing recognition that resistance training methods can be as effective as aerobic training for reducing body weight, improving metabolic heath, and reducing the risk of various chronic noncommunicable diseases (Sigal et al. 2007; Winett and Carpinelli 2001). Furthermore, resistance training may confer greater benefits than aerobic exercise for reducing risk of falls and maintaining functional mobility among elderly people, which confers significant benefits for population health (Davis et al. 2011).

Effect of Resistance Exercise on Cognitive Functioning and the Brain

The benefits of resistance training for physical functioning have been shown to extend to cognitive functioning in aging populations. For instance, in their "Brain Power" study, Liu-Ambrose et al. (2010) randomly assigned 155 older adults in Vancouver to receive either resistance training or balance training once or twice per week over 12 months. Results showed that the executive functioning capacities of those receiving balance training decreased by 0.5% over the 12 months, as would be expected in an aging population. However, the participants who received resistance training increased their executive functioning by 11%–13% over the same time period. Furthermore, these improvements in cognition from just once-weekly resistance training were sustained for a further 12 months after completion of resistance training (Davis et al. 2010). Subsequent trials comparing aerobic and resistance training for cognitive outcomes have shown that both of these types of exercise are equally effective among individuals with age-related cognitive impairments, and improvements in spatial memory were significantly greater in individuals receiving aerobic and resistance training than in inactive control groups (Nagamatsu et al. 2013).

Given these promising early findings, a seminal study (Study of Mental Activity and Resistance Training [SMART]) was recently conducted in Sydney, Australia to establish whether or not resistance training (which targets muscular function) can be as effective as computerized brain training (which targets cognitive functioning directly) for treating cognitive deficits in aging populations (Suo et al. 2016). The study recruited 100 older participants (approximately age 70 years) with subjective memory complaints and randomly assigned them into one of four groups—twice-weekly resistance training, computerized cognitive training (CCT), both, or neither—for 26 weeks. Notably, participants not receiving CCT were given sham (inactive) computer training, whereas those not receiving resistance training were provided with balance training in order to completely match all groups for the types and amount of attention received during the trial. Remarkably, results showed that the resistance training produced greater benefits for overall cognitive functioning than did the cognitive training itself. The study also used brain scans (functional magnetic resonance imaging) before and after the training interventions to explore the neurological mechanisms underlying these cognitive effects. Comparisons between the experimental groups showed that resistance training significantly increased gray matter of the brain. Additionally, the resistance training reversed aging-related white matter degradation (identified by white matter hyperintensities) in various areas across the brain, and these improvements were not observed in the CCT group (Suo et al. 2016).

Outside experimental settings, the connection between muscular function and cognitive or brain functioning can also be observed from an epidemiological perspective. Population-scale research has shown that individuals with greater muscular strength (measured as maximal force outputs from various muscle groups in the upper and lower limbs) perform better across a range of cognitive tasks and are at lower risk of developing cognitive impairments (Boyle et al. 2009; Narazaki et al. 2014). These effects are noted even when controlling for other putative factors that may influence the relationship between muscle strength and cognitive function, such as age, adiposity, and physical activity.

Indeed, maximal handgrip strength (a simple and inexpensive measure of muscular fitness) is now recognized as a clinically useful functional marker of cognitive decline and impaired daily functioning in older adults (Fritz et al. 2017). A powerful example of the connection between handgrip and cognition is provided by a study by Sternäng et al. (2016). This study assessed the maximal handgrip strength and cognitive performance of 708 adults across six time points over a 20-year period and found consistently strong links between grip and cognition at all time points. The reason as to why grip strength predicts cognition is not fully understood, although white matter integrity has been proposed as the potential underlying factor because this aspect of neuronal health is involved in performing a range of physical and mental tasks (Silbert et al. 2008). However, recent studies have also shown that the correlation between changes in handgrip and cognition that consistently occur over time in aging adults cannot be accounted for by white matter degradation alone (Viscogliosi et al. 2017).

Can the Brain Benefits of Resistance Training Apply in Psychiatric Samples?

Despite the mounting evidence of increased strength relating to improved cognition in aging populations, the question still remains whether resistance training has any place in resolving cognitive deficits and other symptoms associated with psychiatric disorders. Until recently, the associations between muscular and cognitive functioning in people with mental health conditions were unexplored. However, two large-scale, population-based studies have recently demonstrated that handgrip strength relates to cognitive performance across multiple domains of cognition. The two studies surveyed 1,162 individuals with schizophrenia (Firth et al. 2018c), 1,475 with bipolar disorder, and 22,699 with major depression (Firth et al. 2018d). The relationships observed between weakened grip strength and poor cognitive performance in psychiatric samples were found to exist independently of potentially confounding factors, such as differences in education, body mass index, and social deprivation between groups.

Some of the relationships between grip strength and certain cognitive tasks, such as reaction time, could feasibly be explained by performance in both requiring muscular function of the hand. However, given that relationships also persisted in tasks of fluid intelligence (reasoning) and delayed recall (prospective memory), which are measured using tasks that do not require hand speed or dexterity, the associations between grip strength and cognition in psychiatric populations cannot be attributed simply to better motor coordination boosting cognitive task performance.

Thus, these recent studies suggest that muscular strength may also provide a useful proxy of cognitive deficits caused by psychiatric conditions. This finding also suggests that interventions that increase muscular strength (i.e., resistance training) may be capable of targeting cognitive symptoms of severe mental illness. Again, however, although this correlation has been shown extensively in healthy aging samples, the effects of resistance training in psychiatric populations is relatively unexplored.

Resistance Training Interventions in People With Mental Illness

A recent systematic review found no randomized controlled trials that have examined cognitive outcomes of strength training interventions in people with schizophrenia (Keller-Varady et al. 2018). However, one small-scale single-arm study (i.e., a study in which all participants receive the intervention) did assess the impact of an 8-week high-intensity strength-based circuit training program for individuals with severe mental illnesses, including bipolar disorder and schizophrenia. Results showed significant improvements in cognitive functioning following the strength-training program—particularly for verbal memory and processing speed. This is an important finding because these domains are often not improved by aerobic exercise in individuals with schizophrenia (Firth et al. 2018a). Interestingly, another small study that used resistance exercise within a mixed training regime for 31 younger patients with early psychosis also observed significant improvements in verbal memory and processing speed after just 12 weeks (Firth et al. 2018a).

Collectively, these studies suggest that resistance training may confer different, but complementary, cognitive benefits for patients with severe mental illness. Feasible neurological mechanisms by which resistance training could exert these effects have also been indicated by other studies in patients with schizophrenia, showing increases in procognitive proteins (such as BDNF) from training programs that incorporate resistance exercise (Kim et al. 2014) and decreases in hormones that potentially impede cognition, such as cortisol (Leone et al. 2015). However, given the small samples and lack of control groups, it is difficult to draw any firm conclusions until further studies of strength training in psychosis have been conducted. Nonetheless, given the emerging evidence in psychosis samples and a strong body of research from nonpsychiatric populations, it is possible to envisage how resistance training could soon become one of the most promising interventions for improving neurocognitive outcomes in people with psychiatric disorders.

One randomized controlled trial has examined the cognitive effects of resistance training in people with major depression. Krogh et al. (2009) randomly assigned patients to resistance versus aerobic versus relaxation training and found no difference in cognition between groups. However, strength training outperformed both aerobic and relaxation groups for real-world functioning: participants receiving resistance training significantly increased time at work over 12 months, taking 12% fewer days off than did patients in the relaxation group. This is an important finding because although the cognitive impairments observed in depressed patients are less severe than in people with psychosis, real-world functional disability (i.e., unemployment and work absence) from major depression still confers a huge social and economic burden (Greenberg et al. 2015). Thus, if resistance training can improve these aspects of major depression, it would prove to be a highly valuable intervention, even without direct cognitive effects.

Indeed, other clinical trials have also shown functional benefits of strength training in people with depression (Singh et al. 1997). Furthermore, greater functional benefits are observed from strength-training regimens with high-intensity rather than low-intensity resistance exercise, strongly suggesting that these benefits are tied to improvements in muscular fitness rather than nonspecific intervention effects (Singh et al. 2005). Thus, resistance training may soon have a place in improving functional capacities among people with psychiatric disorders.

MOVING FORWARD WITH MOVING MORE: CONCLUSION AND CLINICAL CONSIDERATIONS

In this chapter, we discussed the effectiveness and mechanisms of physical exercise as a cognitive enhancement intervention in both healthy and clinical populations. Overall, there is now incredibly compelling evidence that aerobic exercise has procognitive effects. Indeed, the strong ties between aerobic activity and cognitive functioning may even have an evolutionary basis. This is because the rapid growth in brain matter among the *Homo* genus occurred at around the same time in evolutionary history as an accompanying increase in aerobic activity, due to the dawn of the hunter-gatherer lifestyle among our ancestors (Raichlen and Polk 2013). Because certain neurotrophic factors (such as BDNF) not only increase cognition or brain volume but also improve muscular energy regulation, it is possible that the great demand for aerobic capacity in hunter-gatherer times drove selection toward favoring individuals with better energy regulation (from higher levels of neurotrophic factors) and thus greater neural plasticity (Raichlen and Polk 2013). Additionally, the joint role of signaling mechanisms such as BDNF in both neuroplasticity and exercise performance could have conferred further selective benefit through the acute upregulation of BDNF that occurs in response to exercise. This upregulation temporarily boosted cognitive capacities, such as memory and attention, that were critical to success during long endurance runs undertaken for hunting or gathering purposes (Mattson 2012).

Thus, a key aspect of our nature may require the human body to engage in regular physical activity for both physical and cognitive health. However, it should also be considered that our evolution as a species occurred over extended time frames of food scarcity—thus encouraging humans to avoid unnecessary physical exertion. This may explain the extreme levels of sedentary behavior and exercise avoidance observed in today's society and the continued efforts of human beings to make key survival resources (such as food, information, and social networks) as easily and readily available as possible without the requirement to move. Thus, even from an evolutionary perspective, exercise interventions must be developed to be intrinsically motivating and compelling if we are to successfully engage human beings in the types of physically exerting activities required to improve health (Lieberman 2015).

These motivational factors are particularly important to consider for individuals with severe mental illness, who are generally less active and face additional personal and social barriers to exercise engagement (Firth et al. 2016; Vancampfort et al. 2017). Allowing individuals to choose their idealized type of physical activity may help to promote both the uptake and maintenance of exercise over time. Importantly, as detailed throughout this chapter, all sorts of exercise (especially resistance training) can confer cognitive benefits; thus, the optimal modality of exercise for any given patient is most likely to be simply the type of activity he or she will engage with regularly and fully. With this in mind, introducing variation into individuals' training regimes may further promote adherence—and even maximize the cognitive benefits—because recent studies have shown that both aerobic and resistance exercise act together on the brain through independent yet complementary neural mechanisms (Cassilhas et al. 2012).

A final important consideration regarding the evidence presented here is whether the increases in neural connectivity, brain structure, and cognitive task performance that occur from exercise actually translate to improvements in real-world capacities among people with mental illness. Specifically, longer-term studies are required to examine whether individuals who undertake regular exercise as part of their psychiatric care have better personal and social outcomes than that of those who do not—for instance, quicker return to work or education, reduced need for psychiatric medications, or sustained long-term recovery over time. The subsequent chapters in this book will provide further information on how physical exercise, and, indeed, other aspects of a healthy lifestyle, can be used to promote recovery from psychiatric disorders.

DISCUSSION QUESTIONS

1. It is broadly accepted that cardiovascular health cannot be maintained without regular physical activity. Why is brain health viewed differently?
2. An innate link between aerobic activity and cognitive health in human beings may have developed from millennia of environmental demands in hunter-gatherer times. What effects could millennia of sedentary societies and food abundance have on this connection?
3. Our understanding of the specific effects and neurobiological mechanisms of exercise for cognitive functioning is rapidly growing and increasingly refined. How is this of use to our patients?

RECOMMENDED READINGS

Firth J, Stubbs B, Rosenbaum S, et al: Aerobic exercise improves cognitive functioning in people with schizophrenia: a systematic review and meta-analysis. Schizophr Bull 43(3):546–556, 2017

Hillman CH, Erickson KI, Kramer AF: Be smart, exercise your heart: exercise effects on brain and cognition. Nat Rev Neurosci 9(1):58–65, 2008

Suo C, Singh MF, Gates N, et al: Therapeutically relevant structural and functional mechanisms triggered by physical and cognitive exercise. Mol Psychiatry 21(11):1633–1642, 2016

REFERENCES

Bora E, Harrison BJ, Yücel M, et al: Cognitive impairment in euthymic major depressive disorder: a meta-analysis. Psychol Med 43(10):2017–2026, 2013 23098294

Boyle PA, Buchman AS, Wilson RS, et al: Association of muscle strength with the risk of Alzheimer disease and the rate of cognitive decline in community-dwelling older persons. Arch Neurol 66(11):1339–1344, 2009 19901164

Brondino N, Rocchetti M, Fusar-Poli L, et al: A systematic review of cognitive effects of exercise in depression. Acta Psychiatr Scand 135(4):285–295, 2017 28110494

Cassilhas RC, Lee KS, Fernandes J, et al: Spatial memory is improved by aerobic and resistance exercise through divergent molecular mechanisms. Neuroscience 202:309–317, 2012 22155655

Colcombe SJ, Erickson KI, Scalf PE, et al: Aerobic exercise training increases brain volume in aging humans. J Gerontol A Biol Sci Med Sci 61(11):1166–1170, 2006 17167157

Convit A, Wolf OT, Tarshish C, et al: Reduced glucose tolerance is associated with poor memory performance and hippocampal atrophy among normal elderly. Proc Natl Acad Sci USA 100(4):2019–2022, 2003 12571363

Cotman CW, Berchtold NC, Christie L-A: Exercise builds brain health: key roles of growth factor cascades and inflammation. Trends Neurosci 30(9):464–472, 2007 17765329

Davis JC, Marra CA, Beattie BL, et al: Sustained cognitive and economic benefits of resistance training among community-dwelling senior women: a 1-year follow-up study of the Brain Power study. Arch Intern Med 170(22):2036–2038, 2010 21149764

Davis JC, Marra CA, Robertson MC, et al: Economic evaluation of dose-response resistance training in older women: a cost-effectiveness and cost-utility analysis. Osteoporos Int 22(5):1355–1366, 2011 20683707

Erickson KI, Voss MW, Prakash RS, et al: Exercise training increases size of hippocampus and improves memory. Proc Natl Acad Sci USA 108(7):3017–3022, 2011 21282661

Erickson KI, Leckie RL, Weinstein AM: Physical activity, fitness, and gray matter volume. Neurobiol Aging 35(suppl 2):S20–S28, 2014 24952993

Etnier JL, Salazar W, Landers DM, et al: The influence of physical fitness and exercise upon cognitive functioning: a meta-analysis. J Sport Exerc Psychol 19(3):249–277, 1997

Evans VC, Iverson GL, Yatham LN, et al: The relationship between neurocognitive and psychosocial functioning in major depressive disorder: a systematic review. J Clin Psychiatry 75(12):1359 1370, 2014 25551235

Fett A-KJ, Viechtbauer W, Dominguez MD, et al: The relationship between neurocognition and social cognition with functional outcomes in schizophrenia: a meta-analysis. Neurosci Biobehav Rev 35(3):573–588, 2011 20620163

Firth J, Rosenbaum S, Stubbs B, et al: Motivating factors and barriers towards exercise in severe mental illness: a systematic review and meta-analysis. Psychol Med 46(14):2869–2881, 2016 27502153

Firth J, Stubbs B, Rosenbaum S, et al: Aerobic exercise improves cognitive functioning in people with schizophrenia: a systematic review and meta-analysis. Schizophr Bull 43(3):546–556, 2017a 27521348

Firth J, Cotter J, Carney R, et al: The pro-cognitive mechanisms of physical exercise in people with schizophrenia. Br J Pharmacol 174(19):3161–3172, 2017b 28261797

Firth J, Carney R, Elliott R, et al: Exercise as an intervention for first-episode psychosis: a feasibility study. Early Interv Psychiatry 12(3):307–315, 2018a 26987871

Firth J, Stubbs B, Vancampfort D, et al: Effect of aerobic exercise on hippocampal volume in humans: a systematic review and meta-analysis. Neuroimage 166:230–238, 2018b 29113943

Firth, J, Stubbs, B, Vancampfort, D, et al: Grip strength is associated with cognitive performance in schizophrenia and the general population: a UK Biobank study of 476,559 participants. Schizophr Bull 44(4):728–736, 2018c

Firth J, Firth JA, Stubbs B, et al: Association between muscular strength and cognition in major depression or bipolar disorder and healthy controls. JAMA Psychiatry 75(7):740–746 2018d 29710135

Fritz NE, McCarthy CJ, Adamo DE: Handgrip strength as a means of monitoring progression of cognitive decline—a scoping review. Ageing Res Rev 35:112–123, 2017 28189666

Goldberg TE, Goldman RS, Burdick KE, et al: Cognitive improvement after treatment with second-generation antipsychotic medications in first-episode schizophrenia: is it a practice effect? Arch Gen Psychiatry 64(10):1115–1122, 2007 17909123

Grassmann V, Alves MV, Santos-Galduróz RF, et al: Possible cognitive benefits of acute physical exercise in children with ADHD. J Atten Disord 21(5):367–371, 2017 24621460

Green MF, Kern RS, Braff DL, et al: Neurocognitive deficits and functional outcome in schizophrenia: are we measuring the "right stuff"? Schizophr Bull 26(1):119–136, 2000 10755673

Greenberg PE, Fournier A-A, Sisitsky T, et al: The economic burden of adults with major depressive disorder in the United States (2005 and 2010). J Clin Psychiatry 76(2):155–162, 2015 25742202

Keller-Varady K, Varady PA, Röh A, et al: A systematic review of trials investigating strength training in schizophrenia spectrum disorders. Schizophr Res 192:64–68, 2018 28602648

Kim HJ, Song BK, So B, et al: Increase of circulating BDNF levels and its relation to improvement of physical fitness following 12 weeks of combined exercise in chronic patients with schizophrenia: a pilot study. Psychiatry Res 220(3):792–796, 2014 25446461

Kimhy D, Vakhrusheva J, Bartels MN, et al: The impact of aerobic exercise on brain-derived neurotrophic factor and neurocognition in individuals with schizophrenia: a single-blind, randomized clinical trial. Schizophr Bull 41(4):859–868, 2015 25805886

Kimhy D, Lauriola V, Bartels MN, et al: Aerobic exercise for cognitive deficits in schizophrenia—the impact of frequency, duration, and fidelity with target training intensity. Schizophr Res 172(1–3):213–215, 2016 26852401

Kotecki JE: Physical Activity and Health: An Interactive Approach. Burlington, MA, Jones and Bartlett, 2011

Krogh J, Saltin B, Gluud C, et al: The DEMO trial: a randomized, parallel-group, observer-blinded clinical trial of strength versus aerobic versus relaxation training for patients with mild to moderate depression. J Clin Psychiatry 70(6):790–800, 2009 19573478

Leone M, Lalande D, Thériault L, et al: Impact of an exercise program on the physiologic, biologic and psychologic profiles in patients with schizophrenia. Schizophr Res 164(1–3):270–272, 2015 25784171

Lieberman DE: Is exercise really medicine? An evolutionary perspective. Curr Sports Med Rep 14(4):313–319, 2015 26166056

Lin J, Chan SK, Lee EH, et al: Aerobic exercise and yoga improve neurocognitive function in women with early psychosis. NPJ Schizophr 1(0):15047, 2015 27336050

Liu-Ambrose T, Nagamatsu LS, Graf P, et al: Resistance training and executive functions: a 12-month randomized controlled trial. Arch Intern Med 170(2):170–178, 2010 20101012

Lu BY, Ahmed I: The mind-body conundrum: the somatopsychic perspective in geriatric depression. Am J Geriatric Psychiatry 18(5):378–381, 2010 20429082

Malchow B, Keeser D, Keller K, et al: Effects of endurance training on brain structures in chronic schizophrenia patients and healthy controls. Schizophr Res 173(3):182–191, 2016 25623601

Martins C, Kazakova I, Ludviksen M, et al: High-intensity interval training and isocaloric moderate-intensity continuous training result in similar improvements in body composition and fitness in obese individuals. Int J Sport Nutr Exerc Metab 26(3):197–204, 2016 26479856

Mattson MP: Evolutionary aspects of human exercise—born to run purposefully. Ageing Res Rev 11(3):347–352, 2012 22394472

Monti JM, Hillman CH, Cohen NJ: Aerobic fitness enhances relational memory in preadolescent children: the FITKids randomized control trial. Hippocampus 22(9):1876–1882, 2012 22522428

Nagamatsu LS, Chan A, Davis JC, et al: Physical activity improves verbal and spatial memory in older adults with probable mild cognitive impairment: a 6-month randomized controlled trial. J Aging Res 2013:861893, 2013 23509628

Narazaki K, Matsuo E, Honda T, et al: Physical fitness measures as potential markers of low cognitive function in Japanese community-dwelling older adults without apparent cognitive problems. J Sports Sci Med 13(3):590–596, 2014 25177186

Niemann C, Godde B, Voelcker-Rehage C: Not only cardiovascular, but also co-ordinative exercise increases hippocampal volume in older adults. Front Aging Neurosci 6:170, 2014 25165446

Nuechterlein KH, Ventura J, McEwen SC, et al: Enhancing cognitive training through aerobic exercise after a first schizophrenia episode: theoretical conception and pilot study. Schizophr Bull 42(suppl 1):S44–S52, 2016 27460618

Pajonk FG, Wobrock T, Gruber O, et al: Hippocampal plasticity in response to exercise in schizophrenia. Arch Gen Psychiatry 67(2):133–143, 2010 20124113

Pereira AC, Huddleston DE, Brickman AM, et al: An in vivo correlate of exercise-induced neurogenesis in the adult dentate gyrus. Proc Natl Acad Sci USA 104(13):5638–5643, 2007 17374720

Raichlen DA, Polk JD: Linking brains and brawn: exercise and the evolution of human neurobiology. Proc Biol Sci 280(1750):20122250, 2013 23173208

Rosenbaum S, Lagopoulos J, Curtis J, et al: Aerobic exercise intervention in young people with schizophrenia spectrum disorders; improved fitness with no change in hippocampal volume. Psychiatry Res 232(2):200–201, 2015 25862528

Sexton CE, Betts JF, Demnitz N, et al: A systematic review of MRI studies examining the relationship between physical fitness and activity and the white matter of the ageing brain. Neuroimage 131:81–90, 2016 26477656

Sibley BA, Etnier JL: The relationship between physical activity and cognition in children: a meta-analysis. Pediatr Exerc Sci 15(3):243–256, 2003

Sigal RJ, Kenny GP, Boulé NG, et al: Effects of aerobic training, resistance training, or both on glycemic control in type 2 diabetes: a randomized trial. Ann Intern Med 147(6):357–369, 2007 17876019

Silbert LC, Nelson C, Howieson DB, et al: Impact of white matter hyperintensity volume progression on rate of cognitive and motor decline. Neurology 71(2):108–113, 2008 18606964

Singh NA, Clements KM, Fiatarone MA: A randomized controlled trial of progressive resistance training in depressed elders. J Gerontol A Biol Sci Med Sci 52(1):M27–M35, 1997 9008666

Singh NA, Stavrinos TM, Scarbek Y, et al: A randomized controlled trial of high versus low intensity weight training versus general practitioner care for clinical depression in older adults. J Gerontol A Biol Sci Med Sci 60(6):768–776, 2005 15983181

Smith D, Bruce-Low S: Strength training methods and the work of Arthur Jones. J Exerc Physiol Online 7(6):52–68, 2004

Smith PJ, Blumenthal JA, Hoffman BM, et al: Aerobic exercise and neurocognitive performance: a meta-analytic review of randomized controlled trials. Psychosom Med 72(3):239–252, 2010 20223924

Sofi F, Valecchi D, Bacci D, et al: Physical activity and risk of cognitive decline: a meta-analysis of prospective studies. J Intern Med 269(1):107–117, 2011 20831630

Sternäng O, Reynolds CA, Finkel D, et al: Grip strength and cognitive abilities: associations in old age. J Gerontol B Psychol Sci Soc Sci 71(5):841–848, 2016 25787083

Suo C, Singh MF, Gates N, et al: Therapeutically relevant structural and functional mechanisms triggered by physical and cognitive exercise. Mol Psychiatry 21(11):1633–1642, 2016 27001615

Svatkova A, Mandl RC, Scheewe TW, et al: Physical exercise keeps the brain connected: Biking increases white matter integrity in patients with schizophrenia and healthy controls. Schizophr Bull 41(4):869–878, 2015 25829377

Szuhany KL, Bugatti M, Otto MW: A meta-analytic review of the effects of exercise on brain-derived neurotrophic factor. J Psychiatr Res 60:56–64, 2015 25455510

Vakhrusheva J, Marino B, Stroup TS, et al: Aerobic exercise in people with schizophrenia: neural and neurocognitive benefits. Curr Behav Neurosci Rep 3(2):165–175, 2016 27766192

van Praag H: Neurogenesis and exercise: past and future directions. Neuromolecular Med 10(2):128–140, 2008 18286389

van Praag H, Shubert T, Zhao C, et al: Exercise enhances learning and hippocampal neurogenesis in aged mice. J Neurosci 25(38):8680–8685, 2005 16177036

Vancampfort D, Probst M, De Hert M, et al: Neurobiological effects of physical exercise in schizophrenia: a systematic review. Disabil Rehabil 36(21):1749–1754, 2014 24383471

Vancampfort D, Firth J, Schuch FB, et al: Sedentary behavior and physical activity levels in people with schizophrenia, bipolar disorder and major depressive disorder: a global systematic review and meta-analysis. World Psychiatry 16(3):308–315, 2017 28941119

Viscogliosi G, Di Bernardo MG, Ettorre E, et al: Handgrip strength predicts longitudinal changes in clock drawing test performance: an observational study in a sample of older non-demented adults. J Nutr Health Aging 21(5):593–596, 2017 28448092

Voss MW, Heo S, Prakash RS, et al: The influence of aerobic fitness on cerebral white matter integrity and cognitive function in older adults: results of a one-year exercise intervention. Hum Brain Mapp 34(11):2972–2985, 2013 22674729

Winett RA, Carpinelli RN: Potential health-related benefits of resistance training. Prev Med 33(5):503–513, 2001 11676593

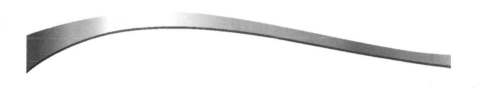

PART II

Exercise in the Prevention and
Management of Specific
Psychiatric Disorders

CHAPTER 3

Physical Exercise in the Management of Major Depressive Disorders

Kayla Fair, Dr.P.H., R.N., M.P.H.

Madhukar H. Trivedi, M.D.

KEY POINTS

- Physical activity has several benefits for patients with major depression and other depressive disorders, including effectiveness for mood symptoms, prevention of other medical conditions, and improvement in psychosocial functioning.
- Benefits have been reported at even small doses of activity, but greater reduction in symptoms seems to be related to higher exercise intensity.
- Medical and public health professionals can better promote physical activity among patients with depression by recognizing changes in motivation, addressing common barriers to exercising, providing psychoeducation regarding evidence-based strategies, and using behavioral activation.
- Opportunities for future research in the field of depression and physical activity include studies of postpartum depression, bipolar disorder, and patients from all socioeconomic and demographic backgrounds.

BACKGROUND

In an epidemiological study, Farmer et al. (1988) linked depressive symptoms to physical activity. In the decades since then, numerous longitudinal and cross-sectional studies have provided additional evidence to suggest that physical activity protects against the development of major depressive disorder (MDD) and may help reduce the severity of symptoms among patients with depression (Harvey et al. 2018; Mammen and Faulkner 2013). The inverse relationship between physical activity and symptoms of depression has been observed across a wide range of sociodemographic factors, including age and gender, and among people residing in low- to middle-income countries (Dishman et al. 2012; Farmer et al. 1988; Galper et al. 2006; Harris et al. 2006; Harvey et al. 2018).

Several randomized controlled trials have explored the effect of exercise as a treatment for MDD, both as a standalone treatment and as an adjuvant to pharmacological treatment and/or psychotherapy (Hallgren et al. 2015; Helgadóttir et al. 2017; Mota-Pereira et al. 2011; Trivedi et al. 2011). In this chapter, we describe recent research findings on the effect of exercise on symptoms of MDD, provide strategies for medical professionals to promote increased physical activity among patients with MDD, and highlight research opportunities in the field of exercise and depression. Table 3–1 provides an overview of key randomized controlled trials discussed in this chapter.

EXERCISE AS TREATMENT FOR DEPRESSION

In an effort to deliver more effective treatments for depressive disorders, researchers have explored alternatives to pharmacological treatment and psychotherapy. One evidence-based treatment option that has been explored is exercise. The evidence suggests that exercise is an effective treatment for MDD, both as a monotherapy and in conjunction with psychotherapy and/or pharmacological therapy (Cooney et al. 2013; Dunn et al. 2005; Rethorst et al. 2009; Schuch et al. 2016a). Patients who engage in physical activity as a way to treat their depressive symptoms may experience a reduction in symptoms similar to the response observed in patients taking antidepressants and/or receiving psychotherapy (Cooney et al. 2013; Rethorst et al. 2009; Schuch et al. 2016a). Therefore, mental health care providers are encouraged to consider exercise as a treatment for their patients with MDD (Rethorst and Trivedi 2013). Exercise is another option for patients who have treatment-resistant depression and has been shown to reduce symptoms and increase psychosocial and cognitive functioning among this population (Blumenthal et al. 2012; Greer et al. 2015, 2016; Mota-Pereira et al. 2011; Trivedi et al. 2006). Some studies show that as little as 1 hour of physical activity a week can be protective against depressive symptoms (Harvey et al. 2018).

Exercise as a treatment for depression offers many potential benefits for patients. One major benefit to exercise as a treatment for depression is that several types of exercise, such as yoga, aerobics, and resistance training, have been shown to be effective (Helgadóttir et al. 2017; Rethorst et al. 2009). Patients who would like to avoid or stop taking medication may be more receptive to engaging in exercise as an alternative to antidepressants (Searle et al. 2011). Furthermore, exercise may prevent the onset of other medical conditions that depressed patients are at increased risk of developing, such as diabetes or heart disease (Warburton et al. 2006).

Exercise Type, Intensity, and Duration

Recent randomized controlled trials have compared the effect of different types, duration, and intensities of physical activity on both self-reported and clinician-measured symptoms of depression (Hallgren et al. 2015; Helgadóttir et al. 2016, 2017). As noted earlier, several types of exercise have been shown to be effective at reducing symptoms of depression, including

TABLE 3–1. Intervention components of exercise trials

Study	Population	Depression criteria	Preintervention criteria	Intervention components	Summary of key findings
Dunn et al. (2005)	80 patients between ages 20 and 45 years	Score between 12 and 25 on the HRSD and diagnosis through SCID	Activity level: fewer than 3 days of physical activity per week with no session ≥20 minutes Treatment: none	Length: 12 weeks Treatment groups: Low dose (7 kcal/kg/week) 3 days/week Low dose (7 kcal/kg/week) 5 days/week High dose (17.5 kcal/kg/ week) 3 days/week Low dose (17.5 kcal/kg/ week) 5 days/week	Public health dose (17.5 kcal/ kg/week) of physical activity can reduce symptoms of depression (Dunn et al. 2005).
Mota-Pereira et al. (2011)	150 patients between ages 18 and 60 years	Nonremitted depression diagnosed through interview with psychiatrist and score of >7 on the HRSD	Activity level: must be engaging in regular aerobic activity Treatment: failure to reach remission after two antidepressant trials and must have received no psychotherapy	Length: 12 weeks Exercise dose: 30–45 minutes of walking 5 days/ week; one walking session a week supervised by exercise professional	Home-based exercise program can promote reduced depressive symptoms and remission among patients with treatment-resistant MDD (Mota-Pereira et al. 2011).

TABLE 3–1. Intervention components of exercise trials *(continued)*

Study	Population	Depression criteria	Preintervention criteria	Intervention components	Summary of key findings
Regassa Trial (Hallgren et al. 2015; Helgadóttir et al. 2016, 2017)	946 patients between ages 18 and 67 years	Score of ≥10 on the PHQ-9	Activity level: all levels of activity Treatment: no limitations	Length: 12 weeks Treatment groups: 3×/week 12 weeks Light exercise: yoga or stretching class Moderate physical activity: moderate-intensity aerobics class Vigorous exercise condition: higher-intensity aerobics class ICBT: online modules monitored by clinician Treatment as usual: determined by primary care physician (usually CBT)	Participants assigned to exercise conditions and ICBT had more reduced depressive symptoms than patients receiving treatment as usual (Hallgren et al. 2015). Low-intensity, moderate-intensity, and vigorous-intensity physical activity can be just as effective on depressive symptoms as treatment as usual posttreatment (Helgadóttir et al. 2016) and at 1-year follow-up (Helgadóttir et al. 2017).

TABLE 3–1. Intervention components of exercise trials (*continued*)

Study	Population	Depression criteria	Preintervention criteria	Intervention components	Summary of key findings
Standard Medical Intervention and Long-Term Exercise Studies I (Babyak et al. 2000)	156 patients ages 50 years and older	Score of ≥13 on the HRSD	Activity level: not engaging in physical activity Treatment: no current psychiatric medications	Length: 16 weeks Intervention groups: Exercise group: 45 minutes of aerobics activity 3×/week (10-minute warm-up, 30 minutes walking/jogging on treadmill to reach target HR, and 5-minute cool down) Medication group: sertraline titrated to therapeutic dosage Combination group: both exercise and sertraline	Exercise during follow-up period was associated with reduced depressive symptoms at 10-month follow-up (Babyak et al. 2000).

TABLE 3–1. Intervention components of exercise trials (*continued*)

Study	Population	Depression criteria	Preintervention criteria	Intervention components	Summary of key findings
Standard Medical Intervention and Long-Term Exercise Studies II (Blumenthal et al. 2007; Hoffman et al. 2011)	202 patients ages 40 years and older	Score of ≥12 on the BDI	Activity level: not engaging in regular physical activity Treatment: no current psychiatric medications	Intervention length: 16 weeks Exercise group: 45 minutes aerobic activity 3×/week (10-minute warm-up, 30 minutes walking/jogging on treadmill to reach target HR, and 5-minute cool down) Treatment groups: Supervised aerobics group: physical activity in group setting with exercise physiologist Home-based session: initial session supervised by exercise physiologist, exercise prescription at home, and supervised follow-up sessions after months 1 and 2 Medication group: sertraline titrated until therapeutic dosage achieved Placebo condition: placebo only	Remission rates were higher among patients assigned to both exercise groups and medication than patients assigned to placebo condition (Blumenthal et al. 2007). There was no significant difference in remission between exercise groups (Blumenthal et al. 2007). Exercise during follow-up period was associated with reduced depressive symptoms during 10-month and 1-year follow-up (Hoffman et al. 2011).

TABLE 3–1. Intervention components of exercise trials (*continued*)

Study	Population	Depression criteria	Preintervention criteria	Intervention components	Summary of key findings
Treatment with Exercise Augmentation for Major Depression (TREAD)	122 patients between ages 18 and 70 years	Score of ≥14 on the HRSD	Activity level: fewer than 3 days of physical activity per week with no session ≥20 minutes Treatment: concurrently taking SSRI at therapeutic dosage for at least 6 months	Intervention length: 12 weeks Treatment groups: participants received supervised and home exercise sessions using treadmills, cycle ergometers, or a combination. Dosage of SSRI remained constant throughout trial. High-dose group: 16 kcal/kg/week of physical activity Low-dose group: 4 kcal/kg/week of physical activity	Higher dose of exercise may promote remission among men and women without a family history of mental illness (Trivedi et al. 2011). Exercise as a treatment for depression can also improve psychosocial and cognitive function (Greer et al. 2015, 2016). Positive affect after exercise is associated with treatment response for patients with MDD (Rethorst et al. 2017b; Suterwala et al. 2016).

TABLE 3–1. Intervention components of exercise trials *(continued)*

Study	Population	Depression criteria	Preintervention criteria	Intervention components	Summary of key findings
Treatment with Exercise Augmentation for Major Depression (TREAD) *(continued)*					Low levels of IL-6 and BDNF, reduced levels of cardiorespiratory fitness, and lower post-exercise positive affect are associated with lower response to exercise as a treatment for depression (Rethorst et al. 2017b).

Abbreviations. BDI=Beck Depression Inventory; BDNF=brain-derived neurotrophic factor; CBT=cognitive-behavioral therapy; HR=heart rate; HRSD=Hamilton Rating Scale for Depression; ICBT=Internet-based cognitive-behavioral therapy; I-6L=interleukin 6; MDD=major depressive disorder; PHQ-9=Patient Health Questionnaire-9; SCID=Structured Clinical Interview for Depression; SSRI=selective serotonin reuptake inhibitor.

resistance training, supervised sessions, group exercise, and even light exercise such as yoga (Blumenthal et al. 2007; Hallgren et al. 2015; Helgadóttir et al. 2017; Rethorst et al. 2009). Providers should recommend that patients engage in physical activity at least three times a week for 45–60 minutes per session as a treatment for depression (Rethorst and Trivedi 2013). Patients and providers should also note that it may take up to 10–12 weeks for symptoms to respond to treatment (Rethorst and Trivedi 2013).

A pilot study exploring exercise as an augmentative treatment had patients participate in an exercise program with tapered supervised sessions with an exercise professional for the first 3 weeks and engage in a home-based exercise program for the final 9 weeks (Trivedi et al. 2006). Patients experienced reductions in posttreatment Hamilton Rating Scale for Depression and Inventory of Depression Symptomology–Self-Report scores. This pilot study led to the Treatment with Exercise Augmentation for Depression (TREAD) study, which evaluated the effect of exercise on patients with non-remitted depression who were prescribed a selective serotonin reuptake inhibitor (Trivedi et al. 2011). TREAD researchers randomly assigned 122 patients into either a low-dose (4 kcal/week) or high-dose (16 kcal/week) exercise group for 12 weeks (Trivedi et al. 2011). Although patients in both groups experienced a reduction in depressive symptoms, remission appeared to be dose dependent, with patients who received a higher dose of exercise experiencing higher remission rates (Trivedi et al. 2011). The study also found that family history was a moderating variable for patients receiving exercise as an augmentation to antidepressant therapy. Specifically, women without a family history of depression and men both with and without family histories of depression were more likely to experience remission in depressive symptoms with a higher dose of exercise than a lower dose (Trivedi et al. 2011).

Another analysis of this same study population measured psychosocial functioning scores and health-related quality of life (Greer et al. 2016). Although both low- and high-dose groups experienced an improvement in psychosocial functioning scores, the high-dose group may have experienced improvements at a faster rate than did the low-dose group (Greer et al. 2016). Positive affect following the initial exercise session in the TREAD study was also investigated as a potential predictor of treatment response. Participants randomly assigned to the high-dose group who experienced positive affect after their first session were more likely to respond to exercise as a treatment and/or experience remission (Suterwala et al. 2016).

Two separate analyses of the Swedish Regassa trial (Hallgren et al. 2015; Helgadóttir et al. 2017) evaluated the effects of exercise intensity on depressive symptoms. Researchers from this trial randomly assigned patients to a low-intensity yoga and stretching class, a moderate-intensity aerobics course, or a high-intensity aerobics course for a 12-week intervention. Depression outcomes were then compared with those of patients receiving Internet-based cognitive-behavioral therapy (ICBT) and standard treatment for depression delivered by their primary care physician: antidepressants and/or cognitive-behavioral therapy (Hallgren et al. 2015; Helgadóttir et al. 2016, 2017). At the 12-week postintervention follow-up, patients in any of the exercise groups or the ICBT group experienced a greater reduction in depressive symptoms than patients assigned to the standard treatment group (Hallgren et al. 2015). Later analysis of the study also found that all levels of exercise were effective in either reducing depression severity or preventing depression severity from increasing (Helgadóttir et al. 2017). In fact, patients in the low-dose exercise condition experienced the greatest reduction in depressive symptoms. The results of this study suggest that all types and intensities of exercise should be encouraged, depending on patient preference (Helgadóttir et al. 2017).

Even though some studies suggest a dose-response relationship with physical activity (Galper et al. 2006), other studies report that patients can experience a reduction in symptoms of depression with even small doses of aerobic activity (Rethorst et al. 2009, 2017b; Teychenne et al. 2008). Findings such as these have prompted researchers to take into account moderating factors and patient characteristics that may provide insight into delivering the most effective exercise-based interventions to treat depression.

Predictors and Moderators of Treatment Efficacy

In addition to learning more about the role that exercise type and intensity plays in preventing depression and reducing the symptoms of depression, several investigations have sought to identify potential moderators, which are variables that may strengthen the relationship between exercise and symptoms of depression (Rethorst et al. 2017b; Schuch et al. 2016b). In a meta-analysis conducted by Schuch et al. (2016b), the authors reported that baseline depression symptoms, demographic variables, medication, frequency of exercise, and duration of trial did not moderate the effect of exercise on depressive symptoms. However, Rethorst et al. (2017b) and Suterwala et al. (2016) found a positive relationship between positive post-exercise affect and a reduction in depression symptoms.

A recent meta-analysis (Stubbs et al. 2016a) evaluated factors that contributed to adherence to exercise programs among patients with depression. This meta-analysis reported several findings that may help with the development of tailored exercise programs to meet the needs of patients with MDD. When compared with depressed patients randomly assigned to control conditions, patients randomly assigned to exercise conditions had better retention rates (Stubbs et al. 2016a). Research participants were more likely to complete exercise sessions when these sessions were supervised by an exercise professional (Stubbs et al. 2016a). The finding suggesting the benefit of supervised sessions was also supported in a meta-analysis conducted by Schuch et al. (2016a). Stubbs et al. (2016a) also found in their meta-analysis that patients who experienced more severe depressive symptoms at baseline were more likely to drop out of exercise trials. This meta-analysis also found that using a combination of both aerobic and strength-training interventions was associated with dropping out of study.

Glowacki et al. (2017) explored barriers to exercise among patients with depression in a scoping review and found that patients who felt exercise was a low priority or who had low self-efficacy, limited time, and/or limited resources (access to facilities or equipment) found it more challenging to engage in physical activity. However, patients who held positive beliefs about the benefits of exercise, established a routine, had adequate social support, and/or had access to tools to monitor their health behaviors and progress (e.g., pedometers, diaries) were more likely to engage in physical activity (Glowacki et al. 2017).

Short-Term Versus Long-Term Benefits

The majority of studies that explore the effects of exercise on depression have focused on short-term benefits; however, a recent analysis of the Regassa trial (Helgadóttir et al. 2017) found that patients with depression can experience a reduction in symptoms 12 months postintervention. This promising finding provides even more encouragement for patients and providers interested in using exercise as a treatment for depression. However, further research on this topic is needed to gather greater insight into the long-term benefits of exercise as a treatment for MDD. A follow-up study on the Standard Medical Intervention and Long-term Exercise (SMILE) trial (Babyak et al. 2000) found that patients randomly assigned to an exercise intervention experienced higher remission rates than patients assigned to a group receiving pharmacological therapy. Investigators later explored the 1-year follow-up for the SMILE trial and reported that engaging in exercise during the follow-up period was associated with reduced depressive symptoms (Hoffman et al. 2011).

EXERCISE AND PREVENTION OF CHRONIC MEDICAL CONDITIONS AMONG INDIVIDUALS WITH DEPRESSION

Patients with a diagnosis of MDD experience a multitude of negative effects on their health as well as negative economic complications from comorbidities of depression and other medical conditions (Greenberg et al. 2015; Sin et al. 2016). Given that patients with depression tend to be less physically active than patients without depression (Farmer et al. 1988; Galper et al. 2006; Harvey et al. 2018), this population is at increased risk of experiencing poor overall health as a result of their lack of physical activity (Warburton et al. 2006). Physical inactivity increases one's risk of developing chronic medical conditions such as type II diabetes, heart disease, and osteoporosis (see Chapter 16, "Lifestyle Interventions for Cardiometabolic Health in People With Psychiatric Disorders").

Unfortunately, patients with depression are not only at increased risk for developing other chronic medical conditions; they also are at increased risk for having poorer health as a result of comorbid conditions than are patients without MDD (Bryan et al. 2010; Katon et al. 2007; Warburton et al. 2006). Inactive patients with depression may experience increased symptoms related to their chronic medical conditions, higher mortality rates if their depression symptoms are poorly managed, and increased economic burden of disease (Bryan et al. 2010; Greenberg et al. 2015; Katon et al. 2007; Rethorst et al. 2017a). Patients with depression and heart disease are at especially high risk for complications associated with heart disease (Sin et al. 2016). Among patients with heart disease, those who have severe symptoms of depression are more likely to be physically inactive, adhere less to their treatment plan, engage in unhealthy behaviors such as smoking, and have increased body mass index and hip-to-waist ratios (Sin et al. 2016). In addition to being at increased risk for experiencing poorer health outcomes than patients with heart disease who do not have depression, these patients are also are more likely to report more symptoms associated with heart disease, such as chest pain and shortness of breath (Katon et al. 2007).

Medical providers who prescribe physical activity to patients with depression can help reduce their patients' depressive symptoms and relieve or reduce symptoms from other chronic medical conditions (Blumenthal et al. 2012; Katon et al. 2007; Warburton et al. 2006). Promoting physical activity among patients with depression may serve the dual purpose of helping to reduce the patient's depressive symptoms while also providing patients with another prevention and reduction strategy for complications from other chronic medical conditions.

Individuals with cancer are also at increased risk for experiencing symptoms of depression during and after treatment (Krebber et al. 2014). Both a systematic literature review (Craft et al. 2012) and a meta-analysis (Brown et al. 2012) found that physical activity can improve the symptoms of depression among patients who are being treated or have been treated for cancer. The meta-analysis also found that cancer survivors had a greater reduction in depressive symptoms when exercise sessions were supervised by an exercise professional (Brown et al. 2012).

Another area that has been explored is the relationship between obesity and depression (Rivenes et al. 2009; Stunkard et al. 2003; Xiang and An 2015). A systematic review and meta-analysis of longitudinal studies observed a bidirectional relationship between obesity and depression (Luppino et al. 2010). Another longitudinal study that followed middle-age adults for 16 years found that overweight and obese patients had a higher incidence of depression than did patients who were not overweight (Xiang and An 2015). Obesity, like many other chronic medical conditions, has a positive association with depressive symptomatology (Rivenes et al. 2009; Stunkard et al. 2003; Xiang and An 2015). Given the increasing number of patients who are classified as overweight or obese, promoting physical activity may help to reduce the risk of depression as well as reduce the prevalence of obesity.

CONCLUSION AND IMPLICATIONS FOR MEDICAL PROVIDERS AND PUBLIC HEALTH PROFESSIONALS

A study conducted by Janney et al. (2017) found that although most patients who used mental health services reported that exercise improved their mood, they reported that their mental health provider did not consistently discuss strategies to increase their physical activity as a way to improve their mood (Janney et al. 2017). Mental health providers and primary care providers may experience several personal, structural, and organizational barriers to delivering physical activity counseling in their setting (Glowacki et al. 2017; Hébert et al. 2012; Searle et al. 2011). One of the most common concerns among medical and public health professionals is the benefit of promoting physical activity to a population of patients who may struggle with motivation; however, providers should note the cyclical nature of depression symptoms, which may result in changes in motivation throughout treatment (Blumenthal et al. 2012). Patients who receive exercise as a treatment for depression have treatment adherence rates that are comparable to those of patients who receive pharmacological treatment and/or psychotherapy (Rethorst et al. 2009). In order to promote adherence, providers should consider some of the most common barriers to engaging in physical activity (e.g., time, resources, motivation) and address them before and throughout treatment (Glowacki et al. 2017; Janney et al. 2017; Searle et al. 2011; Stubbs et al. 2016a).

Given that patients with depression are at increased risk for other chronic conditions, it is especially important to provide consistent education on the benefits of physical activity to this population. One study found that depressed patients with several chronic medical conditions were more likely to regularly access mental health services than were patients with MDD who did not have a comorbid chronic medical condition (Puyat et al. 2017). It may be of benefit for physicians to discuss physical activity with their patients with depression and other chronic medical conditions on a regular basis as a way to promote mental and physical health.

Health behaviors are complex and not easily changed. Even though patients can take small, incremental steps to increase their physical activity, these behaviors require a change in lifestyle. When counseling patients with MDD on increasing their physical activity and maintaining positive health behavior change, providers should use evidence-based strategies and should consider using behavioral activation to promote exercise adherence (Schneider et al. 2016). One method of counseling that providers may want to consider is using the 5 As: ask, advise, assess, assist, arrange (Carroll et al. 2011). Figure 3–1 describes the topics that medical providers should cover when counseling patients on increasing their physical activity using the 5 As, which consider barriers, preferences, and readiness to change (Carroll et al. 2011).

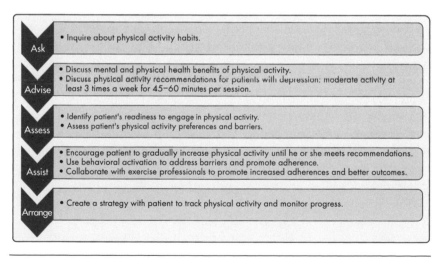

FIGURE 3–1. Key strategies for counseling patients on exercise as treatment for depression using the 5 As.

OPPORTUNITIES FOR FUTURE RESEARCH

The complex nature of the relationship between physical activity and symptoms of depression provides many opportunities for researchers to explore the effect of exercise among special patient populations. In recent years, there has been some discussion about how physical activity can help reduce the symptoms of postpartum depression (Da Costa et al. 2009; Fjeldsoe et al. 2010). A recent meta-analysis demonstrated small effect sizes for exercise interventions for treating postpartum depression, although the authors noted that most of the studies were comparing exercise to usual care, and additional high-quality randomized controlled trials comparing exercise with an active control condition are warranted (Carter et al. 2018). Another recent study explored the effects of physical activity on depressive symptoms in patients from low- and middle-income countries, a less-researched patient population (Stubbs et al. 2016b). Future studies should expand on this work and evaluate interventions for patient populations from all socioeconomic and demographic backgrounds. Future trials should further assess the impact of exercise intensity and duration and the long-term benefits of exercise as a treatment for depression to provide additional insight into how researchers and providers can adapt more tailored interventions that meet the patient's needs and avoid a one-size-fits-all approach (Blumenthal et al. 2012; Glowacki et al. 2017; Rethorst and Trivedi 2013; Searle et al. 2011; Stubbs et al. 2016b; Trivedi et al. 2011). It will be particularly interesting to explore the psychological and neurobiological basis for long-term effects of exercise on depression.

Another area of research that needs further exploration is the effect of exercise on patients with bipolar disorder. Recent systematic reviews have highlighted some of the potential benefits that patients with bipolar disorder may experience from engaging in physical activity, which include reduced symptoms of depression, improved physical health, and improved sleep quality (Melo et al. 2016; Thomson et al. 2015). Because patients with bipolar disorder are at increased risk of experiencing medical comorbidities, a sedentary lifestyle, and negative mental health effects related to poor sleep quality, exercise may provide benefits for this patient population (Melo et al. 2016; Thomson et al. 2015).

Although research findings support that exercise can provide some mental and physical health benefits for patients with bipolar disorder, there is still very little scientific understanding of the relationship between exercise and bipolar disorder (Melo et al. 2016; Thomson et al. 2015). Gaining insight into how exercise affects the mood of patients with bipolar disorder is further complicated by methodological concerns related to study design that hinder generalizability of existing studies (Melo et al. 2016; Thomson et al. 2015). Future studies should seek to gain a better understanding of mechanisms of action, the effect of exercise on sleep-wake cycles of patients with bipolar disorder, the relationship between exercise and states of hypomania and mania, and how exercise type, intensity, and duration affect the mood of patients with bipolar disorder (Thomson et al. 2015).

Case Example

Olivia is a 32-year-old woman who has been prescribed exercise as a treatment for MDD. She meets three times a week with an exercise professional, Sarah, to walk on a treadmill and has gradually increased her activity level to 150 minutes a week. In addition to her three supervised sessions, Olivia is to exercise at least once a week on her own. Each week, Olivia and Sarah meet to plan the next week's exercise sessions and discuss any barriers Olivia encountered during the previous week. Olivia reports that she has not been motivated to complete her home-based exercise sessions. As the weather becomes cooler, she reports that she is less motivated to walk in her neighborhood and has become discouraged that her depressive symptoms have not responded after 4 weeks of consistent exercise. Sarah and Olivia develop a plan to help address barriers and promote adherence.

Sarah starts the discussion by praising Olivia for consistently attending her supervised sessions. She then reinforces that it may take up to 10–12 weeks for symptoms to respond to exercise and encourages Olivia to continue to work out. During the discussion about barriers, Olivia mentions that she is becoming bored with walking and wants to try another type of exercise. After Olivia and Sarah brainstorm different types of exercise, Olivia expresses interest in a Zumba class that her coworkers attend every Saturday but is unsure if it is an acceptable form of physical activity. Sarah encourages Olivia to attend a Zumba class with her coworkers this week, and during the planning session the following week, they will discuss if it is something Olivia would like to continue.

At the next planning session, Olivia reports that she enrolled in the Zumba class and was looking forward to attending every Saturday. Olivia mentions that social support and having someone hold her accountable are motivating factors to exercise. Sarah and Olivia discuss potential barriers to Olivia's consistently attending the class and strategies to address these barriers. At the end of the planning session, Olivia lists two strategies that she will use to promote consistent attendance: 1) She will enlist the social support of a coworker who consistently attends the class every Saturday, and this coworker will be her accountability partner. 2) She will track her exercise on an exercise log and address barriers each week with Sarah.

DISCUSSION QUESTIONS

1. In addition to evidence-based recommendations, what other tools and/or resources can clinicians use to help identify patients who may

benefit from exercise as a treatment for depression and to promote exercise among this patient population?

2. During a routine visit, a patient with MDD requests information about exercise as a treatment for depressive symptoms. What information and resources would you provide this patient?

3. A patient who has been engaging in 150 minutes of physical activity per week for 3 weeks comes in for a follow-up visit to evaluate depressive symptoms. During her visit, she expresses discouragement that she has not noticed any positive changes in her mood since starting the exercise program. What recommendations would you give this patient?

RECOMMENDED READINGS

Blumenthal JA, Smith PJ, Hoffman BM: Is exercise a viable treatment for depression? ACSM's Health Fit J 16(4):14–21, 2012

Carroll JK, Antognoli E, Flocke SA: Evaluation of physical activity counseling in primary care using direct observation of the 5As. Ann Fam Med 9(5):416–422, 2011

Rethorst CD, Trivedi MH: Evidence-based recommendations for the prescription of exercise for major depressive disorder. J Psychiatr Pract 19(3):204–212, 2013

Seime RJ, Vickers KS: The challenges of treating depression with exercise: from evidence to practice. Clin Psychol Sci Pract 13(2):194–197, 2006

REFERENCES

Babyak M, Blumenthal JA, Herman S, et al: Exercise treatment for major depression: maintenance of therapeutic benefit at 10 months. Psychosom Med 62(5):633–638, 2000 11020092

Blumenthal JA, Babyak MA, Doraiswamy PM, et al: Exercise and pharmacotherapy in the treatment of major depressive disorder. Psychosom Med 69(7):587–596, 2007 17846259

Blumenthal JA, Smith PJ, Hoffman BM: Is exercise a viable treatment for depression? ACSM's Health Fit J 16(4):14–21, 2012 23750100

Brown JC, Huedo-Medina TB, Pescatello LS, et al: The efficacy of exercise in reducing depressive symptoms among cancer survivors: a meta-analysis. PLoS One 7(1):e30955, 2012 22303474

Bryan C, Songer T, Brooks MM, et al: The impact of diabetes on depression treatment outcomes. Gen Hosp Psychiatry 32(1):33–41, 2010 20114126

Carroll JK, Antognoli E, Flocke SA: Evaluation of physical activity counseling in primary care using direct observation of the 5As. Ann Fam Med 9(5):416–422, 2011 21911760

Carter T, Bastounis A, Guo B, Morrell JC: The effectiveness of exercise-based interventions for preventing or treating postpartum depression: a systematic review and meta-analysis. Arch Womens Ment Health, 2018 [Epub ahead of print] 29682074

Cooney GM, Dwan K, Greig CA, et al: Exercise for depression. Cochrane Database Syst Rev (9):CD004366, 2013 24026850

Craft LL, Vaniterson EH, Helenowski IB, et al: Exercise effects on depressive symptoms in cancer survivors: a systematic review and meta-analysis. Cancer Epidemiol Biomarkers Prev 21(1):3–19, 2012 22068286

Da Costa D, Lowensteyn I, Abrahamowicz M, et al: A randomized clinical trial of exercise to alleviate postpartum depressed mood. J Psychosom Obstet Gynaecol 30(3):191–200, 2009 19728220

Dishman RK, Sui X, Church TS, et al: Decline in cardiorespiratory fitness and odds of incident depression. Am J Prev Med 43(4):361–368, 2012 22992353

Dunn AL, Trivedi MH, Kampert JB, et al: Exercise treatment for depression: efficacy and dose response. Am J Prev Med 28(1):1–8, 2005 15626549

Farmer ME, Locke BZ, Mo?cicki K ,et al: Physical activity and depressive symptoms: the NHANES I Epidemiologic Follow-up Study. Am J Epidemiol 128(6):1340–1351, 1988 3264110

Fjeldsoe BS, Miller YD, Marshall AL: MobileMums: a randomized controlled trial of an SMS-based physical activity intervention. Ann Behav Med 39(2):101–111, 2010 20174902

Galper DI, Trivedi MH, Barlow CF, et al: Inverse association between physical inactivity and mental health in men and women. Med Sci Sports Exerc 38(1):173–178, 2006 16394971

Glowacki K, Duncan MJ, Gainforth H, et al: Barriers and facilitators to physical activity and exercise among adults with depression: a scoping review. Ment Health Phys Act 13:108–119, 2017

Greenberg PE, Fournier AA, Sisitsky T, et al: The economic burden of adults with major depressive disorder in the United States (2005 and 2010). J Clin Psychiatry 76(2):155–162, 2015 25742202

Greer TL, Grannemann BD, Chansard M, et al: Dose-dependent changes in cognitive function with exercise augmentation for major depression: results from the TREAD study. Eur Neuropsychopharmacol 25(2):248–256, 2015 25453481

Greer TL, Trombello JM, Rethorst CD, et al: Improvements in psychosocial functioning and health-related quality of life following exercise augmentation in patients with treatment response but nonremitted major depressive disorder: results from the TREAD study. Depress Anxiety 33(9):870–881, 2016 27164293

Hallgren M, Kraepelien M, Öjehagen A, et al: Physical exercise and internet-based cognitive-behavioural therapy in the treatment of depression: randomised controlled trial. Br J Psychiatry 207(3):227–234, 2015 26089305

Harris AH, Cronkite R, Moos R: Physical activity, exercise coping, and depression in a 10-year cohort study of depressed patients. J Affect Disord 93(1–3):79–85, 2006 16545873

Harvey SB, Øverland S, Hatch SL, et al: Exercise and the prevention of depression: results of the HUNT cohort study. Am J Psychiatry 175(1):28–36, 2018 28969440

Hébert ET, Caughy MO, Shuval K: Primary care providers' perception of physical activity counselling in a clinical setting: a systematic review. Br J Sports Med 46(9):625–631, 2012 22711796

Helgadóttir B, Hallgren M, Ekblom Ö, et al: Training fast or slow? Exercise for depression: a randomized controlled trial. Prev Med 91:123–131, 2016 27514246

Helgadóttir B, Forsell Y, Hallgren M, et al: Long-term effects of exercise at different intensity levels on depression: a randomized controlled trial. Prev Med 105:37–46, 2017 28823684

Hoffman BM, Babyak MA, Craighead WE, et al: Exercise and pharmacotherapy in patients with major depression: one-year follow-up of the SMILE study. Psychosom Med 73(2):127–133, 2011 21148807

Janney CA, Brzoznowski KF, Richardson CR, et al: Moving towards wellness: physical activity practices, perspectives, and preferences of users of outpatient mental health service. Gen Hosp Psychiatry 49:63–66, 2017 29122150

Katon W, Lin EH, Kroenke K: The association of depression and anxiety with medical symptom burden in patients with chronic medical illness. Gen Hosp Psychiatry 29(2):147–155, 2007 17336664

Krebber AM, Buffart LM, Kleijn G, et al: Prevalence of depression in cancer patients: a meta-analysis of diagnostic interviews and self-report instruments. Psychooncology 23(2):121–130, 2014 24105788

Luppino FS, de Wit LM, Bouvy PF, et al: Overweight, obesity, and depression: a systematic review and meta-analysis of longitudinal studies. Arch Gen Psychiatry 67(3):220–229, 2010 20194822

Mammen G, Faulkner G: Physical activity and the prevention of depression: a systematic review of prospective studies. Am J Prev Med 45(5):649–657, 2013 24139780

Melo MC, Daher EdeF, Albuquerque SG, et al: Exercise in bipolar patients: a systematic review. J Affect Disord 198:32–38, 2016 26998794

Mota-Pereira J, Silverio J, Carvalho S, et al: Moderate exercise improves depression parameters in treatment-resistant patients with major depressive disorder. J Psychiatr Res 45(8):1005–1011, 2011 21377690

Puyat JH, Kazanjian A, Wong H, et al: Comorbid chronic general health conditions and depression care: a population-based analysis. Psychiatr Serv 68(9):907–915, 2017 28457213

Rethorst CD, Trivedi MH: Evidence-based recommendations for the prescription of exercise for major depressive disorder. J Psychiatr Pract 19(3):204–212, 2013 23653077

Rethorst CD, Wipfli BM, Landers DM: The antidepressive effects of exercise: a meta-analysis of randomized trials. Sports Med 39(6):491–511, 2009 19453207

Rethorst CD, Leonard D, Barlow CE, et al: Effects of depression, metabolic syndrome, and cardiorespiratory fitness on mortality: results from the Coopercenter Longitudinal Study. Psychol Med 47(14):2414–2420, 2017a 28414015

Rethorst CD, South CC, Rush AJ, et al: Prediction of treatment outcomes to exercise in patients with nonremitted major depressive disorder. Depress Anxiety 34(12):1116–1122, 2017b 28672073

Rivenes AC, Harvey SB, Mykletun A: The relationship between abdominal fat, obesity, and common mental disorders: results from the HUNT study. J Psychosom Res 66(4):269–275, 2009 19302883

Schneider KL, Panza E, Handschin B, et al: Feasibility of pairing behavioral activation with exercise for women with type 2 diabetes and depression: the Get It study pilot randomized controlled trial. Behav Ther 47(2):198–212, 2016 26956652

Schuch FB, Vancampfort D, Richards J, et al: Exercise as a treatment for depression: a meta-analysis adjusting for publication bias. J Psychiatr Res 77:42–51, 2016a 26978184

Schuch FB, Dunn AL, Kanitz AC, et al: Moderators of response in exercise treatment for depression: a systematic review. J Affect Disord 195:40–49, 2016b 26854964

Searle A, Calnan M, Lewis G, et al: Patients' views of physical activity as treatment for depression: a qualitative study. Br J Gen Pract 61(585):149–156, 2011 21439172

Sin NL, Kumar AD, Gehi AK, et al: Direction of association between depressive symptoms and lifestyle behaviors in patients with coronary heart disease: the Heart and Soul study. Ann Behav Med 50(4):523–532, 2016 26817654

Stubbs B, Vancampfort D, Rosenbaum S, et al: Dropout from exercise randomized controlled trials among people with depression: a meta-analysis and meta regression. J Affect Disord 190:457–466, 2016a 26551405

Stubbs B, Koyanagi A, Schuch FB, et al: Physical activity and depression: a large cross-sectional, population-based study across 36 low- and middle-income countries. Acta Psychiatr Scand 134(6):546–556, 2016b 27704532

Stunkard AJ, Faith MS, Allison KC: Depression and obesity. Biol Psychiatry 54(3):330–337, 2003 12893108

Suterwala AM, Rethorst CD, Carmody TJ, et al: Affect following first exercise session as a predictor of treatment response in depression. J Clin Psychiatry 77(8):1036–1042, 2016 27561137

Teychenne M, Ball K, Salmon J: Physical activity and likelihood of depression in adults: a review. Prev Med 46(5):397–411, 2008 18289655

Thomson D, Turner A, Lauder S, et al: A brief review of exercise, bipolar disorder, and mechanistic pathways. Front Psychol 6:147, 2015 25788889

Trivedi MH, Greer TL, Grannemann BD, et al: Exercise as an augmentation strategy for treatment of major depression. J Psychiatr Pract 12(4):205–213, 2006 16883145

Trivedi MH, Greer TL, Church TS, et al: Exercise as an augmentation treatment for nonremitted major depressive disorder: a randomized, parallel dose comparison. J Clin Psychiatry 72(5):677–684, 2011 21658349

Warburton DE, Nicol CW, Bredin SS: Health benefits of physical activity: the evidence. CMAJ 174(6):801–809, 2006 16534088

Xiang X, An R: Obesity and onset of depression among U.S. middle-aged and older adults. J Psychosom Res 78(3):242–248, 2015 25553601

CHAPTER 4

Physical Exercise in the Management of Anxiety Disorders and Obsessive-Compulsive Disorder

Neil A. Rector, Ph.D.

Margaret A. Richter, M.D.

Bethany Lerman, B.A.

The authors thank Preeya Laxman and Vanessa Montemarano for their editorial assistance on this chapter. This chapter was supported in part by the Canadian Institutes of Health Research (CIHR).

KEY POINTS

- Structured physical exercise can be a helpful adjunctive and stand-alone treatment in anxiety disorders and obsessive-compulsive disorder.
- Potential mechanisms of action of exercise include reductions in anxiety sensitivity, improved feelings of self-efficacy, and improved cognitive functioning.
- Clinical approaches to introducing and maintaining physical exercise include addressing key motivational variables and disorder-specific barriers and integrating exercise into cognitive-behavioral therapy.

Anxiety disorders are highly prevalent, with approximately one-quarter of the population suffering from a diagnosable condition sometime in their lifetime (Kessler et al. 2005). Anxiety disorders are also highly comorbid with other psychiatric and medical conditions, with up to one-third of people with an anxiety disorder meeting criteria for two or more additional anxiety or other psychiatric disorders and a range of physical disorders (Toft et al. 2005). Each disorder is distinct in some ways, but they all share the same hallmark features reflecting excessive and irrational fear: feeling tense and apprehensive and a range of other physical symptoms of discomfort and experiencing significant impairment and/or distress as a result of the cognitive, behavioral, or emotional aspects of the condition. The personal and societal costs (e.g., health care costs, underemployment, disability) associated with the anxiety disorders are staggering, with estimated annual costs exceeding $40 billion (Greenberg et al. 1999).

The main anxiety disorders considered in the current *Diagnostic and Statistical Manual of Mental Disorders*, 5th Edition (DSM-5; American Psychiatric Association 2013) include panic disorder, agoraphobia, specific phobia, social anxiety disorder (social phobia) (SAD), and generalized anxiety disorder (GAD). Although previously grouped together, posttraumatic stress disorder (PTSD; see Chapter 5, "Physical Exercise as a Potentially Useful Component of Posttraumatic Stress Disorder Treatment") and obsessive-compulsive disorder (OCD) have become separate but related conditions in DSM-5. Although OCD is consistently identified as the least prevalent of the anxiety disorders, it is a severe and debilitating condition afflicting about 2% of the population (Kessler et al. 2005), and, in most cases, if untreated, tends to run a chronic and deteriorating course, making it among the top 10 leading causes of disability worldwide (Brundtland 2000). In light of the prevalence and associated personal and societal costs, anxiety and OCD conditions are a significant public health concern, which makes the identification, development, and dissemination of effective, evidence-based treatment approaches extremely important.

International practice guidelines (e.g., guidelines from the National Institute for Health and Care Excellence [NICE], the American Psychiatric Association, and the Canadian Psychiatric Association) focus on the role of pharmacotherapy, particularly antidepressants, and short-term psychological treatments, particularly cognitive-behavioral therapy (CBT), and a combination of the two. Although there is strong empirical support for the role of psychological and biological treatments for the anxiety disorders, there continue to be difficulties associated with access to treatment, adherence, premature termination, nonresponsiveness, persistent impairing symptoms for treatment responders and nonresponders alike, and relapse and recurrence following successful treatment. Thus, there is great need for low-cost, easily accessible, and effective alternative treatments. Increasingly, empirical support is accruing for the role of exercise as a legitimate, evidence-based intervention for anxiety disorders and psychiatric disorders in general, both as adjuncts to pharmacotherapy and CBT and as stand-alone interventions. Exercise training is a healthy and easily accessible, low-cost behavior with minimal risk of adverse events. In the remainder of this chapter, we review the empirical evidence for aerobic exercise in the anxiety disorders, discuss the integration of exercise with first-line treatments, and address clinical aspects associated with dropout from or discontinuation of exercise.

CROSS-SECTIONAL ASSOCIATIONS BETWEEN EXERCISE AND GENERAL MENTAL WELL-BEING

It is recommended that adults ages 18–64 years accumulate at least 150 minutes per week of moderate to vigorous aerobic physical activity, in bouts of 10 minutes or more (Piercy et al. 2018). However, only 20% of adults report meeting these guidelines for weekly moderate to vigorous physical activity (Statistics Canada 2015). Higher levels of fitness have been linked to reduced all-cause mortality (e.g., stroke, cardiovascular disease, certain cancers) (Warburton et al. 2010), but the putative link between exercise and emotional well-being has only recently been systematically tested with clinical populations, resulting in growing empirical support for regular exercise as a treatment option for people with psychiatric disorders. The evidence has emerged from two major sources: 1) naturalistic large-scale epidemiology studies that examine rates of psychiatric conditions and amount of naturally occurring physical exercise and 2) laboratory-based studies that examine the direct impact of short-term exercise programs to reduce psychiatric symptoms. Regarding the former, general population studies have found significant cross-sectional associations between physical activity levels and the presence and severity of mental health disorders (Goodwin 2003; Harvey et al. 2010; Ten Have et al. 2011), with increased physical exercise being associated with reduced levels of depression, anxiety, substance use disorders, and somatoform disorders.

In terms of experimental studies, the most widely assessed benefits of exercise on mental health have focused on depression (see Chapter 3, "Physical Exercise in the Management of Major Depressive Disorders"). There is now substantive empirical evidence for the benefits of exercise for depression, although there is considerable variation in the components of the exercise interventions tested across the extant literature. The duration of exercise varies from 1 to 16 weeks, the type of exercise varies from aerobic to strength training at varying levels of intensity, exercise can be home based or center based, and studies are split between individual and group exercise modalities with or without monitored interventions (Rimer et al. 2012).

When these issues have been directly addressed in meta-analytic reviews, a positive treatment effect for exercise has still been observed. For instance, a Cochrane review examined 23 trials with 907 participants and found a large treatment effect for depression (Cohen's *d*) of 0.82 (Mead et al. 2008). More recently, 28 trials (1,101 participants) comparing exercise with no treatment or a control intervention found an effect size of 0.67 at posttreatment analysis, indicating a robust moderate clinical effect on symptoms of depression (Rimer et al. 2012). The NICE treatment guidelines for depression now recommend structured, supervised exercise programs three times a week (45 minutes to 1 hour) over 10–14 weeks as a low-intensity intervention for mild to moderate depression (National Institute for Health and Care Excellence 2009).

BENEFITS OF EXERCISE IN THE ANXIETY DISORDERS

Although depression and anxiety disorders are frequently comorbid, there are significant differences in phenomenology; onset patterns; course of illness; and putative underlying biological, psychological, and psychosocial risk factors that suggest that anxiety disorders require their own examination with exercise separate from depression. Studies have now begun to examine the direct impact of structured exercise on anxious states and the symptoms of common anxiety disorders. Early randomized controlled trial research and meta-analyses (e.g., Petruzzello et al. 1991) focused on the examination of exercise on acute *anxiety states*. A meta-analysis (Wipfli et al. 2008) with nonclinical participants across 49 exercise studies observed significant change on various self-report measures of anxiety in the moderate effect size (0.48) range. In this review, the typical exercise regimen was three or four times per week of aerobic exercise. In another meta-analytic review, Herring et al. (2010) examined the literature between 1995 and 2007 and found 40 studies of sedentary adults with a chronic illness (e.g., cancer, cardiovascular disease, multiple sclerosis) participating in structured aerobic exercise programs. These studies demonstrated significant moderate effects of aerobic exercise sessions of 30 minutes or more for 3–12 weeks on measures of trait anxiety (0.56) and significant small effects on self-reported state anxiety measures (0.31).

Beyond the impact of exercise on reducing acute anxiety, more recent reviews (Asmundson et al. 2013; Zschucke et al. 2013) have focused on a small number of studies (fewer than a dozen) with promising therapeutic effects of exercise for bona fide anxiety disorders. Studies now demonstrate the ability of aerobic exercise to do the following:

1. Significantly reduce the frequency and severity of panic attacks for participants diagnosed with panic disorder beyond placebo conditions, although this effect is not equal to the benefits of medications or CBT
2. Significantly reduce social anxiety symptoms and improve subjective well-being at posttreatment and follow-up in a manner equivalent to mindfulness-based stress reduction for patients diagnosed with social anxiety disorder
3. Significantly reduce worry and anxious arousal in people with GAD in response to combined aerobic and resistance training compared with waitlist control subjects.

There have also been several preliminary studies testing the efficacy of exercise for OCD. In a study of 15 patients with OCD receiving treatment as usual, Brown et al. (2007) found that a 12-week program of moderate-intensity aerobic exercise (55%–69% maximum heart rate, three or four times weekly, increasing from 20 to 40 minutes in duration) led to significant reductions in OCD symptoms. Large effects were observed from baseline to posttreatment ($d=1.69$) and were still evident at 6-month follow-up ($d=1.11$). In a follow-up analysis of this sample (Abrantes et al. 2009), the acute effects of exercise on anxiety, obsessions, and compulsions were also observed with reductions in pre-exercise to post-exercise anxiety ($d=-0.73$) and compulsions ($d=-0.77$), with a medium effect for reductions in obsessions ($d=0.62$) in the first week of exercise. Furthermore, Lancer et al. (2007) reported that in a sample of individuals with treatment-resistant OCD ($n=11$), a 6-week aerobic exercise intervention significantly reduced self-reported obsessive-compulsive symptoms at postintervention and at 1-month follow-up.

Finally, a pilot study was conducted by our group (Rector et al. 2015) to investigate the utility and efficacy of integrating a structured physical exercise program with standard group CBT for OCD. Participants ($n=11$) completed 12 weeks of group CBT along with thrice-weekly exercise sessions. Exercise regimens were tailored to each participant's fitness level on the basis of peak heart rate captured via an incremental maximal exercise test. Change in Yale-Brown Obsessive Compulsive Scale scores from pretreatment to posttreatment in CBT-group cohorts was very large ($d=2.55$) and surpassed previously established effects of CBT for OCD. We have recently completed a large-scale multisite randomized controlled trial (N. A. Rector et al., in preparation, 2019) that will permit examination of the relative efficacy of aerobic exercise, CBT, and a combination of both versus a nontreatment waitlist control condition for OCD symptoms and underlying cognitive vulnerabilities.

An alternative approach to examining the impact of exercise on distinct anxiety disorders is to cluster together participants with varying anxiety disorders and then determine the effects of exercise on transdiagnostic anxiety symptoms, disorder-specific symptoms, and shared underlying psychological vulnerabilities. In a recent study by LeBouthillier and Asmundson (2017), 42 patients with anxiety disorders were randomly assigned to a 4-week intervention of aerobic exercise, resistance training, or waitlist control. Both exercise modalities were found to be efficacious in producing improvements in anxiety-related disorder symptoms. In addition, resistance training produced significant reductions in underlying psychological vulnerabilities associated with risk for anxisety disorders, including anxiety sensitivity, distress tolerance, and intolerance of uncertainty.

The direct impact of exercise on cognitive vulnerabilities in anxiety disorders has been tested in experimental conditions of a single bout of aerobic exercise. For instance, Broman-Fulks et al. (2015) demonstrated that a single 20-minute moderate-intensity aerobic exercise session significantly reduced anxiety sensitivity (although not distress tolerance). Similarly, LeBouthillier and Asmundson (2015) found that a single 30-minute session of aerobic exercise led to significant reductions with moderate effect sizes across all dimensions of anxiety sensitivity, although, as in the study by Broman-Fulks and colleagues, no impact on distress tolerance was observed.

MECHANISMS OF ACTION

The mechanisms by which physical exercise may improve anxiety symptoms have yet to be fully deduced, although multiple potential mechanisms of action have been postulated. Asmundson et al. (2013) put forth several possible mechanisms underlying the anxiolytic effects of exercise, such as reductions in anxiety sensitivity; inadvertent exposure therapy to feared bodily sensations induced by exercise; improvement in physiological resilience to stressful mood states (e.g., endocrine adaptations, endorphin boosts); changes to isolated routines and inclusion of social interaction; and improvements in sleep, positive affect, and feelings of mastery and self-efficacy.

Given the large empirical literature documenting the positive benefits of physical exercise on depressed mood as noted, as well as the high comorbidity rates between depressive and anxiety disorders (Kessler et al. 2015), it may also be possible that improvement in anxiety symptoms during exercise are a result of acute improvement in accompanying negative mood. For example, the associations between obsessive-compulsive symptoms and depression are well described (Rector et al. 2017), and Abrantes et al. (2009) found that both mood ratings and obsessive-compulsive symptom ratings showed improvement from single pre-exercise to post-exercise sessions in patients with OCD. However, the mechanisms by which exercise may improve negative mood states and psychopathology are still ambiguous and are confounded further by the findings that although improvements in mood should be expected to occur in conjunction with improvements in fitness, only half of exercise studies demonstrate such a positive correlation (Rimer et al. 2012).

Another possibility is that exercise impacts mood and anxiety symptoms via changes in underlying cognitive vulnerabilities. A substantive amount of research supports the existence of positive associations between regular exercise and changes in the brain that improve memory and learning, including neurogenesis, angiogenesis, and enhanced central nervous system metabolism (Prakash et al. 2010). The level of impact of exercise within clinical samples remains largely unexamined, although relatively recent research in depression and other disorders is promising. Déry et al. (2013) demonstrated the opposing effects of aerobic exercise as compared with depression on a putative hippocampal neurogenesis-dependent learning task, with those participants who significantly increased their fitness achieving higher scores. Similarly, Pajonk et al. (2010) reported that after an exercise program, significant increases in hippocampal volume were observed in patients with schizophrenia (12%) and healthy control subjects (16%) compared with a nonexercise group (–1%), along with a

34% improvement in short-term memory test scores for patients with schizophrenia (see Chapter 6, "Physical Exercise in the Management of Schizophrenia Spectrum Disorders"). Erickson et al. (2011) also demonstrated that hippocampal volume increased by 2% after aerobic exercise training, resulting in improvements in spatial memory in older adults (see Chapter 7, "Physical Exercise in the Cognitive Protection and Management of Neurocognitive Disorders"). Brain imaging studies have linked several anxiety disorders with decreased hippocampal volume, such as PTSD (Kitayama et al. 2005) and SAD (Irle et al. 2010). Some studies have also suggested that decreased hippocampal volume may serve as a vulnerability to the development of such disorders (Dannlowski et al. 2012; Gilbertson et al. 2002; Kheirbek et al. 2012), indicating a potential route by which exercise may decrease cognitive vulnerability to anxiety disorders, although more investigation is required in this field before any such conclusions may be drawn.

The potential impact of exercise on improvement of cognitive vulnerabilities may be further moderated by the presence of genes associated with cognitive vulnerability and plasticity, specifically the gene encoding for brain-derived neurotrophic factor (BDNF). BDNF has been found to influence neurogenesis, neuronal survival, synaptic activity, and neurotransmitter synthesis (Gupta et al. 2013) and is identified as the most significant known regulator of synaptic plasticity in adults, underlying memory acquisition and consolidation (e.g., Lu et al. 2008). Gene expression of BDNF in the brain has been shown to increase after exercise, and these increases have been linked to improved learning and memory formation, although the mechanisms behind this increase remain unclear (Sleiman et al. 2016). Thus, BDNF could be hypothesized to relate as well to potential cognitive changes occurring in treatments for anxiety, including exercise.

PROMOTING ADHERENCE AND THE EFFICACY OF EXERCISE IN ANXIETY DISORDERS AND OBSESSIVE-COMPULSIVE DISORDER

The foregoing review points to positive results for the effectiveness of physical exercise to reduce anxiety, anxiety disorder, and OCD symptoms. Studies also demonstrate that tailored exercise regimens with enhanced structure and monitoring may increase the likelihood of achieving optimal clinical outcomes. Although exercise appears to be a promising intervention for the anxiety and OCD disorders, very few studies to date have addressed the barriers to engagement or variables that enhance exercise adherence in persons with anxiety disorders or OCD. The examination of exercise adherence in the broader physical fitness literature has tended to focus on a set of key motivational variables that can be easily culled and used by clinicians attempting to introduce and promote exercise in patient clinical care, such as the following:

- Degree of pleasure or enjoyment experienced during exercise
- Professional supervision by an assistant or coach with positive attitudes toward exercise
- Flexible program times and flexible exercise regimens to meet personal needs and interests
- Social supports for promoting adherence and providing positive reinforcements
- Expectations about becoming efficacious with specific exercise tasks (e.g., ability to perform exercises with relative ease) based on exercise history

This research would suggest that helping patients with anxiety find exercise tasks that are structured, pleasurable, supervised, and idiosyncratic to their abilities and preferences and providing ongoing support are likely to promote adherence and improved outcomes with exercise.

In addition to enhancing motivation, clinicians must also identify active barriers to engaging in consistent exercise. These can include the following:

- Low self-efficacy beliefs regarding the ability to complete exercise and/ or the ability to "stick with it" over time
- Scheduling difficulties and time pressures
- Lack of finances for gym memberships
- Pain and fatigue following workouts
- Fear of injury
- Lack of transportation or time lost to travel to gym
- Social discomfort in gyms

Beyond generic barriers to motivation and adherence, there may be specific barriers to maintaining exercise adherence in people with anxiety disorders and OCD. A number of reviews (e.g., Asmundson et al. 2013) have focused on anxiety-related vulnerabilities such as high anxiety sensitivity and low emotional distress tolerance that may constitute a barrier to facing and experiencing physical feelings of discomfort that mimic symptoms of anxiety. Importantly, preliminary research demonstrates that these cognitive vulnerabilities can be reduced in short-term structured exercise interventions of 4–8 weeks; further research is required to determine whether early reduction of these variables predicts long-term, sustained adherence to exercise.

There may also be disorder-specific barriers to exercise adherence that are unique to the fears of each condition. For instance, patients with panic disorder frequently avoid exercise out of the fear of experiencing similar interoceptive cues, including full panic attacks. Furthermore, a large, busy gym may trigger agoraphobic avoidance. Patients with a primary diagnosis of SAD may fear embarrassing themselves and/or being judged for making mistakes on the equipment, bumping into someone they know and being required to make small talk, or just feeling self-conscious of others watching while they are working out. An obvious possibility for disorder-specific barriers due to disorder-specific anxiety triggers would be whether patients with OCD might have concerns regarding contamination (e.g., touching and using the gym equipment, using the gym showers), harming (e.g., intrusive images of seeing people drop weights on their head, tripping on the treadmill), sexual implications (e.g., unwanted same-sex intrusions in the changing room), or somatic sensations (e.g., preoccupation with breathing rate or swallowing during autonomic arousal) and be prompted to avoid exercise. Exercising in public may constitute an anxiety exposure task for many patients with an anxiety or OCD condition and will require identification and management by the clinician.

INTEGRATING EXERCISE INTO COGNITIVE-BEHAVIORAL THERAPY TREATMENT OF ANXIETY DISORDERS AND OBSESSIVE-COMPULSIVE DISORDER

A number of studies have aimed to integrate exercise into CBT treatment so that the CBT clinician can easily guide patients toward exercise involvement, promote engagement, and work to reduce barriers that may disrupt long-term adherence. For instance, in one study by Brown et al. (2007) that tested the benefits of exercise in OCD, before each of the 12 weekly aerobic sessions, group members participated in cognitive-behavioral sessions focused on increasing motivation aimed at improving initiation and maintenance of the exercise regimen. These sessions included some of the following elements:

- Discussing the benefits of exercise
- Discussing the direct benefits of exercise in managing anxiety and OCD symptoms
- Outlining the specific goals for that particular exercise session
- Discussing how to stay motivated and overcome setbacks

- Coping with negative moods during and after exercise
- Addressing specific barriers for that session

The latter item may require the clinician to fit certain exercise contexts (e.g., gym) and specific behaviors (e.g., allowing oneself to exercise at the front of a class) into the overall graded-exposure hierarchy. To minimize nonadherence due to anxiety triggers, it may be that clinicians can start with items low on the hierarchy to promote early engagement with exercise (e.g., walking or jogging outside alone) and then enhance exposure to more demanding tasks (e.g., joining a gym, committing to spinning class three times per week) as needed. Brown et al. (2007) used CBT strategies to enhance exercise adherence, and our recent trial work, which aimed to integrate structured exercise into standard CBT interventions for OCD (N.A. Rector et al., "An examination of structured physical exercise in OCD: treatment efficacy, additive benefits to CBT, and cognitive correlates of change," in preparation, 2019), attempted to weave in a focus on exercise at the beginning of each session as part of the routine CBT session for OCD and included the following elements:

1. Starting each session with a review of exercise homework since the previous session
2. Discussion and troubleshooting of barriers to completing specific homework tasks
3. Use of motivational enhancement to promote engagement with exercise as part of the CBT rationale of personal responsibility, commitment, and engagement in discomfort
4. Ending each session with a review of homework goals, including exercise goals and OCD exposure or cognitive restructuring goals
5. Weekly check-ins with identified support to promote social support and encouragement

In our pilot study of patients with moderate to severe OCD with representation from all of the major OCD symptom presentations (contamination/washing, doubting/checking, "bad thoughts," and order/symmetry), none of the participants reported OCD symptom triggers as a barrier to completing the exercise, although the majority of participants had exercise at the gym as an item on their hierarchy (Rector et al. 2015). The overall exercise adherence rate was found to be approximately 80% across the 12 weeks of treatment. Other studies have reported on the seamless use of exercise, particularly running, as an interoceptive exposure task in the context of CBT for panic disorder, showing that it contributes to decreases in catastrophic thinking, feelings of anxiety, and reduced anxiety sensitivity, and these effects are greatest for individuals with heightened anxiety sensitivity (Sabourin et al. 2015).

In some instances, patients may have multiple interactive barriers to exercise that need to be identified and targeted directly to reduce avoidance behavior and promote engagement with exercise. For instance, a patient in our program avoided the gym because of contamination concerns regarding the equipment (e.g., bodily fluids, disinfectant residue) and heightened anxiety sensitivity around the anxious feelings that routinely occurred in the obsessional cycle, often to the point of bona fide panic attacks. In the first several sessions of CBT treatment, anxiety sensitivity was addressed with psychoeducation about the causes and consequences of anxiety. Over the first week, interoceptive exposure tasks included hyperventilation in session and as part of daily homework. This was followed by running exercises in session, with psychoeducation and decatastrophization of autonomic nervous system arousal in the office and as part of homework over the second week. Concurrently, CBT strategies were introduced to identify, examine, and reframe exaggerated threat appraisals pertaining to contamination from the gym equipment (e.g., sickness, infections, toxins) in session and as part of homework. By targeting both the OCD symptom and anxiety sensitivity barriers early in CBT treatment, the patient felt ready to start attending the gym with permitted use of safety behaviors (e.g., 20-minute time frame, not holding the handles of the treadmill, continuation of exercise only to the point of moderate anxiety). Then, beyond the third week, homework routinely involved exposure tasks that identified a range of items from the patient's OCD contamination hierarchy but also included reducing safety behaviors at the gym until the patient was fully able to touch and use the equipment and elevate heart rate to 80% of maximum heart rate efficiency, with the attendant autonomic nervous system arousal symptoms.

SUMMARY AND CONCLUSION

Anxiety disorders are among the most prevalent forms of mental illness. CBT and pharmacotherapy have demonstrated efficacy as empirically supported first-line interventions for all of the anxiety and OCD disorders, although the vast majority of individuals with anxiety or OCD will never receive these treatments (Mohr et al. 2010). Given the problems with access to efficacious treatments, the potential for physical exercise to contribute to the successful management of anxiety and OCD disorders is extremely promising. Although preliminary, there is emerging evidence from randomized controlled trials that aerobic exercise and resistance training programs have an impact on acute anxious states and reactivity and longer-term transdiagnostic and disorder-specific symptom functioning, with positive studies reported in panic disorder, GAD, SAD, and OCD. There are also a small number of studies that show the ability of exercise to reduce underlying cognitive and emotional vulnerabilities associated with the development and maintenance of anxious states and anxiety disorders. For instance, high anxiety sensitivity has been shown to constitute vulnerability for the development and maintenance of various anxiety disorders, including panic disorder and agoraphobia. Exercise, particularly high-intensity aerobic exercise, appears to reduce anxiety sensitivity even in a single-dose exercise session. This suggests that anxiety sensitivity may be an important mechanism of change in exercise, as it has been shown to be in CBT.

The small extant literature examining the clinical benefits of exercise on anxiety symptoms and disorders has employed varying exercise regimens with different types of exercise, levels of intensity, duration, and periods of follow-up. Similar to that observed in exercise interventions for depression, there has been considerable variability in the timing, format, and duration of exercise interventions in the anxiety disorders. However, the majority of research has focused on and supported the benefits of aerobic exercise, typically at three times per week between 8 and 12 weeks in duration, which is in line with the current NICE treatment guidelines for depression with structured, aerobic exercise programs three times a week for duration of 10–14 weeks (National Institute for Health and Care Excellence 2009). At the present time, the NICE guidelines for the use of structured exercise in the management of depression recommend that exercise occur optimally within groups with a competent professional to provide guidance, monitoring, and troubleshooting of exercise-related problems and barriers (National Institute for Health and Care Excellence 2009). There are also a range of other factors that treating clinicians can recommend for increasing physical activity and facilitating long-term persistence with structured exercise programs (e.g., use of schedules).

Finally, from a scientific perspective, there are numerous research opportunities that warrant further attention. First, it is very important to determine the long-term maintenance of gains achieved in short-term 10- to 14-week structured exercise programs, including determination of what maintenance dose of exercise will be required to sustain gains. Second, specific identification of the key aspects of exercise protocols is needed, along with how protocols may be adjusted to achieve best results (e.g., which type of exercise, at what type of intensity, for what period of time), as tailored to the individual on the basis of fitness level, physical health, and exercise interests. Third, more research is required that tests exercise as a stand-alone intervention versus an augmentation to other first-line interventions such as CBT and pharmacotherapy. Fourth, a focus on the psychological, biological, and social mechanisms of action in exercise will contribute to the refinement of exercise interventions and to the broader understanding of the etiology and treatment of anxiety disorders.

DISCUSSION QUESTIONS

1. What are the main anxiety disorders for which structured physical exercise has demonstrated clinical efficacy?
2. Anxiety sensitivity has been shown to constitute vulnerability to the development and maintenance of various anxiety disorders. What is the ability of exercise to reduce this vulnerability in single-dose exercise sessions and more fulsome exercise regimens?
3. As the treating clinician of a patient presenting with an anxiety disorder or OCD, how will you aim to introduce, integrate, and monitor physical exercise as part of your overall management strategy?

RECOMMENDED READINGS

Asmundson GJ, Fetzner MG, Deboer LB, et al: Let's get physical: a contemporary review of the anxiolytic effects of exercise for anxiety and its disorders. Depress Anxiety 30(4):362–373, 2013

LeBouthillier DM, Asmundson GJ: The efficacy of aerobic exercise and resistance training as transdiagnostic interventions for anxiety-related disorders and constructs: a randomized controlled trial. J Anxiety Disord 52:43–52, 2017

National Institute for Health and Clinical Excellence: Depression: The Treatment and Management of Depression in Adults. Leicester, UK, British Psychological Society, 2009

Rector NA, Richter MA, Lerman B, Regev R: A pilot test of the additive benefits of physical exercise to CBT for OCD. Cogn Behav Ther 44(4):328–340, 2015

REFERENCES

Abrantes AM, Strong DR, Cohn A, et al: Acute changes in obsessions and compulsions following moderate-intensity aerobic exercise among patients with obsessive-compulsive disorder. J Anxiety Disord 23(7):923–927, 2009 19616916

American Psychiatric Association: Diagnostic and Statistical Manual of Mental Disorders, 5th Edition. Arlington, VA, American Psychiatric Association, 2013

Asmundson GJ, Fetzner MG, Deboer LB, et al: Let's get physical: a contemporary review of the anxiolytic effects of exercise for anxiety and its disorders. Depress Anxiety 30(4):362–373, 2013 23300122

Broman-Fulks JJ, Kelso K, Zawilinski L: Effects of a single bout of aerobic exercise versus resistance training on cognitive vulnerabilities for anxiety disorders. Cogn Behav Ther 44(4):240–251, 2015 25789738

Brown RA, Abrantes AM, Strong DR, et al: A pilot study of moderate-intensity aerobic exercise for obsessive compulsive disorder. J Nerv Ment Dis 195(6):514–520, 2007 17568300

Brundtland GH: Mental health in the 21st century. Bull World Health Organ 78(4):411, 2000 10885158

Dannlowski U, Stuhrmann A, Beutelmann V, et al: Limbic scars: long-term consequences of childhood maltreatment revealed by functional and structural magnetic resonance imaging. Biol Psychiatry 71(4):286–293, 2012 22112927

Déry N, Pilgrim M, Gibala M, et al: Adult hippocampal neurogenesis reduces memory interference in humans: opposing effects of aerobic exercise and depression. Front Neurosci 7:66, 2013 23641193

Erickson KI, Voss MW, Prakash RS, et al: Exercise training increases size of hippocampus and improves memory. Proc Natl Acad Sci USA 108(7):3017–3022, 2011 21282661

Gilbertson MW, Shenton ME, Ciszewski A, et al: Smaller hippocampal volume predicts pathologic vulnerability to psychological trauma. Nat Neurosci 5(11):1242–1247, 2002 12379862

Goodwin RD: Association between physical activity and mental disorders among adults in the United States. Prev Med 36(6):698–703, 2003 12744913

Greenberg PE, Sisitsky T, Kessler RC, et al: The economic burden of anxiety disorders in the 1990s. J Clin Psychiatry 60(7):427–435, 1999 10453795

Gupta VK, You Y, Gupta VB, et al: TrkB receptor signalling: implications in neurodegenerative, psychiatric and proliferative disorders. Int J Mol Sci 14(5):10122–10142, 2013 23670594

Harvey SB, Hotopf M, Overland S, et al: Physical activity and common mental disorders. Br J Psychiatry 197(5):357–364, 2010 21037212

Herring MP, O'Connor PJ, Dishman RK: The effect of exercise training on anxiety symptoms among patients: a systematic review. Arch Intern Med 170(4):321–331, 2010 20177034

Irle E, Ruhleder M, Lange C, et al: Reduced amygdalar and hippocampal size in adults with generalized social phobia. J Psychiatry Neurosci 35(2):126–131, 2010 20184810

Kessler RC, Berglund P, Demler O, et al: Lifetime prevalence and age-of-onset distributions of DSM-IV disorders in the National Comorbidity Survey Replication. Arch Gen Psychiatry 62(6):593–602, 2005 15939837

Kessler RC, Sampson NA, Berglund P, et al: Anxious and non-anxious major depressive disorder in the world health organization world mental health surveys. Epidemiol Psychiatr Sci 24(3):210–226, 2015 25720357

Kheirbek MA, Klemenhagen KC, Sahay A, et al: Neurogenesis and generalization: a new approach to stratify and treat anxiety disorders. Nat Neurosci 15(12):1613–1620, 2012 23187693

Kitayama N, Vaccarino V, Kutner M, et al: Magnetic resonance imaging (MRI) measurement of hippocampal volume in posttraumatic stress disorder: a meta-analysis. J Affect Disord 88(1):79–86, 2005 16033700

Lancer R, Motta R, Lancer D: The effect of aerobic exercise on obsessive-compulsive disorder, anxiety, and depression: a preliminary investigation. Behav Ther 30(3):53, 57–62, 2007

LeBouthillier DM, Asmundson GJ: A single bout of aerobic exercise reduces anxiety sensitivity but not intolerance of uncertainty or distress tolerance: a randomized controlled trial. Cogn Behav Ther 44(4):252–263, 2015 25874370

LeBouthillier DM, Asmundson GJG: The efficacy of aerobic exercise and resistance training as transdiagnostic interventions for anxiety-related disorders and constructs: A randomized controlled trial. J Anxiety Disord 52:43–52, 2017 29049901

Lu Y, Christian K, Lu B: BDNF: a key regulator for protein synthesis-dependent LTP and long-term memory? Neurobiol Learn Mem 89(3):312–323, 2008 17942328

Mead GE, Morley W, Campbell P, et al: Exercise for depression. Cochrane Database Syst Rev (4):CD004366, 2008 18843656

Mohr DC, Ho J, Duffecy J, et al: Perceived barriers to psychological treatments and their relationship to depression. J Clin Psychol 66(4):394–409, 2010 20127795

National Institute for Health and Clinical Excellence: Depression: The Treatment and Management of Depression in Adults. Leicester, UK, British Psychological Society, 2009

Pajonk FG, Wobrock T, Gruber O, et al: Hippocampal plasticity in response to exercise in schizophrenia. Arch Gen Psychiatry 67(2):133–143, 2010 20124113

Petruzzello SJ, Landers DM, Hatfield BD, et al: A meta-analysis on the anxiety-reducing effects of acute and chronic exercise. Outcomes and mechanisms. Sports Med 11(3):143–182, 1991 1828608

Piercy KL, Troiano RP, Ballard RM, et al: The Physical Activity Guidelines for Americans. JAMA 320(19):2020–2028, 2018 30418471

Prakash RS, Snook EM, Motl RW, et al: Aerobic fitness is associated with gray matter volume and white matter integrity in multiple sclerosis. Brain Res 1341:41–51, 2010 19560443

Rector NA, Richter MA, Lerman B, et al: A pilot test of the additive benefits of physical exercise to CBT for OCD. Cogn Behav Ther 44(4):328–340, 2015 25738234

Rector NA, Wilde JL, Richter MA: Obsessive compulsive disorder and comorbidity: rates, models, and treatment approaches, in The Wiley Handbook of Obsessive-Compulsive Disorders, Vol 2. Edited by Abramowitz JS, McKay D, Storch EA. Hoboken, NJ, Wiley-Blackwell, 2017, pp 697–725

Rimer J, Dwan K, Lawlor DA, et al: Exercise for depression. Cochrane Database Syst Rev (7):CD004366, 2012 22786489

Sabourin BC, Stewart SH, Watt MC, et al: Running as interoceptive exposure for decreasing anxiety sensitivity: replication and extension. Cogn Behav Ther 44(4):264–274, 2015 25730341

Sleiman SF, Henry J, Al-Haddad R, et al: Exercise promotes the expression of brain derived neurotrophic factor (BDNF) through the action of the ketone body beta-hydroxybutyrate. eLife 5:e15092, 2016 27253067

Statistics Canada: Directly measured physical activity of Canadian adults, 2012 to 2013. Ottawa, ON, Statistics Canada, 2015. Available at: www150.statcan.gc.ca/n1/pub/82-625-x/2015001/article/14136-eng.htm. Accessed December 10, 2018.

Ten Have M, de Graaf R, Monshouwer K: Physical exercise in adults and mental health status findings from the Netherlands Mental Health Survey and Incidence Study (NEMESIS). J Psychosom Res 71(5):342–348, 2011 21999978

Toft T, Fink P, Oernboel E, et al: Mental disorders in primary care: prevalence and co-morbidity among disorders. results from the Functional Illness in Primary Care (FIP) study. Psychol Med 35(8):1175–1184, 2005 16116943

Warburton DE, Charlesworth S, Ivey A, et al: A systematic review of the evidence for Canada's Physical Activity Guidelines for Adults. Int J Behav Nutr Phys Act 7:39, 2010 20459783

Wipfli BM, Rethorst CD, Landers DM: The anxiolytic effects of exercise: a meta-analysis of randomized trials and dose-response analysis. J Sport Exerc Psychol 30(4):392–410, 2008 18723899

Zschucke E, Gaudlitz K, Ströhle A: Exercise and physical activity in mental disorders: clinical and experimental evidence. J Prev Med Public Health 46(suppl 1):S12–S21, 2013 23412549

Physical Exercise as a Potentially Useful Component of Posttraumatic Stress Disorder Treatment

Matthew J. Friedman, M.D., Ph.D.

KEY POINTS

- Limited evidence suggests that physical exercise may improve symptoms of posttraumatic stress disorder (PTSD) directly and may augment other treatments for PTSD.
- Hyperarousal cluster symptoms may be particularly responsive to physical exercise.
- Exercise may improve symptoms of PTSD via desensitization to autonomic arousal; supporting neuroplasticity and neurogenesis in memory centers; stimulating endocannabinoids; and/or having an impact on mastery, trust, and social connection.
- Specific research is needed to confirm these relationships in people with PTSD.

There is no question that exercise is good for you. The question that I have been asked to address is whether exercise has a specific benefit for individuals with posttraumatic stress disorder (PTSD). At the outset, I shall complain about the question: There are many different kinds of exercise. Some are solitary, whereas others have a social/cooperative/competitive component. Among the latter, some require major reliance on other people, as in rock climbing, where you must trust the individual at the other end of the rope, in contrast to certain team sports, where the major challenge is communication and coordination. Thus, the question of the benefits of exercise is by no means a straightforward one. If it turns out that certain exercises are beneficial, it will be important to figure out whether the therapeutic ingredient is primarily due to aerobic and fitness factors; the social, emotional, and character-building context in which the exercise is carried out; and/or the neurobiological benefits that directly affect brain function.

In this chapter, I first review what little research has been published on exercise as a component of PTSD treatment. Then, I provide a case example from my own experience when I directed a psychiatric inpatient program many years ago. Next, I review some relevant neuroscientific findings regarding exercise and indicate how such results might be relevant to the therapeutic value of exercise. I finish up with some suggestions for a future research agenda that might advance our knowledge so that we can ask better questions about the potential therapeutic role for exercise in the treatment of PTSD.

REVIEW OF THE LITERATURE

A Cochrane review published in 2010 (Lawrence et al. 2010) concluded that there was no published research that was sufficiently rigorous and free of bias on the subject of "sports and games" for PTSD. Since that time, there have been a few randomized clinical trials and other reports on exercise and PTSD.

Motta and colleagues did much of the early work. They published three small studies with children, adolescents, and adults, mostly female and often institutionalized, in which the major intervention was predicated on the benefits of aerobic exercise (Diaz and Motta 2008; Manger and Motta 2005; Newman and Motta 2007). In all studies, participants engaged in a protocol in which they maintained 60%–90% maximum heart rate for 20–30 minutes over a 4- to 10-week period. There were no control groups, so post-exercise outcomes were compared with each participant's pre-exercise baseline. Assessments were carried out at termination of the exercise protocol and 1 month later.

Manger and Motta (2005) reported that 9 men and women who participated in twelve 20-minute solitary treadmill sessions exhibited significant reductions in both PTSD and depressive symptom severity after 10 weeks and that such benefits were still evident 1 month later. Newman and Motta (2007) tested 11 adolescent females (ages 14–17) on a 20-minute aerobic exercise routine that was repeated at least 20 times during an 8-week period. Again, improvement was observed in both PTSD and depressive symptom severity, as well as loss of the PTSD diagnosis in 10 of the 11 participants. Finally, Diaz and Motta (2008) performed a similar study with 12 adolescent girls in a residential treatment facility. Marked improvement, which was maintained for 1 month, was again observed with regard to PTSD symptom severity. The authors attributed all of these positive results to the benefits of repeated aerobic exercise.

Taken together, these results are promising but certainly not conclusive. All three studies are limited by small sample size, nonrandomization, no control group, high risk of bias, and lack of standardization of the exercise protocol itself. Several of these concerns have been addressed in subsequent randomized clinical trials, some of which focused on the efficacy of exercise itself, whereas others evaluated exercise as an adjunct to ongoing PTSD treatment.

Fetzner and Asmundson (2015) conducted a randomized controlled trial that sought to understand the active ingredient in aerobic exercise that might account for its beneficial effects on PTSD, depression, and anxiety sensitivity. They also explored the importance of attentional focus during exercise as the therapeutic mechanism by randomly assigning participants to 1) a cognitive distraction group where attention was directed away from "uncomfortable and potentially distressing somatic symptoms" generated during exercise, 2) a group instructed to increase attention to such somatic symptoms, or 3) a control group given no instructions in this regard. Thirty-three adults (mostly women) recruited through newspaper ads were randomly assigned to one of these three groups (11 in each). Each participant exercised on a stationary bicycle at 60%–80% heart rate for six 20-minute aerobic exercise sessions over 2 weeks. All three groups showed significant improvement in total PTSD symptom severity as measured by the PTSD Checklist and in all four DSM-IV (American Psychiatric Association 1994) PTSD symptom clusters (re-experiencing, avoidance, numbing, and hyperarousal). They also improved in anxiety sensitivity but not in depression. However, gains were not well maintained at 1 week or at 1 month, suggesting that improvement was transient and that more exercise and/or sustained exercise is needed for stable positive outcomes.

Contrary to the hypothesis about the importance of attentional focus, there was no difference between the cognitive distraction, somatic focus, and control groups. The authors speculated that rather than shifting attentional focus, exercise might have been beneficial because participants "gained a sense of accomplishment...rexperienced behavioral activation, or [had] undergone neurochemical changes" (Fetzner and Asmundson 2015, p. 310).

Kim et al. (2013) reported a randomized controlled trial showing the effectiveness of a mindfulness-based stretching and deep breathing exercise program. Eleven female nurses randomly assigned to this intervention showed significant improvement in PTSD symptoms compared with a control group of 11 nurses. Goldstein et al. (2018) incorporated this approach into a much more elaborate approach that combined aerobic and resistance exercise with yoga movements and postures that also included mindfulness-based stress reduction. The intervention itself was called a group-based integrative exercise program, and it was administered to 47 veterans who were randomly assigned either to integrative exercise or to a waitlist control group. The integrative exercise group exhibited greater reduction in overall PTSD symptom severity, although such improvement was due primarily to a reduction in PTSD hyperarousal symptoms; the PTSD re-experiencing and avoidance or numbing clusters showed much less improvement. Other benefits from integrative exercise were improved psychological, but not physical, quality of life. The integrative exercise intervention was also both feasible and acceptable to veterans. The authors emphasized the practicability of this approach and the fact that as an exercise or yoga intervention, it was not hampered by the stigma associated with seeking mental health treatment for PTSD.

Babson et al. (2015) took a very different approach, focusing on prior research showing the benefits of exercise among individuals with poor sleep. They hypothesized that individuals with anxiety and co-occurring sleep problems might benefit most from exercise. Participants were 217 male veterans admitted to a 60- to 90-day Veterans Administration (VA) residential PTSD program in which they all received cognitive-behavioral therapy (CBT). Exercise was defined as the total distance cycled while engaged in a group bicycling program; all cycling activity was monitored throughout the hospitalization. Sleep was assessed by the Pittsburgh Sleep Quality Index (PSQI), a well-regarded self-report scale. Although neither sleep nor exercise per se were directly related to changes in PTSD symptom severity, there was a significant interaction between sleep and exercise. Those veterans with the poorest sleep and the highest cycling mileage exhibited significant reductions in the hyperarousal clusters of PTSD symptoms. There was no benefit for good sleepers, nor did other PTSD symptom clusters improve. Major limitations of this study are that it was retrospective, there was no random assignment (veterans self-selected to participate in the cycling program), and sleep measures on the PSQI were self-report rather than polysomnographic. It is intriguing to note that in both the Goldstein et al. (2018) study and this study, exercise-related PTSD improvement was primarily in the hyperarousal cluster and not in other symptom categories.

Rosenbaum et al. (2015a) conducted a randomized clinical trial in which 81 participants with PTSD were randomly assigned to either usual inpatient care (psychotherapy, medication, and group therapy) or usual care plus exercise. Exercise involved three 30-minute resistance training sessions per week plus a pedometer-based walking program. Participants in the exercise group exhibited significant improvement in PTSD symptom severity, depression, waist circumference, body weight, and body fat percentage. A major limitation of the study was that follow-up data were compromised because many participants could not be located for follow-up assessments.

Endocannabinoids were the focus of a very innovative study by Crombie et al. (2018), who monitored pre-exercise and post-exercise mood and endocannabinoid levels in 12 individuals with PTSD and in 12 healthy control subjects. Exercise consisted of a 30-minute moderate-intensity aerobic exercise session, after which participants were provided with an accelerometer to quantify their physical activity during the next 7 days; participants also filled out activity logs in conjunction with the accelerometer. Both groups exhibited increases in endocannabinoid levels following this procedure, but the magnitude of such increases were significantly less in the PTSD group (suggesting, perhaps, a blunted endocannabinoid system in PTSD; see discussion that follows). On the other hand, the PTSD group exhibited greater mood improvement and pain reduction than did the healthy control subjects. The authors pointed out that the preliminary findings from this small pilot study need to be replicated in a larger, randomized, more rigorous trial.

Two studies assessed the impact of exercise as adjunctive treatment for individuals receiving CBT. Liedl et al. (2011) randomly assigned 30 traumatized refugees in three groups of 10 to biofeedback-based CBT (CBT-BF), CBT-BF plus exercise, or a waitlist control. This cohort was heavily traumatized physically as well as psychologically, and participants also reported many pain complaints. Exercise was individualized by a physiotherapist to address chronic headache, neck ache, and back pain. In addition to 10 sessions of CBT-BF, the CBT-BF plus exercise group received ten 20-minute sessions of exercise. There was no significant difference between the CBT-BF and CBT-BF plus exercise groups with respect to PTSD symptom severity; both groups showed modest improvement. The major outcome was that the CBT-BF plus exercise group did have more improvement with regard to the Pain Coping Questionnaire.

Finally, in a very interesting theoretically driven pilot study, Powers et al. (2015) randomly assigned nine patients to 12 sessions of prolonged exposure therapy versus prolonged exposure plus exercise. Participants completed a 30-minute treadmill exercise immediately prior to each prolonged exposure session. In addition to measuring PTSD and other symptoms, the investigators measured plasma brain-derived neurotrophic factor (BDNF), a neurotropin that promotes neurogenesis, synaptic plasticity, and long-term potentiation in the hippocampus. Prolonged exposure plus exercise produced greater reduction in PTSD symptoms than prolonged exposure therapy alone, but the difference was not significant because of low statistical power due to small sample size. Most notably, prolonged exposure plus exercise produced a marked elevation in plasma BDNF that was not exhibited by individuals in the prolonged exposure group. The authors cautioned readers that peripheral (e.g., plasma) BDNF levels may not reflect brain BDNF levels and mentioned that exercise may also enhance other brain mechanisms that more directly ameliorate PTSD symptoms. This is a groundbreaking study that shifted the focus of research to neurobiological mechanisms that might mediate positive outcomes in PTSD treatment.

CLINICAL EXAMPLE

During the late 1970s and early 1980s, I directed the inpatient psychiatric unit at the VA Medical Center in White River Junction, Vermont. The hospital is one of the two major teaching hospitals of the Geisel School of Medicine at Dartmouth College. At that time, Outward Bound had established a pilot project for disturbed adolescents based at the Dartmouth-Hitchcock Medical Center (Plakun et al. 1981). It took little persuasion to interest Outward Bound staff in exercise programs for veteran patients who had been diagnosed primarily with PTSD, depression, schizophrenia, or some combination. Activities included rock climbing, cross-country skiing, high and low ropes courses, problem-solving exercises, hiking, orienteering, and canoeing. Psychiatric nursing and activities therapy staff accompanied Outward Bound staff on all exercises. Although we never measured PTSD, depression, or other symptoms, we did gather data showing that the intervention was well received by patients, who indicated that the process had increased their self-esteem. Efforts on my part to design and conduct a randomized clinical trial ran into a number of institutional barriers, especially a disinclination to use randomization for fear of depriving any patient of such a popular intervention.

Despite the lack of quantitative data, I was so favorably impressed by such activities that later, after completion of the Dartmouth Outward Bound Mental Health Project, I hired my own activities therapist, who continued to carry out such outdoor activities for veterans for many years (Roland et al. 1987). We even built a low ropes course on the VA hospital campus that could be used by veterans with physical disabilities. Our approach differed from that of other experiential challenge programs in that it paid less attention to activities that involve physical risks. Instead, we focused more attention on activities that involve social, cognitive, and emotional risks.

Exercise programs for patients with PTSD have benefits in three PTSD-specific symptom domains: mastery, trust, and social connection.

1. *Mastery:* PTSD develops when an individual is unable to cope successfully with an extremely stressful event. Helplessness during the occurrence of the trauma has long been recognized as a contributing factor. The most successful CBT approaches are built partially on the fact that PTSD patients not only feel weak, helpless, and inadequate but also perceive the world as an overwhelming and malevolent environment with which they cannot cope (Gillihan et al. 2014; Resick et al. 2014). Therefore, recognizing the acquisition of mastery, or even competence, regarding rock climbing, cross-country skiing, or other physical activities during an Outward Bound exercise has specific meaning for a PTSD patient who believes himself or herself to be weak, incompetent, cowardly, or a failure.

2. *Trust:* Loss of trust is a frequent symptom among patients with PTSD. Such loss may have occurred because a trusted person perpetrated rape or sexual violence, a trusted military leader gave orders that resulted in many deaths or injuries, or assurances of safety by trusted authorities preceded a terrorist attack or natural disaster that produced mass casualties. For such individuals to trust another individual with their personal safety—as in rock climbing, when someone tied to their rope is responsible for their personal safety—is a vivid opportunity for experiencing and processing such trust issues with a skilled therapist.

3. *Social connection:* People with PTSD often isolate themselves from other people. It is a protective posture to ensure that they never find themselves in situations where they are vulnerable and can potentially be exposed to another traumatic event. The mutual dependence, team problem solving, and general socialization inherent in the outdoor activities are clearly an antidote to the isolation and social withdrawal associated with PTSD.

In other words, beyond the neurobiological impact of exercise, the social parameters of an exercise intervention may be relevant in targeting some very specific PTSD symptoms.

HOW MIGHT EXERCISE REDUCE POSTTRAUMATIC STRESS DISORDER SYMPTOMS?

There is very little literature specifically addressing the potential benefits of exercise in PTSD treatment. I was unable to find any PTSD-specific research on exercise-based enhancement of feelings of mastery, trust, or social connectedness, which I speculated might be therapeutic for my veteran psychiatric inpatients 35–40 years ago. Fetzner and Asmundson's (2015) results indicate that shifting attentional focus does not appear to be important. Rosenbaum et al. (2015b) observed simultaneous reductions of waist circumference, body weight, and body fat percentage along with PTSD symptom severity due to physical activity and called to attention the positive association between PTSD and obesity, metabolic syndrome, and type 2 diabetes. They have called for more research on the importance of reducing cardiometabolic risk factors when treating PTSD and other psychiatric disorders.

For me, the most exciting putative mechanism of action is neurobiological. Powers et al. (2015) showed that exercise increased BDNF among PTSD patients receiving prolonged exposure therapy. Their small pilot study is consistent with a number of findings regarding the benefits of exercise on brain structure and function, especially with respect to neurogenesis and synaptic plasticity (see Chapter 2, "Physical Exercise and the Brain"). It is beyond the scope of this chapter to review this topic in depth, and readers are referred to a number of excellent reviews on this topic (Eadie et al. 2005; Greenwood and Fleshner 2011; Kempermann et al. 2010; Krystal et al. 2017; Silverman and Deuster 2014). Briefly stated, it is well known that chronic stress has deleterious effects on neuronal cytoarchitecture, marked by defoliation of dendritic spines, reduction in synaptic density, and loss of neurons, resulting in reduction of hippocampal volume. Under such circumstances, treatments that promote neurogenesis might be expected to have therapeutic effects. Indeed, the selective serotonin reuptake inhibitor paroxetine (one of two such drugs with U.S. Food and Drug Administration approval as a treatment for PTSD) produced an increase in hippocampal volume that was associated with recovery from PTSD (Vermetten et al. 2003). (Among other actions, selective serotonin reuptake inhibitors increased BDNF; Duman 2004.)

There is abundant evidence that exercise enhances neuroplasticity, promotes neurogenesis, increases dendritic complexity, and increases synaptic connectivity. Such effects are associated with increased levels of BDNF (see Krystal et al. 2017). Voluntary exercise has been shown to increase neurogenesis in the dentate gyrus of the hippocampus, where it also enhances long term potentiation (Eadie et al. 2005). Kempermann et al. (2010) have shown in preclinical studies that locomotion stimulates hippocampal neurogenesis. Greenwood and Fleshner (2011) reviewed the evidence showing that exercise-mediated neuroplasticity within the central serotonergic system facilitates stress resistance and resilience. Silverman and Deuster (2014) suggested the following sequence of positive psychological and resilience-enhancing benefits: exercise 1) serves as a buffer against stress and stress-related disorders, 2) blunts and optimizes neuroendocrine and physiological responses to physical and psychosocial stressors, 3) promotes an anti-inflammatory state, and 4) enhances neuroplasticity and growth factor expression.

Another postulated neurobiological system through which the benefits of exercise are mediated is the endocannabinoid system. The rationale for the finding that aerobic exercise increases endocannabinoid levels, improves mood, and reduces pain in individuals with PTSD (Crombie et al. 2018) is found in evidence that the endocannabinoid system is dysregulated in PTSD (Hill et al. 2013; Neumeister et al. 2013), exercise increases endocannabinoids in healthy individuals (see Crombie et al. 2018 for references), and augmentation of the endocannabinoid system improves fear extinction in animals and humans (Lutz et al. 2015; Rabinak et al. 2014). Crombie et al. (2018) found further evidence of such a deficiency. In their study, the exercise response was blunted in individuals with PTSD because their exercise-mediated elevation in endocannabinoids was significantly less than that observed in healthy control subjects. Clearly, this is a very important area for further research.

LOOKING AHEAD

Results certainly suggest that exercise may have a beneficial role in improving the functional status and feelings of well-being among individuals with PTSD. It is now important to identify key questions and design studies that will address them specifically. Because my area of focus is PTSD and not other psychiatric disorders (which are addressed elsewhere in this book), I do not know how well the PTSD literature reflects what has been published regarding exercise and mental health in general. I was frankly surprised to find that most PTSD-related research addressing exercise-mediated mechanisms of action has focused primarily on neurobiological questions (e.g., synaptic plasticity, BDNF, and neurogenesis as well as on the endocannabinoid system) rather than the physiological (e.g., aerobic), cognitive (e.g., mastery), interpersonal (e.g., trust), or social aspects (e.g., alienation) of exercise. My own belief is that some exercises may be better suited to address some problems than others. It is important to understand nonspecific benefits of exercise compared with benefits that may address specific psychiatric problems (e.g., PTSD vs. depression vs. substance use disorder).

There are several areas of inquiry that should be included in future research on exercise in PTSD:

- Identify which types of exercise or exercise formats (e.g., solitary vs. group) are most likely to produce which benefits for which individuals and under which conditions
- Distinguish the general, nonspecific benefits of exercise from the mechanisms that might be particularly indicated in PTSD; a spectrum of hypothesized exercise-related mechanisms might be relevant, ranging from enhanced BDNF or neurogenesis and endocannabinoid levels to enhanced trust and social connectedness
- Address the timing and dosage of specific exercises as adjuncts to more traditional evidence-based PTSD treatments
- Identify which exercises might benefit which PTSD symptom clusters (e.g., the PTSD hyperarousal symptoms, but not other symptom clusters, have shown the greatest improvement following exercise in the small body of research published to date)

Clearly, we have a great deal to learn. Exercise is cheap, freely available, physically beneficial, satisfying, and usually enjoyable. We know that exercise is good for us, but we need to have a better understanding of such benefits for both personal well-being and, possibly, as a useful component of treatment for people with PTSD and other psychiatric disorders. It's time to get to work.

DISCUSSION QUESTIONS

1. What forms of exercise might be most likely to be helpful for specific PTSD symptom clusters or specific subgroups of patients with PTSD?
2. How might the effects of exercise on BDNF and neuroplasticity in memory circuits work synergistically with other treatments for PTSD? What might be the best timing for using them together?
3. How might the accessibility of exercise benefit people with PTSD?

RECOMMENDED READINGS

Greenwood BN, Fleshner M: Exercise, stress resistance, and central serotonergic systems. Exerc Sport Sci Rev 39(3):140–149, 2011

Krystal JH, Abdallah CG, Averill LA, et al: Synaptic loss and the pathophysiology of PTSD: Implications for ketamine as a prototype novel therapeutic. Curr Psychiatry Rep 19(10):74, 2017

Silverman MN, Deuster PA: Biological mechanisms underlying the role of physical fitness in health and resilience. Interface Focus 4(5):20140040, 2014

REFERENCES

American Psychiatric Association: Diagnostic and Statistical Manual of Mental Disorders, 4th Edition. Washington, DC, American Psychiatric Association, 1994

Babson KA, Heinz AJ, Ramirez G, et al: The interactive role of exercise and sleep on veteran recovery from symptoms of PTSD. Ment Health Phys Act 8:15–20, 2015

Crombie KM, Brellenthin AG, Hillard CJ, et al: Psychobiological responses to aerobic exercise in individuals with posttraumatic stress disorder. J Trauma Stress 31(1):134–145, 2018 29388710

Diaz AB, Motta R: The effects of an aerobic exercise program on posttraumatic stress disorder symptom severity in adolescents. Int J Emerg Ment Health 10(1):49–59, 2008 18546759

Duman RS: Role of neurotrophic factors in the etiology and treatment of mood disorders. Neuromolecular Med 5(1):11–25, 2004 15001809

Eadie BD, Redila VA, Christie BR: Voluntary exercise alters the cytoarchitecture of the adult dentate gyrus by increasing cellular proliferation, dendritic complexity, and spine density. J Comp Neurol 486(1):39–47, 2005 15834963

Fetzner MG, Asmundson GJ: Aerobic exercise reduces symptoms of posttraumatic stress disorder: a randomized controlled trial. Cogn Behav Ther 44(4):301–313, 2015 24911173

Gillihan SJ, Cahill SP, Foa EB: Psychological theories of PTSD, in Handbook of PTSD: Science and Practice, 2nd Edition. Edited by Friedman MJ, Keane TM, Resick PA. New York, Guilford, 2014, pp 166–184

Goldstein LA, Mehling WE, Metzler TJ, et al: Veterans group exercise: a randomized pilot trial of an integrative exercise program for veterans with posttraumatic stress. J Affect Disord 227:345–352, 2018 29145076

Greenwood BN, Fleshner M: Exercise, stress resistance, and central serotonergic systems. Exerc Sport Sci Rev 39(3):140–149, 2011 21508844

Hill MN, Bierer LM, Makotkine I, et al: Reductions in circulating endocannabinoid levels in individuals with post-traumatic stress disorder following exposure to the World Trade Center attacks. Psychoneuroendocrinology 38(12):2952–2961, 2013 24035186

Kempermann G, Fabel K, Ehninger D, et al: Why and how physical activity promotes experience-induced brain plasticity. Front Neurosci 4:189, 2010 21151782

Kim SH, Schneider SM, Bevans M, et al: PTSD symptom reduction with mindfulness-based stretching and deep breathing exercise: randomized controlled clinical trial of efficacy. J Clin Endocrinol Metab 98(7):2984–2992, 2013 23720785

Krystal JH, Abdallah CG, Averill LA, et al: Synaptic loss and the pathophysiology of PTSD: implications for ketamine as a prototype novel therapeutic. Curr Psychiatry Rep 19(10):74, 2017 28844076

Lawrence S, De Silva M, Henley R: Sports and games for post-traumatic stress disorder (PTSD). Cochrane Database Syst Rev (1):CD007171, 2010 20091620

Liedl A, Müller J, Morina N, et al: Physical activity within a CBT intervention improves coping with pain in traumatized refugees: results of a randomized controlled design. Pain Med 12(2):234–245, 2011 21223501

Lutz B, Marsicano G, Maldonado R, et al: The endocannabinoid system in guarding against fear, anxiety and stress. Nat Rev Neurosci 16(12):705–718, 2015 26585799

Manger TA, Motta RW: The impact of an exercise program on posttraumatic stress disorder, anxiety, and depression. Int J Emerg Ment Health 7(1):49–57, 2005 15869081

Neumeister A, Normandin MD, Pietrzak RH, et al: Elevated brain cannabinoid CB1 receptor availability in post-traumatic stress disorder: a positron emission tomography study. Mol Psychiatry 18(9):1034–1040, 2013 23670490

Newman CL, Motta RW: The effects of aerobic exercise on childhood PTSD, anxiety, and depression. Int J Emerg Ment Health 9(2):133–158, 2007 17725082

Plakun E, Tucker G, Harris P: Outward Bound: an adjunctive psychiatric therapy. J Psychiatr Treat Eval 3(1):33–37, 1981

Powers MB, Medina JL, Burns S, et al: Exercise augmentation of exposure therapy for PTSD: rationale and pilot efficacy data. Cogn Behav Ther 44(4):314–327, 2015 25706090

Rabinak CA, Angstadt M, Lyons M, et al: Cannabinoid modulation of prefrontal-limbic activation during fear extinction learning and recall in humans. Neurobiol Learn Mem 113:125–134, 2014 24055595

Resick PA, Monson CM, Gutner CA, et al: Psychosocial treatments for adults with PTSD, in Handbook of PTSD: Science and Practice, 2nd Edition. Edited by Friedman MJ, Keane TM, Resick PA. New York, Guilford, 2014, pp 419–436

Roland CC, Summers S, Friedman MJ, et al: Creation of an experiential challenge program. Ther Recreation J 21(2):54–63, 1987

Rosenbaum S, Sherrington C, Tiedemann A: Exercise augmentation compared with usual care for post-traumatic stress disorder: a randomized controlled trial. Acta Psychiatr Scand 131(5):350–359, 2015a 25443996

Rosenbaum S, Tiedemann A, Berle D, et al: Exercise as a novel treatment option to address cardiometabolic dysfunction associated with PTSD. Metabolism 64(5):e5–e6, 2015b 25681009

Silverman MN, Deuster PA: Biological mechanisms underlying the role of physical fitness in health and resilience. Interface Focus 4(5):20140040, 2014 25285199

Vermetten E, Vythilingam M, Southwick SM, et al: Long-term treatment with paroxetine increases verbal declarative memory and hippocampal volume in post-traumatic stress disorder. Biol Psychiatry 54(7):693–702, 2003 14512209

CHAPTER 6

Physical Exercise in the Management of Schizophrenia Spectrum Disorders

Shuichi Suetani, B.Sc., M.B., Ch.B., FRANZCP

Davy Vancampfort, Ph.D.

KEY POINTS

- People with schizophrenia suffer from a significant physical health burden that contributes to the differential mortality gap compared with the general population.
- Physical activity can help reduce this burden as well as improve both psychological and physical well-being of people living with schizophrenia.
- The main challenge that we now face is the implementation of effective physical activity interventions for people with schizophrenia long term.

In recent years, there has been much research and clinical attention on physical activity as a safe, cost-effective, and efficacious intervention to reduce cardiometabolic risk factors and symptom severity in people with schizophrenia, with evidence that physical activity may restore brain volume (Dauwan et al. 2016; Firth et al. 2017b; Vancampfort et al. 2010). As a result, there is now an increased acknowledgment among psychiatry professionals of the importance of physical health and associated lifestyle modifications for people with schizophrenia (Suetani et al. 2017).

Using examples from Australia, we describe how physical activity interventions may be implemented widely within everyday clinical practice in public mental health services. We have divided the chapter into three main sections. In the first section, we briefly describe unmet needs for symptom management, brain recovery, and functional restoration as well as the magnitude of problems associated with the physical health and treatment response of people with schizophrenia. In the second section, which is the core section of this chapter, we describe how physical activity can help reduce these problems and outline some successful examples of physical activity intervention studies around the world. In the final section, we discuss potential future directions for this field, in particular, how we may able to implement physical activity treatment in a sustainable manner in everyday clinical practice.

PSYCHIATRIC AND PHYSICAL HEALTH OF PEOPLE WITH SCHIZOPHRENIA

Pharmacotherapy and Psychiatric Symptoms of Schizophrenia

Broadly, there are three main domains of symptoms that characterize schizophrenia: positive symptoms (delusions and hallucinations; so-called psychotic symptoms in which contact with reality is lost), negative symptoms (particularly impaired motivation, reduction in spontaneous speech, and social withdrawal), and cognitive symptoms (poorer performance than control subjects over a wide range of cognitive functions) (Kahn et al. 2015). Although antipsychotic medications remain the cornerstone of treatment for positive symptoms (Galletly et al. 2016; Leucht et al. 2017), the discontinuation rates for most antipsychotic medications remain high, with a substantial minority (around one in five; Agid et al. 2011) developing treatment resistance. In such situations, clozapine demonstrates superior efficacy compared with other antipsychotic medications, though one systematic review estimated the number needed to treat to be nine (i.e., eight out of nine individuals do not display adequate response even with clozapine; Siskind et al. 2016).

Antipsychotic medications have less efficacy for negative symptoms (Leucht et al. 2017), and other medication options also have relatively limited effects (Arango et al. 2013; Kahn et al. 2015). This is in spite of research suggesting that negative symptoms generate greater burden on the functional status of people with schizophrenia (Rabinowitz et al. 2012). Moreover, after controlling for potential biases, a systematic review (Jauhar et al. 2014) found limited benefits of psychotherapy in both positive and negative symptoms of schizophrenia. Furthermore, there is currently very little effective pharmacological treatment for cognitive symptoms—deficits that often precede the diagnosis and persist throughout the course of illness for many people with schizophrenia (Kahn and Keefe 2013).

In addition to these phenotypes, significant reductions are found in total gray matter and white matter volumes, as well as whole brain volume, in people taking antipsychotics for schizophrenia. Reductions are already evident in individuals with first-episode psychosis but are more pronounced in those with a poor prognosis and advanced illness associated with cognitive decline (Kahn et al. 2015). These changes are likely to be related to loss of neuronal connectivity and dendritic spines and reductions in supporting glial cells, leading to alterations in neurotropic factors in the brain (Noordsy et al. 2018). A meta-analysis consisting of 30 longitudinal neuroimaging studies (Fusar-Poli et al. 2013) found that people with schizophrenia had progressive gray matter volume reduction compared with control groups. They also found that higher cumulative exposure to antipsychotic treatment was associated with greater reduction in brain volumes (Fusar-Poli et al. 2013).

A systematic review of data since 1921 from 50 samples and 20 countries estimated that only one in seven individuals with schizophrenia recovers (Jääskeläinen et al. 2013). The definition of *recovery* consisted of improvements in at least two domains—symptoms and social/functional outcomes—and improvements in at least one of these two domains needed to have persisted for longer than 2 years. Perhaps the most striking finding of the review was that in spite of advances in psychiatry over the past decades (e.g., the introduction and use of newer antipsychotic medications, increased attention and efforts given to psychosocial interventions, and major changes in service provision such as deinstitutionalization and early psychosis services; McGrath et al. 2014), there was no evidence that the rate of recovery from schizophrenia had increased over time. Combined together, these findings reflect urgent needs for innovative treatment options that improve psychiatric symptoms and thus recovery rates for people with schizophrenia.

Physical Health Status of People With Schizophrenia

Functional recovery from schizophrenia is further complicated by significant physical comorbidities. People with schizophrenia are known to lose approximately 15 years of potential life to the illness (Hjorthøj et al. 2017), and the majority of this reduced life expectancy is due to preventable physical conditions such as cardiovascular diseases and diabetes mellitus (Olfson et al. 2015). There are many factors that contribute to these mortality and morbidity gaps. For example, most psychotropic medications contribute significantly to deterioration of the cardiometabolic risk profile, mainly through substantial weight gain (Correll et al. 2015). However, cardiometabolic risk is often not adequately monitored under mental health services, and even when people with schizophrenia do present to health services for physical illnesses, they are less likely to receive optimal health care (Kisely et al. 2009). These issues are further exacerbated by the clinical features of schizophrenia itself. For example, positive symptoms such as paranoid ideation may lead to reluctance to seek medical interventions, negative symptoms such as reduced motivation may lead to missed appointments, and cognitive symptoms such as memory impairment may lead to difficulty complying with treatment regimens.

Cardiometabolic risk status for people with schizophrenia was well described in the Survey of High Impact Psychosis (SHIP) study from Australia. With data from more than 1,800 people living with psychosis, the SHIP study found that 1) three-quarters of participants were either overweight or obese, with more than 80% having central abdominal obesity, 2) two-thirds of participants were current cigarette smokers, and 3) more than half of people in the study met the criteria for metabolic syndrome (Galletly et al. 2012). Similarly, a meta-analysis consisting of 136 studies and more than 180,000 individuals found that compared with the general population, people with schizophrenia were 1) four times more likely to have abdominal obesity, 2) 2.4 times more likely to have metabolic syndrome, and 3) twice as likely to have diabetes mellitus (Vancampfort et al. 2013).

PHYSICAL ACTIVITY AND SCHIZOPHRENIA

Physical Activity Among People With Schizophrenia

Improving the physical activity status of people with schizophrenia is rapidly gaining both research and clinical attention as an important, feasible, and efficacious behavior modification target in this population (Suetani et al. 2016a). Data from the SHIP study estimated that nearly 50% of people with psychosis in Australia were insufficiently physically active to obtain health benefits (Suetani et al. 2016b). Likewise, in a cohort of 450 community patients with psychosis in the United Kingdom, 44% were engaged in insufficient levels of physical activity (Gardner-Sood et al. 2015). Furthermore, a landmark meta-analysis consisting of 35 studies with 3,453 people with schizophrenia estimated that people with schizophrenia engaged in 80.4 minutes of light-intensity physical activity, 16.2 minutes of moderate-intensity physical activity, and only 1.1 minutes of vigorous-intensity physical activity per day (Stubbs et al. 2016), with more than 40% of them not meeting the recommended 150 minutes of moderate physical activity per week. In comparison to the general population, people with schizophrenia engaged in significantly less moderate-intensity physical activity (14.2 minutes less per day) and vigorous-intensity physical activity (3.4 minutes less per day), but there was no difference in the amount of light-intensity physical activity per day.

The presence of negative symptoms and cardiometabolic comorbidities such as metabolic syndrome and obesity have been strongly associated with low physical activity status in people with schizophrenia. To a lesser degree, such factors as medication side effects, lack of knowledge regarding cardiometabolic risk profile, low self-efficacy and physical self-perception, unhealthy eating habits, and social isolation were also found to be associated with low physical activity status (Vancampfort et al. 2012). Much like the general population, many people with schizophrenia consider weight loss, improved mood, and reduced stress as major motivating factors for engaging in physical activity (Firth et al. 2016). At the same time, related factors such as low mood and high level of stress, as well as lack of social support, were seen as major barriers to physical activity engagement by people with schizophrenia. These findings were echoed in a recent study by Dahle and Noordsy (2018) that demonstrated that people with schizophrenia identified self-image as the most powerful motivation to exercise. They also reported improved global well-being and fewer depressive and anxiety symptoms as well as improved cognition as important reasons to exercise.

Efficacy of Physical Activity for Symptoms and Functioning

Research evidence for the benefits of physical activity in people with schizophrenia is now overwhelming. Using data from 20 studies with 695 participants, an important systematic review by Firth et al. (2015) found that even though physical activity interventions had no significant effect on body mass index (BMI), they led to improvement in measures of physical fitness as well as reduction of both positive and negative symptoms of schizophrenia. The review found that when the effects of four studies that used moderate to vigorous physical activity were combined, there was significant positive impact (i.e., statistically significant reduction) on total psychiatric symptoms (standardized mean difference [SMD]=–0.72; 95% confidence interval [CI] between –1.14 and –0.29). Furthermore, the benefit was seen in both positive symptoms (SMD=–0.54; 95% CI between –0.95 and –0.13) and negative symptoms (SMD=–0.44; 95% CI between –0.78 and –0.09). The study also found that the *dose* of physical activity is important because the benefits were prominent in those who were engaged in approximately 90 minutes or more per week of moderate to vigorous physical activity.

Another systematic review, consisting of 29 studies and 1,109 individuals with schizophrenia, demonstrated that physical activity interventions can improve both positive and negative symptoms as well as depressive symptoms, quality of life, and global functioning (Dauwan et al. 2016). This review used Hedges' *g* to quantify effect sizes of combined studies using a random effect model. They found that physical activity interventions had significant benefit for the total psychiatric symptoms (Hedges' *g*=0.39; 95% CI 0.19–0.58), positive symptoms (Hedges' *g*=0.49; 95% CI 0.14–0.50), and negative symptoms (Hedges' *g*=0.49; 95% CI 0.31–0.67). Likewise, they showed significant impact on quality of life (Hedges' *g*=0.55; 95% CI 0.35–0.76) and depression (Hedges' *g*=0.71; 95% CI 0.33–1.09).

A third systematic review demonstrated that physical activity is effective in improving global cognition, which was again found to be dose dependent (i.e., the greater the amount of physical activity, the larger the cognitive improvement) (Firth et al. 2017a). Related to this, Firth et al. (2017b) also explored the potential impact of physical activity on brain volume and found five studies that examined the impact of physical activity on brain volume in people with schizophrenia. All five examined volume of the hippocampus, with two reporting an increase and three finding no change in hippocampal volume. Even in the studies that found no change in hippocampal volume, the physical activity intervention group showed other benefits, such as increased cardiorespiratory fitness (CRF) and short-term memory, and two of the studies demonstrated increases in volumes of other regions of brain (left anterior lobe in one and total cerebral volume in another). Also, it should be noted that the particular study that found no association had a small sample number of five (Rosenbaum et al. 2015). In view of these findings, combined with the existing evidence of increased brain volumes in response to physical activity in other populations, the authors of the review postulated that stimulation of neurogenesis may be one of the procognitive mechanisms of physical activity in people with schizophrenia (Firth et al. 2017b).

Related to physical activity, there is an emerging interest in the importance of CRF in people with schizophrenia. CRF is often defined as the ability of the circulatory, respiratory, and muscular systems to supply oxygen during sustained physical activity. There have been studies to suggest that people with schizophrenia have significantly reduced CRF compared with the general population, which in turn may be independently associated with an increased cardiovascular mortality rate (Vancampfort et al. 2017). Lower CRF was associated with a higher level of negative symptoms in some cross-sectional studies (Vancampfort et al. 2015). One randomized controlled study demonstrated that a 6-month exercise intervention improved CRF in people with schizophrenia, with associated significant improvement in positive symptoms but not in negative symptoms (Scheewe et al. 2013). Moreover, a recent cohort study has reported an association between higher CRF and reduced risk of developing psychotic disorders (Kunutsor et al. 2018).

It appears that physical activity interventions with higher intensity or higher frequency are associated with greater improvement in CRF (Vancampfort et al. 2017). Another important observation was that the interventions that were being supervised by qualified professionals such as physiotherapists and exercise physiologists had a much better outcome. In fact, this is a consistent feature found in a systematic review and meta-analysis that included data from 19 randomized controlled trials consisting of 594 individuals with schizophrenia, exploring the factors that influence dropout rates from physical activity intervention studies (Vancampfort et al. 2016). This review demonstrated the importance of the qualification of the professionals delivering the physical activity intervention because patients who were supervised by physical therapists and exercise physiologists had statistically significantly reduced dropout rates from the studies as compared with patients of mental health professionals who were not trained in physical activity intervention.

Efficacy of Physical Activity Interventions

Several notable physical activity intervention studies have been published in recent years. The Achieving Healthy Lifestyles in Psychiatric Rehabilitation (ACHIEVE) trial was an 18-month intervention study in the United States consisting of 291 overweight or obese participants with severe mental disorders. Of these, more than half (58%) of participants had a diagnosis of schizophrenia (Daumit et al. 2013). The intervention of this trial consisted of individual and group physical activity, nutritional counseling, and on-site physical activity sessions. The program had a particular focus on skills building and environmental support. Trained members of the study staff led exercise classes for the first 6 months. After that, exercise sessions were offered using a video specifically prepared for this trial. At the completion of the study, the mean weight loss for the intervention group was 3.4 kg compared with 0.3 kg in the control group. Similarly, 37.8% of people in the intervention group lost 5% or more of their initial weight, compared with 22.7% in the control group ($P=0.009$). However, the study did not explore the effect of physical activity on psychiatric symptom outcomes.

Another randomized controlled trial from the United States, the STRIDE trial (Green et al. 2015), consisted of 200 individuals with severe mental disorders and an initial BMI of higher than 27 (i.e., in the overweight range). Almost all of the participants (98%) had a diagnosis of either schizophrenia or affective psychosis/bipolar disorder. The intervention consisted of two 6-month phases. The first 6 months consisted of weekly 2-hour group meetings covering topics including nutrition, physical activity, and lifestyle changes; each meeting also included a 20-minute physical activity session. The intervention encouraged moderate caloric reduction using Dietary Approaches to Stop Hypertension (DASH). After the initial 6 months, the participants moved on to the maintenance phase for another 6 months. During this second phase of the study, participants engaged in monthly group meetings and individual monthly contacts with intervention group facilitators. At the completion of the active phase (i.e., after the first 6 months), participants in the intervention group lost an average of 4.4 kg more than those in the control group. At the completion of the maintenance phase (i.e., 12 months after the commencement of the study), those in the intervention group lost an average of 2.6 kg more than those in the control group ($P=0.004$). At the end of the study, the participants in the intervention group also had a significant decline in fasting glucose level, whereas those in the control group did not. It is important to acknowledge, however, that most of the weight loss in the intervention group occurred in the first 6 months (i.e., the active phase), and there was no statistically significant difference in the weight loss between the groups in the maintenance phase. There were no differences in psychiatric hospitalizations in either group, with 15.6% of control participants and 15.4% of intervention participants having hospitalizations during the study period.

Compared with ACHIEVE and STRIDE, which included a nutritional counseling component, the Self Health Action Plan for Empowerment (InSHAPE) study focused specifically on the effect of physical activity in reducing weight (Bartels et al. 2013). The study compared the 12-month InSHAPE fitness program (intervention) with a free fitness club membership and education (control). The study included 133 participants with severe mental disorders and a BMI greater than 25, with just over 40% of the participants having a diagnosis of schizophrenia. People in the intervention group received weekly supervised training sessions at a gym with a qualified fitness trainer. The fitness trainers provided education on the principles of healthy eating and physical activity. They were also trained to tailor individual wellness plans to the needs of people with severe mental disorders. After 12 months, 40% of the participants in the intervention group achieved a clinically meaningful improvement in fitness, defined as improvement of more than 50 meters in the 6-minute walk test. This rate was twice that of the control group (20%). There was, however, no significant difference between the groups in terms of clinically meaningful weight loss, defined as loss of more than 5% of initial weight. When this trial was replicated at a larger scale ($N=200$), 51% of the participants in the intervention group achieved clinically meaningful improvement in either fitness or weight loss, compared with only 38% in the control group (Bartels et al. 2015). Moreover, the benefit appeared to be sustained 6 months after the completion of the study, with 48% of people in the intervention group still maintaining the improvement. Another striking finding from this replication study was that its pragmatic design facilitated the participation of a more ethnically diverse (46% nonwhite) and older (mean age 44 years) study sample compared with most other trials—subgroups within the population of people with severe mental disorders that are traditionally more difficult to engage in lifestyle research.

Outside the United States, the Keeping the Body in Mind (KBIM) program run in Sydney, Australia provided a pragmatic example of how lifestyle interventions with an emphasis on physical activity can be integrated within a public mental health service setting. KBIM began with the implementation of routine metabolic screening in a first-episode psychosis service located within a public community mental health center, gradually evolving over a number of years to incorporate a range of interventions to reduce the cardiometabolic risk profile of people with schizophrenia. An in-house gym was built, and an exercise physiologist worked one on one with patients to prescribe and supervise individualized exercise programs. This led to a truly multidisciplinary KBIM mental health team, consisting of a senior nurse, a dietitian, an exercise physiologist, and a peer-support worker, with medical input from both psychiatrists and an endocrinologist. An evaluation of the KBIM program showed that individuals with first-episode psychosis who engaged in the KBIM intervention (a 12-week program of individual sessions with members of the KBIM team and the opportunity to participate in weekly sports groups) experienced significantly less weight gain (1.8 kg) compared with those in the standard-care group, who gained an average of 7.8 kg over the same period of time (Curtis et al. 2016). More recently, the KBIM program has been extended to other vulnerable groups, such as people with a long history of schizophrenia who are taking clozapine, and is now embedded as routine care within the service for more than 550 patients across the KBIM catchment area. The initial success of the KBIM program led to continued wider adoption within the wider community of mental health services in the region.

Combined, the current body of research evidence suggests that 1) physical activity interventions can improve both physical parameters and psychiatric symptoms as well as brain volumes of individuals with schizophrenia, and 2) it appears feasible for physical activity interventions to be incorporated within mental health services, especially with assistance from qualified professionals such as physiotherapists and exercise physiologists. The question we face now is how do we make physical activity intervention part of routine mental health care?

TRANSLATING RESEARCH EVIDENCE INTO CLINICAL PRACTICE

In spite of the promising efficacy of physical activity interventions in research settings, the wider implementation into clinical settings remains a challenge (Lederman et al. 2017; Pratt et al. 2016). In contrast to the findings from the InSHAPE study (Bartels et al. 2015), a recent review of the existing evidence indicated that most of the benefits associated with physical activity interventions disappear once the intervention is finished (Gates et al. 2015). The mental and physical health problems of people with schizophrenia are long-term issues; therefore, they need long-term solutions. The question is no longer about whether or not physical activity interventions are efficacious for people with schizophrenia—we know they are—but rather, the question should now be how can we best implement physical activity interventions and embed them into our day-to-day clinical practice (Bartels 2015; Lederman et al. 2017)?

Translating the principles of short-term randomized controlled trials into practicalities of sustainable daily practice will also allow us to explore some of the questions that have not been adequately answered so far in research. For example, how do we engage people who are hardest to engage (e.g., older individuals, racial minorities, people with pronounced negative symptoms) and are most likely to benefit from such interventions? What is the optimum *dose* of physical activity interventions that would maximize the benefits while minimizing dropouts? How do we best measure physical activity status in people with schizophrenia? Should we use objective measures such as accelerometers rather than subjective reports such as questionnaires? Should we be focusing more on measures of *fitness* such as CRF rather than the amount of physical activity per se?

Lederman et al. (2017) proposed strategies to achieve such sustainable implementation on the basis of some successful examples in Australia. They identified that most successful physical activity interventions for people with schizophrenia included such components as an early intervention approach, routine metabolic monitoring, multidisciplinary team management, and the use of behavioral change strategies as well as programs that were individualized and supervised. They also argued that in order for sustainable implementation of physical activity interventions to occur within mental health services, such factors as creating cultural changes within mental health services (i.e., acknowledgment that physical well-being of our patients is as important as their mental health); building capacity among staff members to allow for facilitation of physical activity interventions; and developing formalized collaboration with community organizations are essential. Furthermore, we need more robust, long-term evaluation of physical activity programs, cost-effectiveness analyses, and wider patient engagement in every step of the implementation for it to be truly sustainable (Lederman et al. 2017).

The Society of Behavioral Medicine and the American College of Sports Medicine reported in their recent joint position statement that lack of funding is often the greatest challenge to broad dissemination of physical activity programs for people with serious mental disorders (Pratt et al. 2016). They argued for adoption of the following recommendations to support the use of physical activity intervention programs in conjunction with community mental health services as a first-line treatment to improve health outcomes and reduce health care costs:

1. Ensure that treatment settings maximize effectiveness by providing programs that are of sufficient duration (i.e., at least 4 months), with adequate frequency of face-to-face contact and support from fitness professionals.
2. Clearly specify standards of professional accreditation for delivering physical activity programs to people with serious mental disorders by establishing minimum training competency standards.
3. Allocate funds to train fitness professionals to deliver physical activity programming in community mental health settings and perhaps more specifically to the U.S. health care setting.
4. Increase the range of disciplines of licensed or certified allied and mental health professionals who are eligible for reimbursement to deliver physical activity programs in mental health settings.

At a more individual patient level, Noordsy et al. (2018) proposed specific steps to incorporate physical activity in individual treatment plans that can be used in day-to-day clinical practice. In essence, these steps consist of assessment of lifetime and current physical activity status, education regarding the role of physical activity as a treatment option, provision of a clear and specific goal-oriented physical activity recommendation, and monitoring of progress and response to physical activity. This formalized process of medical evaluation, recommendation, monitoring, and reinforcement of success is likely to help encourage ongoing physical activity engagement for patients with schizophrenia.

Case Example

Steve was 19 years old when he experienced onset of psychosis early in his sophomore year at college. On intake with the coordinated specialty care (CSC) team, the psychiatrist identified that Steve played team sports through high school and continued playing on intramural teams during his freshman year. He had become inactive over the summer while working long hours at an internship. Steve and his CSC team developed a plan together to reduce his course load, start medication and cognitive-behavioral therapy for psychosis, minimize substance use, and resume regular physical activity. The psychiatrist educated Steve about the potential for exercise to help protect and heal his brain and the potential impact on symptoms and well-being. Noting Steve's passion for basketball, they started with a plan for him to shoot baskets or run for 30 minutes every other day. All team members checked in with Steve on his adherence to the plan at subsequent visits. Initially, Steve went outside a few times and alternated walking and running for 15 minutes. When prompted, he was able to identify reduced anxiety and better energy after exercising. He identified overstimulation as a barrier to basketball at the school gym, so his therapist helped him locate a quiet outdoor court where he could shoot on his own. Through iterative goal setting, reinforcement for achievement, recognition of positive effects, and goal revision, Steve began to enjoy running or shooting baskets daily and noted improved mood, sleep, and concentration. Focusing on basketball also helped him gain distance from paranoia and voices. Steve noted that he was more efficient in school work shortly after exercise, but the effect faded after several hours, so he and his therapist developed a plan to intersperse calisthenics or a brisk walk outside to regain focus during long study sessions. As his paranoia faded, Steve discovered that he could go to the gym before it got crowded and enjoy playing pick-up games with a few peers. Steve and his psychiatrist also identified a local 10-kilometer road race as a target, which created motivation for expanding the duration of his running sessions.

CONCLUSION AND FUTURE DIRECTIONS

People living with schizophrenia have unacceptably higher rates of mortality and morbidity compared with those without schizophrenia. Despite some improvement in care provision over the past decades, many people with schizophrenia continue to have high rates of residual symptoms, especially in negative symptom and cognitive domains, with little improvement in recovery rates. Current treatment options have limited efficacy for these symptoms, and there is an urgent need for novel interventions. There is now an overwhelming body of research evidence demonstrating the short-term benefits of physical activity interventions for both physical and psychological well-being of people with schizophrenia. Physical activity intervention is a feasible, cost-effective, and efficacious treatment option that can potentially reduce the differential mortality and morbidity gaps in people with schizophrenia as well as improve residual symptoms of the illness. For sustainable implementation to occur, however, research evidence alone is unlikely to be sufficient. We urgently need both cultural and policy changes driven by both passionate clinicians and increased funding. We now need to shift our efforts into finding ways to facilitate successful translation of research efficacy of physical activity interventions into clinical effectiveness in our day-to-day practice for people with schizophrenia.

DISCUSSION QUESTIONS

1. Given the amount of research evidence indicating the benefits of physical activity interventions for people with schizophrenia, why are these

interventions not offered routinely to patients? Apart from research evidence, what else is needed for this to happen where you work?

2. Is it better to focus on one lifestyle intervention at a time (e.g., increasing physical activity engagement), or is it better to focus on multiple lifestyle habits at once (e.g., quitting smoking, improving diet, as well as increasing physical activity)?

3. How can we engage people who are not interested in physical activity, and how do we motivate people to stay engaged in physical activity long term?

RECOMMENDED READINGS

Firth J, Cotter J, Elliott R, et al: A systematic review and meta-analysis of exercise interventions in schizophrenia patients. Psychol Med 45(7):1343–1361, 2015. This review summarizes the benefit of physical activity intervention for both psychological and physical well-being of people with schizophrenia.

Kimhy D, Ballon J: The role of aerobic exercise in the treatment of early psychosis, in Early Intervention in Psychosis. Edited by Hardy K, Ballon JS, Noordsy DL, Adelsheim S. Washington, DC, American Psychiatric Association Publishing (in press)

Lederman O, Suetani S, Stanton R, et al: Embedding exercise interventions as routine mental health care: implementation strategies in residential, inpatient and community settings. Australas Psychiatry 25(5):451–455, 2017

Vancampfort D, Wampers M, Mitchell AJ, et al: A meta-analysis of cardiometabolic abnormalities in drug naïve, first-episode and multi-episode patients with schizophrenia versus general population controls. World Psychiatry 12(3):240–250, 2013. This systematic review clearly illustrates the magnitude of cardiometabolic problems in people with schizophrenia at different stages of their illness.

REFERENCES

Agid O, Arenovich T, Sajeev G, et al: An algorithm-based approach to first-episode schizophrenia: response rates over 3 prospective antipsychotic trials with a retrospective data analysis. J Clin Psychiatry 72(11):1439–1444, 2011 21457676

Arango C, Garibaldi G, Marder SR: Pharmacological approaches to treating negative symptoms: a review of clinical trials. Schizophr Res 150(2–3):346–352, 2013 23938176

Bartels SJ: Can behavioral health organizations change health behaviors? The STRIDE study and lifestyle interventions for obesity in serious mental illness. Am J Psychiatry 172(1):9–11, 2015 25553493

Bartels SJ, Pratt SI, Aschbrenner KA, et al: Clinically significant improved fitness and weight loss among overweight persons with serious mental illness. Psychiatr Serv 64(8):729–736, 2013 23677386

Bartels SJ, Pratt SI, Aschbrenner KA, et al: Pragmatic replication trial of health promotion coaching for obesity in serious mental illness and maintenance of outcomes. Am J Psychiatry 172(4):344–352, 2015 25827032

Correll CU, Detraux J, De Lepeleire J, et al: Effects of antipsychotics, antidepressants and mood stabilizers on risk for physical diseases in people with schizophrenia, depression and bipolar disorder. World Psychiatry 14(2):119–136, 2015 26043321

Curtis J, Watkins A, Rosenbaum S, et al: Evaluating an individualized lifestyle and life skills intervention to prevent antipsychotic-induced weight gain in first-episode psychosis. Early Interv Psychiatry 10(3):267–276, 2016 25721464

Dahle D, Noordsy D: Factors motivating spontaneous exercise in individuals with schizophrenia spectrum disorders. Schizophr Res 199:436–437, 2018 29656908

Daumit GL, Dickerson FB, Wang NY, et al: A behavioral weight-loss intervention in persons with serious mental illness. N Engl J Med 368(17):1594–1602, 2013 23517118

Dauwan M, Begemann MJ, Heringa SM, et al: Exercise improves clinical symptoms, quality of life, global functioning, and depression in schizophrenia: a systematic review and meta-analysis. Schizophr Bull 42(3):588–599, 2016 26547223

Firth J, Cotter J, Elliott R, et al: A systematic review and meta-analysis of exercise interventions in schizophrenia patients. Psychol Med 45(7):1343–1361, 2015 25650668

Firth J, Rosenbaum S, Stubbs B, et al: Motivating factors and barriers towards exercise in severe mental illness: a systematic review and meta-analysis. Psychol Med 46(14):2869–2881, 2016 27502153

Firth J, Stubbs B, Rosenbaum S, et al: Aerobic exercise improves cognitive functioning in people with schizophrenia: a systematic review and meta-analysis. Schizophr Bull 43(3):546–556, 2017a 27521348

Firth J, Cotter J, Carney R, et al: The pro-cognitive mechanisms of physical exercise in people with schizophrenia. Br J Pharmacol 174(19):3161–3172, 2017b 28261797

Fusar-Poli P, Smieskova R, Kempton MJ, et al: Progressive brain changes in schizophrenia related to antipsychotic treatment? A meta-analysis of longitudinal MRI studies. Neurosci Biobehav Rev 37(8):1680–1691, 2013 23769814

Galletly C, Castle D, Dark F, et al: Royal Australian and New Zealand College of Psychiatrists clinical practice guidelines for the management of schizophrenia and related disorders. Aust N Z J Psychiatry 50(5):410–472, 2016 27106681

Galletly CA, Foley DL, Waterreus A, et al: Cardiometabolic risk factors in people with psychotic disorders: the second Australian national survey of psychosis. Aust N Z J Psychiatry 46(8):753–761, 2012 22761397

Gardner-Sood P, Lally J, Smith S, et al: Cardiovascular risk factors and metabolic syndrome in people with established psychotic illnesses: baseline data from the IMPaCT randomized controlled trial. Psychol Med 45(12):2619–2629, 2015 25961431

Gates J, Killackey E, Phillips L, et al: Mental health starts with physical health: current status and future directions of non-pharmacological interventions to improve physical health in first-episode psychosis. Lancet Psychiatry 2(8):726–742, 2015 26249304

Green CA, Yarborough BJ, Leo MC, et al: The STRIDE weight loss and lifestyle intervention for individuals taking antipsychotic medications: a randomized trial. Am J Psychiatry 172(1):71–81, 2015 25219423

Hjorthøj C, Stürup AE, McGrath JJ, et al: Years of potential life lost and life expectancy in schizophrenia: a systematic review and meta-analysis. Lancet Psychiatry 4(4):295–301, 2017 28237639

Jääskeläinen E, Juola P, Hirvonen N, et al: A systematic review and meta-analysis of recovery in schizophrenia. Schizophr Bull 39(6):1296–1306, 2013 23172003

Jauhar S, McKenna PJ, Radua J, et al: Cognitive-behavioural therapy for the symptoms of schizophrenia: systematic review and meta-analysis with examination of potential bias. Br J Psychiatry 204(1):20–29, 2014 24385461

Kahn RS, Keefe RS: Schizophrenia is a cognitive illness: time for a change in focus. JAMA Psychiatry 70(10):1107–1112, 2013 23925787

Kahn RS, Sommer IE, Murray RM, et al: Schizophrenia. Nat Rev Dis Primers 1:15067, 2015 27189524

Kisely S, Campbell LA, Wang Y: Treatment of ischaemic heart disease and stroke in individuals with psychosis under universal healthcare. Br J Psychiatry 195(6):545–550, 2009 19949207

Kunutsor SK, Laukkanen T, Laukkanen JA: Cardiorespiratory fitness is associated with reduced risk of future psychosis: A long-term prospective cohort study. Schizophr Res 192:473–474, 2018 28476337

Lederman O, Suetani S, Stanton R, et al: Embedding exercise interventions as routine mental health care: implementation strategies in residential, inpatient and community settings. Australas Psychiatry 25(5):451–455, 2017 28585448

Leucht S, Leucht C, Huhn M, et al: Sixty years of placebo-controlled antipsychotic drug trials in acute schizophrenia: systematic review, Bayesian meta-analysis, and meta-regression of efficacy predictors. Am J Psychiatry 174(10):927–942, 2017 28541090

McGrath JJ, Miettunen J, Jääskeläinen E, et al: The onset and offset of psychosis—and what happens in between—a commentary on 'Reappraising the long-term course and outcome of psychotic disorders: the AESOP-10 Study' by Morgan et al. (2014). Psychol Med 44(13):2705–2711, 2014 25066328

Noordsy DL, Burgess JD, Hardy KV, et al: Therapeutic potential of physical exercise in early psychosis. Am J Psychiatry 175(3):209–214, 2018 29490501

Olfson M, Gerhard T, Huang C, et al: Premature mortality among adults with schizophrenia in the United States. JAMA Psychiatry 72(12):1172–1181, 2015 26509694

Pratt SI, Jerome GJ, Schneider KL, et al: Increasing US health plan coverage for exercise programming in community mental health settings for people with serious mental illness: a position statement from the Society of Behavior Medicine and the American College of Sports Medicine. Transl Behav Med 6(3):478–481, 2016 27146275

Rabinowitz J, Levine SZ, Garibaldi G, et al: Negative symptoms have greater impact on functioning than positive symptoms in schizophrenia: analysis of CATIE data. Schizophr Res 137(1–3):147–150, 2012 22316568

Rosenbaum S, Lagopoulos J, Curtis J, et al: Aerobic exercise intervention in young people with schizophrenia spectrum disorders; improved fitness with no change in hippocampal volume. Psychiatry Res 232(2):200–201, 2015 25862528

Scheewe TW, Backx FJ, Takken T, et al: Exercise therapy improves mental and physical health in schizophrenia: a randomised controlled trial. Acta Psychiatr Scand 127(6):464–473, 2013 23106093

Siskind D, McCartney L, Goldschlager R, et al: Clozapine v. first- and second-generation antipsychotics in treatment-refractory schizophrenia: systematic review and meta-analysis. Br J Psychiatry 209(5):385–392, 2016 27388573

Stubbs B, Firth J, Berry A, et al: How much physical activity do people with schizophrenia engage in? A systematic review, comparative meta-analysis and meta-regression. Schizophr Res 176(2–3):431–440, 2016 27261419

Suetani S, Rosenbaum S, Scott JG, et al: Bridging the gap: what have we done and what more can we do to reduce the burden of avoidable death in people with psychotic illness? Epidemiol Psychiatr Sci 25(3):205–210, 2016a 26768358

Suetani S, Waterreus A, Morgan V, et al: Correlates of physical activity in people living with psychotic illness. Acta Psychiatr Scand 134(2):129–137, 2016b 27218211

Suetani S, Scott JG, McGrath JJ: The importance of the physical health needs of people with psychotic disorders. Aust N Z J Psychiatry 51(1):94–95, 2017 27521576

Vancampfort D, Knapen J, Probst M, et al: Considering a frame of reference for physical activity research related to the cardiometabolic risk profile in schizophrenia. Psychiatry Res 177(3):271–279, 2010 20406713

Vancampfort D, Knapen J, Probst M, et al: A systematic review of correlates of physical activity in patients with schizophrenia. Acta Psychiatr Scand 125(5):352–362, 2012 22176559

Vancampfort D, Wampers M, Mitchell AJ, et al: A meta-analysis of cardio-metabolic abnormalities in drug naïve, first-episode and multi-episode patients with schizophrenia versus general population controls. World Psychiatry 12(3):240–250, 2013 24096790

Vancampfort D, Rosenbaum S, Probst M, et al: Promotion of cardiorespiratory fitness in schizophrenia: a clinical overview and meta-analysis. Acta Psychiatr Scand 132(2):131–143, 2015 25740655

Vancampfort D, Rosenbaum S, Schuch FB, et al: Prevalence and predictors of treatment dropout from physical activity interventions in schizophrenia: a meta-analysis. Gen Hosp Psychiatry 39:15–23, 2016 26719106

Vancampfort D, Rosenbaum S, Schuch F, et al: Cardiorespiratory fitness in severe mental illness: a systematic review and meta-analysis. Sports Med 47(2):343–352, 2017 27299747

CHAPTER 7

Physical Exercise in the Cognitive Protection and Management of Neurocognitive Disorders

J. Kaci Fairchild, Ph.D.

Christie Mead, M.S.

Laura Dunn, M.D.

KEY POINTS

- The widespread benefits of physical activity and exercise extend to the prevention and management of neurocognitive disorders, such as mild cognitive impairment and Alzheimer's disease.

- The beneficial effects of exercise include increased brain volume, reduced β-amyloid (Aβ), and improved cognitive function.

- Potential pathways through which exercise exerts its beneficial effects on cognition include increased neurogenesis, enhanced synaptic plasticity, activation of neurotransmitter systems, and stimulation of growth factors such as brain-derived neurotrophic factor and vascular endothelial growth factor.

- The American College of Sports Medicine/American Heart Association guidelines for physical activity for older adults build on established federal guidelines, with an additional emphasis on the inclusion of activities focused on balance and flexibility as well as the importance of an activity plan or exercise prescription.

The neurocognitive disorders (NCDs) represent a broad category of disorders in which the primary problem is cognitive impairment that is caused by structural or metabolic brain disease (Ganguli et al. 2011). This impairment is acquired, as opposed to developmental; thus, it represents a decline in the person's functioning in one or more cognitive domains (e.g., complex attention, executive function, learning and memory, language, perceptual-motor, social cognition). The NCDs include delirium as well as the syndromes of major and minor NCDs and their subtypes, which include Alzheimer's disease (the most common cause of major NCD), vascular disease, frontotemporal lobar degeneration, Lewy body disease, Parkinson's disease, Huntington's disease, prion disease, HIV infection, and traumatic brain injury (TBI). In addition, substance and/or medication use may cause or contribute to major NCDs (American Psychiatric Association 2013). These subtypes represent the etiologies, or potential causes, of the cognitive and functional impairment. Although the distinction between the major and minor syndromes is somewhat subjective, accurate diagnosis involves careful assessment of both the severity of cognitive impairment and the level of assistance needed in performing activities of daily living (Looi and Velakoulis 2014). Complicating matters further, many patients have mixed etiologies for their disorder.

Physical activity and exercise have long been associated with widespread health benefits, which include primary and secondary prevention as well as management of chronic health problems such as heart disease, diabetes, high blood pressure, obesity, and osteoporosis (Petersen et al. 2018; Warburton and Bredin 2017). The benefits of physical activity and exercise also extend to brain health and cognitive function. Exercise has both immediate and long-term effects on memory and is potentially protective against some NCDs. Although there are many etiological subtypes of NCDs, the bulk of the research exploring exercise as an intervention for the prevention and management of these disorders has focused on age-associated NCDs, namely, mild cognitive impairment (MCI; minor NCD) and dementia presumed due to Alzheimer's disease (major NCD due to Alzheimer's disease).

In this chapter, we provide a brief overview of normal age-related cognitive changes as well as the most common causes of the age-associated NCDs. We then review the literature supporting the role of exercise in the prevention and management of NCDs as well as the current physical activity recommendations for older adults. Finally, we close the chapter with emerging issues in the field of exercise and NCDs and future directions for researchers.

NORMATIVE AGING AND AGE-ASSOCIATED NEUROCOGNITIVE DISORDERS

The prevalence of NCDs increases with age; however, not all older adults will experience age-related pathological changes in cognitive function. Aging is a notoriously heterogeneous process. As individuals age, there is increasing variation in health-related functioning, including cognitive health. Because of the numerous important implications for individuals (e.g., reduced independence and quality of life), families, and society, distinguishing between normative and non-normative aging is extremely relevant.

Although many older adults worry about their memory, some changes in cognitive functioning are extremely common and probably do not represent cause for clinical concern. For instance, processing speed tends to decrease, and divided attention (multitasking) becomes more difficult in most older adults. On the other hand, other cognitive functions should remain stable with age, such that changes noticed by individuals or their family or other close contacts should trigger further evaluation. These cognitive functions include recognition memory (e.g., recalling details of a story when asked yes or no questions) as well as procedural memory (memory for how to do something). There is increasing evidence that subjective cognitive decline, even in the absence of objective evidence of cognitive decline, may signal future cognitive decline (Rabin et al. 2015).

As research on cognitive impairment has progressed, the terminology used to define and describe cognitive disorders has evolved. This terminology can be confusing to patients and families as well as clinicians themselves. One such term is *mild cognitive impairment*. The criteria for MCI are essentially the same as those for mild NCD (Petersen et al. 2014). However, the concept and clinical characterization of MCI have been described over a longer period of time, so clinicians should be familiar with the criteria, evaluation, and management of MCI. The current operationalized MCI criteria require a change in cognitive abilities from a previous level, and this change must be objectively confirmed (e.g., through neuropsychological testing). The decline cannot be severe enough to meet the diagnostic criteria for major NCD (i.e., dementia) and cannot be accompanied by significant functional impairment. Individuals with MCI exhibit reduced performance beyond what would be expected for the individual's age and education in one or more cognitive domains.

MCI is further divided into amnestic (predominantly memory deficits) and nonamnestic (problems in other cognitive domains, such as executive function or language) subtypes, although this classification also is evolving. To date, there are no approved pharmacological treatments for MCI. A great deal of research has focused on the investigation of lifestyle interventions as a means to reverse cognitive impairment or delay conversion to major NCD. Examples include cognitive training protocols, dietary interventions, and physical exercise. Of these interventions, physical exercise has the greatest support for positively impacting cognitive function.

The prevalence of MCI is estimated at 15%–20% in older adults, with the prevalence increasing with age. Petersen and colleagues' (2014) review of the construct of MCI reported that the average prevalence of MCI in the general population is 18.9%. Furthermore, the risk of MCI transitioning to major NCD is approximately 10% per year (with lower rates in general population studies and higher rates in clinic referral samples) (Petersen et al. 2014). Not all persons with MCI develop a major NCD; in fact, in some individuals, the cognitive impairment remains stable or even reverses to normal cognitive function. Although risk factors for MCI have been studied extensively, none have been definitively identified. Some evidence suggests that depression may be a predictor of MCI. Of note, protective factors include physical activity as well as social and cognitive activity (Petersen et al. 2014). Given that persons with MCI, particularly those in whom memory is affected, are more likely to develop a major NCD, a primary focus of research has been to identify strategies to prevent or delay the transition from MCI to major NCD.

Major NCDs, or dementias, have a broad range of etiological subtypes. These disorders are diagnosed when the individual demonstrates significant cognitive decline in at least one cognitive domain, *and* this decline interferes with independent daily functioning. The diagnostic criteria for the subtypes of NCDs are provided in DSM-5 (American Psychiatric Association 2013). Alzheimer's disease is the most common major NCD; it accounts for 60%–80% of all cases of dementia. Yet only about half of major NCDs are due solely to Alzheimer's pathology. Many people experience other pathological changes attributable to other dementias. This mixed pathology is often diagnosed only at autopsy; however, if detected earlier in the disease process it is known as mixed dementia (Alzheimer's Association 2017).

Risk factors for Alzheimer's disease can be divided into nonmodifiable and modifiable types. Examples of nonmodifiable risk factors include age, familial history of the disease, and presence of the ε4 form of the apolipoprotein gene (*APOE*). Of these three nonmodifiable risk factors, age confers the greatest risk. The prevalence of the disease increases from 3% of persons ages 65–74 to 17% of persons ages 75–84 to 32% of persons ages 85 and older (Alzheimer's Association 2017). Although age is the greatest factor, it is insufficient to be the sole cause of Alzheimer's disease. It is more often the case that age, or another nonmodifiable risk factor, interacts with modifiable risk factors to further increase a person's vulnerability to the disease. Modifiable risk factors for Alzheimer's disease include cardiovascular disease risk factors (e.g., hypertension, dyslipidemia, obesity, diabetes, smoking, metabolic syndrome), education, TBI, and cognitive and social engagement. Sedentary behavior, as opposed to a lack of physical activity, has also been linked to numerous chronic health conditions, including late-life cognitive impairment. Given that the majority of risk factors for Alzheimer's disease are modifiable, it would follow that a person could reduce his or her risk of developing Alzheimer's through proper management of these conditions.

Despite extensive research in the public and private sectors, treatment options for Alzheimer's disease remain limited. For mild Alzheimer's disease, there are several approved cholinesterase inhibitors (i.e., donepezil, rivastigmine, galantamine), although their benefits are typically described as modest. For moderate to severe Alzheimer's disease, these same agents, as well as the *N*-methyl-D-aspartate antagonist memantine, are approved. The treatment of Alzheimer's disease has been unfortunately stymied by many failed attempts to develop disease-modifying agents that target the disease's underlying pathology (Khoury et al. 2017). For non-Alzheimer's forms of major NCD, pharmacological treatments are limited to off-label uses. It is important to note that none of these medications have been shown to slow or stop the progression of disease. Therefore, as with MCI, research on lifestyle interventions will continue to be important in addressing the growing population of people with cognitive disorders.

As the U.S. population of older adults increases substantially in the coming years—with a projected 20% of the population being 65 and older by the year 2050—there is a growing need to understand how older adults can optimally maintain and even improve their physical and cognitive health. A growing body of literature suggests that a number of interventions may improve the chances of aging "successfully" (Harmell et al. 2014). Importantly, these interventions include physical activity.

PHYSICAL EXERCISE AND COGNITION IN OLDER ADULTS

Regular exercise leads to improved health outcomes, and these benefits extend to late-life cognitive function. In observational studies of healthy older adults, regular exercise has been associated with preserved ability in a range of cognitive functions, including processing speed, executive function, and memory (Blondell et al. 2014; Teri et al. 2014). There appears to be a dose-response relationship between the intensity of physical activity and cognitive functioning because higher levels of physical activity are associated with better cognitive function, reduced risk of MCI, and reduced risk of dementia (Geda et al. 2010; Kerr et al. 2013; Teri et al. 2014).

Physical activity positively impacts brain volume, particularly in the frontal and temporal regions, including the hippocampus. In the frontal region, some studies have found that greater physical activity is associated with larger brain volume and better executive functioning. In the temporal region, findings from cross-sectional longitudinal studies broadly report that more physical activity is related to larger hippocampal volumes and better spatial memory (Voelcker-Rehage and Niemann 2013). Physical activity has also been related to changes in other brain areas, although results are not as consistent or as well studied (Voelcker-Rehage and Niemann 2013).

In addition to these structural changes to the brain, exercise is also associated with reduced deposition of β-amyloid (Aβ) peptides in both animals and humans (Steen Jensen et al. 2016). Extracellular accumulation of Aβ is one of the neuropathological hallmarks of Alzheimer's disease because it aggregates or "clumps" to form senile plaques throughout the gray matter of the brain. The beneficial effects of exercise on Aβ are all the more promising because traditional pharmacological approaches have been largely unsuccessful in targeting the underlying pathology of Alzheimer's disease.

Clinical trials of physical exercise and its effects on cognition in older adults with and without cognitive decline have noted benefits ranging from significant gains in one-third of the studies of healthy older adults to significant gains in two-thirds of the studies of cognitively impaired older adults (Colcombe and Kramer 2003; van Uffelen et al. 2008). Older adults who engage in aerobic exercise only or combined (i.e., aerobic and resistance exercises) interventions generally experience positive effects on cardiorespiratory fitness, hippocampal volume, and cognition (Erickson et al. 2011). Areas of cognition that have shown greatest improvement include executive functioning, spatial memory, attention, and processing speed (Hötting and Röder 2013; Kramer et al. 2006; Smith et al. 2010; Voelcker-Rehage and Niemann 2013). Importantly, some exercise trials have shown promise in the amelioration of cognitive impairment in persons with MCI (Sofi et al. 2011; Zheng et al. 2016), with the cognitive effects being most pronounced in women (Baker et al. 2010).

HOW DOES EXERCISE IMPACT COGNITIVE FUNCTION?

The underlying mechanisms by which exercise impacts cognition begin at the cellular and molecular levels. The brain has the ability to adapt to change by reorganizing neural connections in response to external demands, a process referred to as *neuroplasticity*. Research suggests that exercise facilitates neuroplasticity, which is associated with cognitive benefits (Hötting and Röder 2013). In order to study neuroplasticity and the neurobiological mechanisms through which exercise influences cognition, researchers turn to animal studies to directly measure such variables as neurogenesis, synaptic plasticity, neurotransmitters, and growth factors. Animal studies are vital to our understanding of molecular and cellular level changes because they provide controlled conditions that both isolate the effects of exercise and allow for direct measurement of effects on the brain. In contrast, human studies of exercise rely on more indirect measures of brain changes, including brain imaging, peripheral growth factor, and cognitive functioning measures. By connecting animal models to human studies, researchers have been able to describe the systemic effects of exercise from the cellular or molecular level through to cognitive functioning (Voss et al. 2013).

The earliest animal studies found that rodents in enriched environments (social, cognitive, and physical stimulation) experienced benefits including increases in each of the following: overall brain weight, dendritic spine growth, neurotrophin levels, and hippocampal neurogenesis. These results have largely been replicated and supported over time. Of note, within the enriched environments studies, exercise (wheel running) alone has been found to have significant positive impacts on neuroplasticity (Hamilton and Rhodes 2015; van Praag 2008; Voss et al. 2013).

Neurogenesis

Exercise is believed to enhance *neurogenesis*, specifically in the dentate gyrus region of the hippocampus. The dentate gyrus is an area that contributes to episodic memory formation as well as other functions. Exercise is thought to contribute to neurogenesis by increasing the survival of proliferating cells. A multitude of studies has shown that voluntary physical activity in rodents predicts neurogenesis, which is associated with cognitive performance. Specifically, increased running distance is correlated with higher levels of hippocampal neurogenesis and improved spatial memory. In addition to increasing adult hippocampal neurogenesis, exercise can also affect the morphology of the dentate gyrus granule cells by increasing dendritic length, spine density, and complexity. Strong support that exercise can augment neurogenesis is particularly meaningful considering that the hippocampus is highly susceptible to age-related problems such as neurodegenerative diseases (Hamilton and Rhodes 2015; van Praag 2008; Voss et al. 2013).

Synaptic Plasticity

Synaptic plasticity, or the ability of synapses to strengthen or weaken, is affected by exercise. Long-term potentiation (LTP) or long-term depression occur with repeated stimulation or understimulation, respectively, and can cause lasting changes in the strength of connection between two neurons. LTP is important for learning and memory, and animal studies have shown physical activity to increase LTP in the dentate gyrus granule cells. This process is likely related to neurogenesis, which occurs in the same region, because young cells have been suggested to have greater plasticity than mature cells. In studies of young rodents, running has a strong positive association to LTP. In studies of mature and aged mice, exercise has been found to have preventive and reversing effects on age-related declines in LTP, neurogenesis, and spatial memory (O'Callaghan et al. 2009; van Praag 2008; Voss et al. 2013).

Neurotransmitter Systems

Exercise also affects neurotransmitters by upregulating glutamatergic (excitatory) and downregulating γ-aminobutyric acid (inhibitory) systems. Within the dentate gyrus, glutamate may play a role in regulating neurogenesis. In animal models, running leads to elevations in certain glutamate receptors in the hippocampus, suggesting that exercise influences glutamatergic systems and thereby neuron function. Similarly, exercise activates the serotonergic, dopaminergic, noradrenergic, and cholinergic systems, each of which is involved in cognition (Hamilton and Rhodes 2015; Kramer et al. 2006; van Praag 2008).

Neurotrophic Factors

Growth factors that stimulate cell growth and regulate proliferation and differentiation are important in synaptic plasticity and neurogenesis. As with other molecular processes, neurotrophin levels decrease with age and are associated with declines in hippocampal volume and memory functioning. Brain-derived neurotrophic factor (BDNF), a specific growth factor in the neurotrophin family, plays a role in several key aspects of neuronal function (e.g., survival, differentiation, growth, synaptic transmission) and is especially prone to exercise-induced changes.

In rodent studies, various forms of exercise, including forced running, voluntary exercise, and strength training, have been found to increase BDNF levels (Hamilton and Rhodes 2015; Kramer et al. 2006; Voss et al. 2013). Both short and long exercise periods have led to increased BDNF expression in the hippocampus, and rodent studies have linked increased hippocampal BDNF levels to better spatial memory and learning. The effects of exercise on BDNF expression may be moderated by age because BDNF levels appear to be more sensitive to physical activity in younger rodents than in aged rodents. Older rodents that undergo longer-term running have shown reduced BDNF decline compared with age-matched sedentary control subjects.

In humans, BDNF can be measured peripherally, and similar to animal studies, physical activity has been found to increase circulating BDNF levels. In a study of older adults who underwent a 12-month exercise program, increased hippocampal volume was associated with greater BDNF changes (Erickson et al. 2011). Other studies have found similar results in older adults, revealing changes in circulating BDNF to be correlated to changes in the parahippocampal and middle temporal gyrus regions of the brain (Voss et al. 2013). Although BDNF has been the main focus in this subsection, it should be noted that other growth factors, such as vascular endothelial growth factor, are also upregulated with exercise and have been found to positively impact brain health.

IMPLICATIONS FOR PRACTICE

In light of the growing evidence highlighting the cognitive benefits of exercise, the American Academy of Neurology updated its practice guidelines to reflect the stance that providers should recommend regular exercise (minimum of twice weekly) to patients diagnosed with MCI (Petersen et al. 2018). Federal guidelines for physical activity recommendations are based on the Centers for Disease Control and Prevention guidelines for physical activity. These recommendations were originally developed for use in healthy adults. The American College of Sports Medicine (ACSM), in collaboration with the American Heart Association (AHA), published specific physical activity recommendations for older adults (Nelson et al. 2007). The second edition of the Federal Guidelines, published in 2018, now also include specific recommendations for older adults (Piercy et al. 2018). These updated recommendations detail the minimum physical activity requirements for two groups: adults ages 65 and older and adults ages 50–64 with "clinically significant" chronic medical conditions or functional limitations that impact their ability to participate in physical activity and exercise.

The current guidelines for physical activity in older adults recommend a minimum of 30 minutes of moderate-intensity aerobic activity 5 days a week (150 minutes total) or 20 minutes of vigorous-intensity aerobic activity 3 days a week. Alternatively, older adults can also choose to engage in an equivalent combination of moderate-intensity and vigorous-intensity aerobic activity each week. Aerobic activity should be performed for at least 10 minutes to obtain the physiological benefits. Thus, for those older adults who have been sedentary or who have limited exercise capacity, the 30 minutes of daily activity can be divided into three 10-minute segments each day and still be sufficient to meet the recommended amounts of physical activity.

Aerobic activity is only one component of the physical activity recommendations. To complement this aerobic activity, older adults should also engage in muscle-strengthening activity or resistance exercises on at least 2 nonconsecutive days each week. Current guidelines recommend the use of weights that allow for 10–15 repetitions performed at a moderate to high effort level and that engage each major muscle group.

These physical activity recommendations for older adults build on guidelines for younger people in several key areas. First, the older adult–specific guidelines acknowledge the importance of flexibility and balance exercises. Older adults should engage in at least 10 minutes of activities designed to increase flexibility and activities to maintain or improve balance 2 days a week. Second, the older adult–specific recommendations address the importance of physical activity and exercise as both treatments for chronic health conditions and as essential interventions to prevent the occurrence of other health conditions. Finally, these recommendations highlight the importance of an activity plan or exercise prescription. An activity plan or exercise prescription should include specific information about the type of exercises to be performed, how and where the exercises are to be performed, how often and how long the exercises should be performed, and the intensity level of the exercise. The activity plan should take into account the older adult's current fitness level and make adjustments accordingly (Nelson et al. 2007).

Physical activity guidelines, including those discussed here, provide recommendations in terms of moderate and vigorous levels of exercise intensity. Exercise intensity is a measure of how hard a person feels he or she is working while engaged in an activity. Providers and patients have both objective and subjective methods of quantifying exercise intensity. Objective measurements of exercise intensity use a person's heart rate to indicate how hard the heart is working during exercise. A person's maximum heart rate can be calculated with the following formula: 220 minus the person's age. Moderate-intensity exercise is 50%–70% of a person's maximum heart rate, and vigorous-intensity exercise is 70%–85% of a person's maximum heart rate. For example, a person who is 84 years old would have an approximate maximum heart rate of 136 beats per minute (bpm). For this person, the moderate intensity level would range from 68 bpm to 95 bpm, and the vigorous intensity level would range from 95 bpm to 116 bpm. Providers should exercise caution when establishing heart rate training zones for older adults because this simple equation does not take into account important factors such as level of physical fitness, medications, and medical conditions. These are important factors to consider because each can raise or lower a person's maximum heart rate. The maximum heart rate can be measured precisely by an exercise physiologist during a cardiac or exercise stress test.

An acceptable alternative to using a person's heart rate is the use of self-report scales of exercise intensity. The most frequently used scale is the Borg Rating of Perceived Exertion (Borg 1982). The Borg scale is a measure of rate of perceived exertion (RPE). The scale ranges from 6 to 20, in which a rating of 20 represents maximum effort (Figure 7–1). The Borg scale is a simple method to estimate heart rate, which is obtained by multiplying the Borg score by a factor of 10. For example, someone may rate brisk walking as a 13 on the Borg scale, which would translate to an approximate heart rate of 130.

Self-report scales of this type use physical markers such as increased perspiration and heart rate and change in breathing to estimate a person's level of effort or exercise intensity. Although this subjective perception of exercise intensity is correlated to objective measurements, such as heart rate, this is not a linear relationship (Borg 1982; Nelson et al. 2007). Older adults with cognitive impairment may also need additional explanation and guidance as to the use of RPEs as a measure of exercise intensity. As such, the ACSM/AHA practice guidelines suggest the use of supervised exercise so that the older adult can better understand the prescribed exercise intensity.

The old adage "Check with your doctor before you start an exercise program" is particularly true for older adults who are concerned about or

Rating	Level of exertion
6	No exertion
7	Very, very light
8	
9	Very light
10	
11	Fairly light
12	
13	Somewhat hard
14	
15	Hard
16	
17	Very hard
18	
19	Very, very hard
20	Maximal exertion

FIGURE 7–1.   Borg Rating of Perceived Exertion.

experiencing late-life cognitive impairment such as MCI or dementia. Older adults are more likely to be sedentary and experience cardiovascular disease (e.g., high blood pressure, atrial fibrillation), respiratory disease (e.g., chronic obstructive pulmonary disease, asthma), or musculoskeletal problems (e.g., arthritis), all of which may impact their ability to safely exercise without appropriate modifications. Modifications to an exercise program may include variations in the frequency and intensity of exercise, rate of titration of physical activity, type of exercise recommended (e.g., aerobic, resistance, balance, flexibility), and level of supervision required. Furthermore, older adults often have medical conditions that must be considered when recommending a physical activity plan.

Generally, exercise prescriptions for older adults include such components as the type of exercise, frequency of exercise, intensity of the exercise, duration of the exercise, and progression. Table 7–1 highlights the components of an exercise prescription for a healthy older adult.

TABLE 7–1. Components of exercise prescription for a healthy older adult

---

Type of exercise

Aerobic, dynamic exercise[a]

Resistance training[b]

Flexibility and balance training[c]

Frequency

Aerobic: 3–5 days per week

Resistance training: at least 2 days per week

Flexibility and balance training: at least 2 days per week

Intensity

Target rate of perceived exertion of 12–14 on Borg scale of 6–20

Heart rate reserve of 60%–80% of maximum heart rate

Duration

Aerobic: 30–40 minutes[d]

Resistance: 8–12 repetitions per exercise, 1–3 sets per exercise

Balance and flexibility: at least 10 minutes

Note. Older adults may present with comorbidities that necessitate the tailoring of the prescription to their specific comorbidities.
[a]Examples of aerobic activity include brisk walking, riding a bicycle, elliptical training, and swimming.
[b]Resistance training should include all major muscle groups and can include resistance bands, free weights, resistance machines, and body weight exercises.
[c]Flexibility and balance training should include static and dynamic techniques for all major muscle groups.
[d]May need to begin with 10-minute sessions to build stamina in sedentary or deconditioned older adults.

FUTURE DIRECTIONS

Although the majority of research into the effects of exercise on the prevention and management of NCDs has focused on age-associated disorders, a small but growing body of research has examined the use of physical exercise as a potential treatment option for TBI. This preliminary research suggests a positive effect on global cognitive function in persons with a TBI (Morris et al. 2016; Vanderbeken and Kerckhofs 2017). Unfortunately, this literature is only suggestive of a positive effect because the research has methodological issues (small, heterogeneous samples and suboptimal measurement of cognitive function) that preclude making stronger conclusions at this point. In light of the evidence supporting the relationship between exercise and cognitive function, there is a clear need for well-designed trials of exercise in persons experiencing cognitive impairment due to TBI.

Physical activity and exercise are widely recommended interventions for protecting, preserving, and even improving cognition. These recommendations are based on copious research supporting the benefits of exercise on various health and cognitive outcomes (e.g., reduced risk of cardiovascular problems, diabetes, stroke, or cognitive impairment). However, although the benefits of exercise—including improvements in cognitive functioning, preservation of cognition, and dementia risk—have been shown in multiple studies, it should be noted that there are mixed findings, and some research on the topic has not produced significant results. This variability may be due to the lack of common and widely used definitions of both exercise and cognition. Exercise is a complex process that affects many modifiable risk factors that could positively impact cognitive health. Thus, more research is needed to better understand the causal mechanisms that underlie the relationship between cognitive function and exercise. This research would be enhanced through improvements in technology that allow for more precise measurement of constructs (e.g., cortical BDNF expression in humans).

DISCUSSION QUESTIONS

1. What might be the evolutionary advantage to humans for the brain to respond to physical exercise with improved memory and cognition?
2. What changes in cognitive function do you notice after you exercise? What do your patients report?
3. A patient presents with subjective memory loss and family history of dementia, asking for treatment to prevent further decline. How would you advise him or her?
4. How would you support an older patient in achieving regular exercise?

RECOMMENDED READING

U.S. Department of Health and Human Services: Physical Activity Guidelines for Americans, 2nd Edition. Washington, DC, U.S. Department of Health and Human Services, 2018

REFERENCES

American Psychiatric Association: Diagnostic and Statistical Manual of Mental Disorders, 5th Edition. Arlington, VA, American Psychiatric Association, 2013

Alzheimer's Association: 2017 Alzheimer's disease facts and figures. Alzheimers Dement 13(4):325–373, 2017

Baker LD, Frank LL, Foster-Schubert K, et al: Effects of aerobic exercise on mild cognitive impairment: a controlled trial. Arch Neurol 67(1):71–79, 2010 20065132

Blondell SJ, Hammersley-Mather R, Veerman JL: Does physical activity prevent cognitive decline and dementia? A systematic review and meta-analysis of longitudinal studies. BMC Public Health 14:510–522, 2014 24885250

Borg GA: Psychophysical bases of perceived exertion. Med Sci Sports Exerc 14(5):377–381, 1982 7154893

Colcombe S, Kramer AF: Fitness effects on the cognitive function of older adults: a meta-analytic study. Psychol Sci 14(2):125–130, 2003 12661673

Erickson KI, Voss MW, Prakash RS, et al: Exercise training increases size of hippocampus and improves memory. Proc Natl Acad Sci USA 108(7):3017–3022, 2011 21282661

Ganguli M, Blacker D, Blazer DG, et al: Classification of neurocognitive disorders in DSM-5: a work in progress. Am J Geriatr Psychiatry 19(3):205–210, 2011 21425518

Geda YE, Roberts RO, Knopman DS, et al: Physical exercise, aging, and mild cognitive impairment: a population-based study. Arch Neurol 67(1):80–86, 2010 20065133

Hamilton GF, Rhodes JS: Exercise regulation of cognitive function and neuroplasticity in the healthy and diseased brain, in Progress in Molecular Biology and Translational Science, Vol 135. Edited by Bouchard C. Amsterdam, the Netherlands, Elsevier, 2015, pp 381–406

Harmell AL, Jeste D, Depp C: Strategies for successful aging: a research update. Curr Psychiatry Rep 16(10):476, 2014 25135776

Hötting K, Röder B: Beneficial effects of physical exercise on neuroplasticity and cognition. Neurosci Biobehav Rev 37(9 pt B):2243–2257, 2013 23623982

Kerr J, Marshall SJ, Patterson RE, et al: Objectively measured physical activity is related to cognitive function in older adults. J Am Geriatr Soc 61(11):1927–1931, 2013 24219194

Khoury R, Patel K, Gold J, et al: Recent progress in the pharmacotherapy of Alzheimer's disease. Drugs Aging 34(11):811–820, 2017 29116600

Kramer AF, Erickson KI, Colcombe SJ: Exercise, cognition, and the aging brain. J Appl Physiol (1985) 101(4):1237–1242, 2006 16778001

Looi JC, Velakoulis D: Major and minor neurocognitive disorders in DSM-5: the difference between the map and the terrain. Aust N Z J Psychiatry 48(3):284–286, 2014 24293049

Morris T, Gomes Osman J, Tormos Munoz JM, et al: The role of physical exercise in cognitive recovery after traumatic brain injury: a systematic review. Restor Neurol Neurosci 34(6):977–988, 2016 27834788

Nelson ME, Rejeski WJ, Blair SN, et al: Physical activity and public health in older adults: recommendation from the American College of Sports Medicine and the American Heart Association. Circulation 116(9):1094–1105, 2007 17671236

O'Callaghan RM, Griffin EW, Kelly AM: Long-term treadmill exposure protects against age-related neurodegenerative change in the rat hippocampus. Hippocampus 19(10):1019–1029, 2009 19309034

Petersen RC, Caracciolo B, Brayne C, et al: Mild cognitive impairment: a concept in evolution. J Intern Med 275(3):214–228, 2014 24605806

Petersen RC, Lopez O, Armstrong MJ, et al: Practice guideline update summary: mild cognitive impairment: report of the Guideline Development, Dissemination, and Implementation Subcommittee of the American Academy of Neurology. Neurology 90(3):126–135, 2018 29282327

Piercy KL, Troiano RP, Ballard RM: The Physical Activity Guidelines for Americans. JAMA 320(19):2020-2028, 2018 30418471

Rabin LA, Smart CM, Crane PK, et al: Subjective cognitive decline in older adults: an overview of self-report measures used across 19 international research studies. J Alzheimers Dis 48(suppl 1):S63–S86, 2015 26402085

Smith PJ, Blumenthal JA, Hoffman BM, et al: Aerobic exercise and neurocognitive performance: a meta-analytic review of randomized controlled trials. Psychosom Med 72(3):239–252, 2010 20223924

Sofi F, Valecchi D, Bacci D, et al: Physical activity and risk of cognitive decline: a meta-analysis of prospective studies. J Intern Med 269(1):107–117, 2011 20831630

Steen Jensen C, Portelius E, Siersma V, et al: Cerebrospinal fluid amyloid beta and tau concentrations are not modulated by 16 weeks of moderate- to high-intensity physical exercise in patients with Alzheimer disease. Dement Geriatr Cogn Disord 42(3–4):146–158, 2016 27643858

Teri L, McCurry SM, Logsdon RG, et al: Exercise and health promotion for older adults with cognitive impairment, in Oxford Handbook of Clinical Geropsychology. Edited by Pachana NA, Laidlaw K. New York, Oxford University Press, 2014, pp 1250–1266

Vanderbeken I, Kerckhofs E: A systematic review of the effect of physical exercise on cognition in stroke and traumatic brain injury patients. NeuroRehabilitation 40(1):33-48, 2017 27814304

van Praag H: Neurogenesis and exercise: past and future directions. Neuromolecular Med 10(2):128–140, 2008 18286389

van Uffelen JG, Chin A Paw MJ, Hopman-Rock M, et al: The effects of exercise on cognition in older adults with and without cognitive decline: a systematic review. Clin J Sport Med 18(6):486–500, 2008 19001882

Voelcker-Rehage C, Niemann C: Structural and functional brain changes related to different types of physical activity across the life span. Neurosci Biobehav Rev 37(9 pt B):2268–2295, 2013 23399048

Voss MW, Vivar C, Kramer AF, et al: Bridging animal and human models of exercise-induced brain plasticity. Trends Cogn Sci 17(10):525–544, 2013 24029446

Warburton DER, Bredin SSD: Health benefits of physical activity: a systematic review of current systematic reviews. Curr Opin Cardiol 32(5):541–556, 2017 28708630

Zheng G, Xia R, Zhou W, et al: Aerobic exercise ameliorates cognitive function in older adults with mild cognitive impairment: a systematic review and meta-analysis of randomised controlled trials. Br J Sports Med 2016 27095745 Epub ahead of print

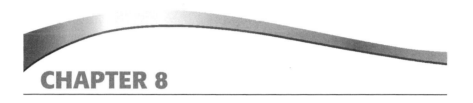

CHAPTER 8

Exercise and Addiction

Anna Lembke, M.D.

Amer Raheemullah, M.D.

KEY POINTS

- The DSM-5 diagnostic criteria for addiction encompass the 4 Cs: (loss of) control, compulsion, craving, and continued use despite consequences.
- Exercise can disrupt drug escalation in animals and humans, making it a promising component of any primary prevention program.
- Exercise ameliorates withdrawal symptoms, decreases cravings, and mitigates the risk of relapse. It is a useful and underused tool in the treatment of addiction and recovery maintenance.
- Motivational interviewing and contingency management are helpful for addressing challenges associated with initiation and maintenance of exercise in people with substance use disorders. Successful initiation and maintenance are associated with social support, self-efficacy, active choices, health contracts, assurances of safety, and positive reinforcement.
- Addiction to exercise has a similar course and symptomatology as addiction to drugs and alcohol. Interventions include a period of abstinence followed by a more moderated and closely monitored exercise program.

Any attempt to discuss the relationship between exercise and addiction must perforce acknowledge the difficulty in defining both exercise and addiction. Exercise might at first glance appear to be the easier of the two constructs to delineate, but it turns out addiction is the term whose meaning has achieved a greater level of clarity to date.

Addiction is the continued use of a substance despite harm to self and others and/or a desire to quit or cut back. The *Diagnostic and Statistical Manual of Mental Disorders* (DSM-5; American Psychiatric Association 2013) uses the term *substance use disorder* to denote addiction, and we use these terms interchangeably here. The DSM-5 diagnostic criteria for addiction encompass the 4 Cs: (loss of) control (e.g., using more than intended), compulsion (mental preoccupation with and automaticity around use), craving (physiological and/or mental states of wanting to use), and continued use despite consequences (future use is not deterred by problems arising from use). The physiological phenomena of tolerance and withdrawal are included in the DSM-5 criteria, but they are not required in order to make the diagnosis.

Exercise, by contrast, eludes a coherent and consistent definition in the medical literature, which makes comparisons across studies challenging.

Some studies let subjects define exercise for themselves. Others group exercise on the basis of type of sport or activity. Others use duration and frequency as the unit of measure. Still others define the concept of *heart rate reserve*, which is the difference between maximal and resting heart rate.

These limitations notwithstanding, we provide a narrative review examining the impact of exercise across chronological stages of the addictive process (escalation, withdrawal, relapse). We also briefly touch on the neurobiology of addiction and exercise, factors associated with successful initiation and maintenance of an exercise program, and addiction *to* exercise. We use the terms *drug* and *substance* interchangeably to encompass all addictive molecules. The animal and human data support the following findings: 1) exercise attenuates escalation of drug use, 2) exercise mitigates withdrawal and de-escalates drug use, and 3) exercise protects against relapse.

ATTENUATED ESCALATION OF DRUG USE THROUGH EXERCISE

Animal studies exploring the impact of exercise on initiation and escalation of drug use have typically used a running wheel and drug self-administration paradigm. Rats given access to a running wheel 6 weeks prior to drug exposure self-administer cocaine later and less often than rats who have not had wheel training prior to drug exposure (Smith and Pitts 2011; Smith et al. 2012). This finding has been replicated with heroin (Smith and Pitts 2012). Rats exposed to methamphetamine concurrently with access to an activity wheel show lower levels of methamphetamine self-administration than rats lacking access to an activity wheel (Miller et al. 2012). Similar findings occur with alcohol (Ehringer et al. 2009). When exercise is not voluntary but rather forced on the animal, it still results in reduced voluntary drug consumption. Forced running reduces morphine self-administration in rats (Hosseini et al. 2009) and prevents the development of a preference for a drug-associated environment (Chen et al. 2008; Fontes-Ribeiro et al. 2011; Thanos et al. 2010).

Human studies exploring the impact of exercise on initiation and escalation of drug use have focused on adolescents and young adults. High levels of physical activity in junior high school, high school, and early adulthood predict lower levels of cigarette and illicit drug use (Lynch et al. 2013). Adolescent twins categorized as persistent exercisers, occasional exercisers, or persistently inactive demonstrate twin discordance for later drug use depending on level of physical activity: persistent physical inactivity predicts illicit drug use and alcohol-related problems during young adulthood (Korhonen et al. 2009). Athletic participation among youth is associated with lower frequency of cigarette, marijuana, and other illicit substance use (Terry-McElrath and O'Malley 2011). When we treat patients who are using substances, especially adolescents experimenting with substances, we recommend a vigorous exercise program as a preventive measure to mitigate the risk of progression to addictive use.

However, not all team participation reduces substance use, serving as a reminder that exercise is just one of many variables affecting substance use. One study showed that male students participating in school-sponsored football, swimming, or wrestling or out-of-school tennis were at increased risk for using at least one substance. Female students participating in out-of-school dance, cheerleading, gymnastics, skateboarding, or surfing were at increased risk for using at least one substance (Moore and Werch 2005). Other variables affecting substance use may include weight requirements, peer dynamics, team cohesion, and team values such as individualism versus identity submersion. The value of individualism across different cultural groups is an independent risk factor for increased alcohol consumption (Inman et al. 2017).

Anecdotal reports have highlighted the risk of opioid use due to sports injuries. Trends show that nonmedical prescription opioid and lifetime heroin use among adolescents who engage in sports and exercise declined between 1997 and 2014 (Veliz et al. 2016). However, there appear to be no differences in heroin and/or nonmedical use of prescription opioids between twelfth graders who participate in sports and twelfth graders who do not participate in sports, suggesting that for opioids, team sport participation may not be protective.

The Icelandic Model of Adolescent Substance Use Prevention (Sigfúsdóttir et al. 2009), a collaboration between policymakers, behavioral scientists, practitioners, and community residents in Iceland, focused on reducing known risk factors for substance use while strengthening community protective factors. Exercise and participation in sports programs were emphasized in this comprehensive prevention initiative along with parental engagement and various extracurricular and recreational activities. During this intervention, annual cross-sectional data demonstrated a gradual decline in substance use among adolescents from 1997 to 2007.

MITIGATED WITHDRAWAL AND DE-ESCALATED DRUG USE DUE TO EXERCISE

In animal studies, access to a running wheel mitigates withdrawal. Voluntary wheel running reduces the severity of withdrawal signs in morphine-dependent rats (Miladi-Gorji et al. 2012). Diarrhea, anxiety, irritability, teeth chattering, and writhing are all significantly decreased in exercising rats compared with sedentary rats dependent on morphine. Voluntary wheel running in rats during alcohol withdrawal also protects against seizures (Devaud et al. 2012).

In human studies, exercise has been shown to help withdrawal and to de-escalate drug use. A systematic review of 14 studies in people with nicotine addiction suggested that compared with a passive condition, a single session of exercise can regulate cravings and withdrawal symptoms, with bouts of exercise as high as 60%–85% of heart rate reserve lasting 30–40 minutes to as low as 24% heart rate reserve lasting 15 minutes (Taylor et al. 2007). Withdrawal symptoms and cigarette cravings decrease rapidly during exercise and remain reduced for up to 50 minutes after exercise (Taylor et al. 2007). Of 20 study participants addicted to a range of substances including opioids, cocaine, amphetamines, and cannabis who completed an exercise program three times a week for 2–6 months, 10 reduced drug intake and 5 stopped using any substance (Roessler 2010). In a cohort of individuals with cannabis use disorder, exercise decreased average daily cannabis use by more than 50% (Buchowski et al. 2011). Longer periods of exercise, namely, 10 supervised 30 minute treadmill sessions reaching 60%–70% of heart rate reserve over 2 weeks, led to reduced levels of cannabis use among adults who met the criteria for cannabis dependence but were not seeking treatment (Buchowski et al. 2011).

In clinical care, exercise is an essential part of managing the protracted abstinence syndrome of withdrawal. In addition to the physiological symptoms of acute withdrawal, protracted abstinence syndrome is characterized by anxiety, irritability, insomnia, and dysphoria, which can continue for months to years. Except in cases of extreme physiological withdrawal (or other clinical scenarios in which exercise is not tolerated), we encourage patients to engage in 30 minutes of exercise daily to mitigate signs and symptoms of withdrawal and help de-escalate drug use.

EXERCISE AS PROTECTION AGAINST RELAPSE

Exercise has been shown to decrease drug-seeking behaviors and drug reinstatement (relapse) in animals who had previously been addicted. A study in laboratory rats demonstrated that only one session of wheel running is sufficient to decrease drug-seeking behavior in the early period of abstinence after daily self-administration of cocaine (Zlebnik et al. 2010). Another study evaluated rats after 10 days of 24-hour access to cocaine (Lynch et al. 2010). These rats subsequently underwent a 14-day period of abstinence and either were given access to a running wheel for 2 hours per day or were placed in similar boxes with the wheel locked. The study found that 2 hours per day of exercise reduced extinction responding (i.e., cocaine seeking during the period of abstinence) by approximately 35%. Furthermore, it reduced cue-induced reinstatement responding (i.e., cocaine seeking triggered by drug cues) by almost 50%.

These effects appear to be dose dependent. In another study, rats were given 24-hour access to relatively high doses of cocaine for 10 consecutive days to produce addictive behavior consistent with that seen under extended access conditions (Peterson et al. 2014). Afterward, they underwent a 14-day period of abstinence and were given either unlocked or locked wheel access for 1, 2, or 6 hours a day. Following the fourteenth day of abstinence, when cocaine seeking is known to be high, rats were evaluated under a 1-hour cue-induced reinstatement session. In these sessions, rats were exposed to a single 5-second presentation of cues formerly associated with cocaine (illumination of stimulus light above the previously active lever and the sound of the infusion pump), and their lever responses (i.e., cocaine seeking) were recorded. The rats showed decreased cocaine intake during the 10-day extended access period in a dose-dependent manner by duration of access to wheel running. One hour per day of access to wheel running does not affect levels of cocaine seeking as compared with locked-wheel access (mean responses of self-administration were greater than 40 per hour for both groups). However, 2 and 6 hours a day of wheel running were effective in decreasing cocaine self-administration, with 6 hours a day suppressing cocaine seeking almost to the point of extinction (fewer than 15 responses per hour).

In humans, craving is a major contributor to resumption of drug use after a period of abstinence. Interventions that decrease craving and drug-seeking behavior have the potential to decrease the probability of relapse in persons recovering from addiction. In a hospital-based alcohol recovery setting, patients endorsed short-term relief from alcohol craving during a brief bout of moderate-intensity exercise (Ussher et al. 2004). Specifically, stationary cycling for 10 minutes of moderate intensity, reaching 40%–60% heart rate reserve, as compared with another session of lighter intensity reaching only 5%–20% of heart rate reserve, decreased urges to drink during but not after exercise. In another study, physical activity of very low intensity and duration, such as isometric exercise or stretching, reduced cravings as compared with a passive condition (Taylor et al. 2007), highlighting a valuable coping strategy in situations where cravings peak quickly or aerobic exercise is impractical. In a third study, treatment-seeking addicted adults who engaged in a weekly 20- to 40-minute aerobic group exercise activity for 12 weeks, reaching 55%–69% of maximal heart rate, experienced an increase in nonusing days at the end of training and at 3-month follow-up (Brown et al. 2010). As previously mentioned, animal studies demonstrate a dose-dependent relationship between exercise and drug seeking. More research is needed in human studies to further delineate the dose of exercise required to mitigate risk of relapse.

For patients in recovery, especially for those who report ongoing craving, we recommend daily exercise to establish a baseline as well as exercise as needed for craving—the more intense the craving, the more intense the exercise needed to combat the craving. Craving is often experienced as an adrenaline surge, accompanied by intense anxiety. In our clinical experience, engaging in exercise in the moment of craving can serve as an antidote to the altered physiology of craving as well as teach nonchemical coping strategies.

NEUROBIOLOGY OF THE IMPACT OF EXERCISE ON DRUG USE

Exercise increases the neurotransmitters dopamine, serotonin, norepinephrine, and epinephrine, as well as endocannabinoids, and endogenous opioid peptides (Linke and Ussher 2015; Lynch et al. 2013). In particular, central concentrations of dopamine are increased by acute bouts of exercise (Linke and Ussher 2015). Through its effects on dopaminergic signaling in the reward pathway, exercise acts as a nondrug reward that competes with drugs (Lynch et al. 2013). These rewards are also achieved though the endogenous opioid peptides released through exercise. Interestingly, when the opioid receptor is blocked in laboratory rats by the opioid antagonist naloxone, the rewarding effects of wheel running are diminished (Lett et al. 2002).

Exercise also affects another neurotransmitter, glutamate. Prolonged exposure to illicit substances decreases basal levels of glutamate but increases the response of glutamate to drug administration (Schmidt and Pierce 2010). These changes in glutamate signaling play a critical role in mediating drug seeking and relapse after chronic drug exposure (Kalivas 2009). Exercise normalizes glutamate signaling and decreases glutamate levels, implying that exercise may decrease drug-seeking behavior by attenuating the response of glutamate produced by drug administration (Smith and Lynch 2012). Taken together, exercise acts as a nondrug reward that competes with drugs through its effects on dopaminergic signaling in the reward pathway (Lynch et al. 2013) and expedites healing and homeostasis in the withdrawal and recovery period.

Beyond neurotransmitters, exercise produces neuroanatomical changes through neurogenesis and gliogenesis (birth of new neurons and supporting glial cells generated from neural stem cells, respectively), which affects drug self-administration and drug-seeking behaviors. Neurogenesis continuously occurs in specific areas in the adult brain and is important for learning, memory, and behavior inhibition. For example, the hippocampus is a major site of neurogenesis and is important in mediating drug taking and drug seeking in animal models. Studies show that reduced adult hippocampal neurogenesis is a risk factor for addiction in animal models, suggesting that interventions that increase hippocampal neurogenesis could prevent addiction (Noonan et al. 2010). Exercise reliably induces neurogenesis in many areas in the hippocampus (see Chapter 2, "Physical Exercise and the Brain," and Smith and Lynch 2012).

Similarly, deficits in prefrontal functioning likely play an important role in the cognitive behavioral and emotional changes that perpetuate drug use (Goldstein and Volkow 2002). Exercise increases gliogenesis in the prefrontal cortex of rats and has positive effects on prefrontal-dependent behaviors in humans (Smith and Lynch 2012), such as future planning and delayed gratification.

FACTORS ASSOCIATED WITH SUCCESSFUL INITIATION AND MAINTENANCE OF AN EXERCISE PROGRAM

Despite the evidence, exercise is seldom implemented as part of a global addiction recovery treatment program. Part of the problem is patient resistance. Patients with substance use disorders often report low motivation to exercise, lack of transportation or time, and financial constraints that make it difficult to purchase exercise equipment or gym membership (Weinstock et al. 2017). Even when these barriers are eliminated in residential addiction treatment settings, adherence and dropout remain challenges (Muller and Clausen 2015).

Factors associated with successful initiation and maintenance of an exercise program in this population include social support, self-efficacy, active choices, health contracts, assurances of safety, and positive reinforcement (Cress et al. 2005). Several studies show that interventions using contingency management can increase exercise adherence (Mitchell et al. 2013). Motivational interviewing improves outcomes in a variety of health conditions and has been used along with contingency management to address challenges associated with initiation and maintenance of exercise in people with substance use disorder (Weinstock et al. 2017).

In our clinical practice, we routinely use motivational interviewing techniques to motivate patients to exercise. We find that patients who are initially resistant will begin to incorporate exercise in their daily routine when we help them reflect on the pros and cons of exercise, barriers to exercise, and so on. We also educate our patients regarding the benefits of exercise—not only the benefits to their overall mental and physical health but also the benefits of improving the odds of staying in recovery and avoiding relapse.

ADDICTION TO EXERCISE

Some people engage in compulsive and destructive exercise in a way that mirrors addiction to drugs. This is not surprising, given exercise's stimulating effects on the dopamine reward pathway and other neuroanatomical structures implicated in addiction. Although exercise addiction appeared in the literature as early as the 1970s, there is still no consensus on how to identify and classify this phenomenon, making it difficult for researchers to study its prevalence and severity (Lichtenstein et al. 2017). Exercise addiction is not yet an accepted diagnosis in the *International Classification of Diseases* (ICD) or DSM. To date, DSM-5 recognizes only gambling as a behavioral addiction. Despite this lack of consensus, making a diagnosis of exercise addiction relies on a thorough history taking, clinical judgment, and an understanding of addiction. Several questionnaires, validated scales, and various measures are available to assist in the clinical assessment of exercise addiction (Adams et al. 2003).

Symptoms of exercise addiction include continued exercise despite negative consequences (serious physical injury, social or interpersonal problems, marital strain, and interference with occupational and social activities); craving; unsuccessful attempts to cut back; tolerance; and withdrawal symptoms such as restlessness, irritability, fatigue, anxiety, and depression (Hausenblas and Downs 2002; Landolfi 2013). Exercise addiction has been linked to eating disorder pathology, mood disorders, and certain personality traits such as perfectionism, narcissism, and obsessive-compulsive traits (Lichtenstein et al. 2017). Common features of therapeutic intervention strategies include individual psychotherapy along with education, building coping skills, and managing triggers (Adams et al. 2003).

Case Example

Lorena is a 32-year-old woman with an addiction to running. She continued to compulsively engage in daily running, up to 100 miles per week, despite musculoskeletal injuries and an adverse impact on her marriage and her ability to care for her children. The weight loss associated with her compulsive running is largely ego-syntonic for her and contributed simultaneously to a nascent co-occurring eating disorder (anorexia). Our intervention consisted of psychoeducation around exercise addiction, a period of abstinence from running (1 month) as a way to reset her reward pathway, and a return to more moderate levels of exercise with restrictions and monitoring. In the early abstinence phase, Lorena experienced withdrawal symptoms, including anxiety, irritability, restlessness, and insomnia. When she returned to moderate exercise after a month of abstinence, she struggled to keep herself to the agreed-on running goals but was able to do so, with some slips, by focusing on her values—that is, her desire to be healthy and available for her family. She also substituted swimming, yoga, and other more moderate (for her) forms of exercise. She benefited from the addition of an antidepressant, which ameliorated persistent anxiety around eating and not exercising.

CONCLUSION

Animal and human studies demonstrate that exercise is effective in preventing escalation of drug use, ameliorating withdrawal and de-escalating drug use, and reducing risk of relapse. By stimulating release of dopamine, endocannabinoids, and endorphins, exercise acts as a competing reinforcer on the brain's reward pathway. It also promotes long-lasting neuroanatomical changes through neurogenesis and gliogenesis. Exercise itself can become an addiction when individuals continue to engage in exercise despite injury and global dysfunction. Nonetheless, the evidence is clear and convincing that exercise is a useful tool at all stages of the addiction cycle. Despite barriers, we encourage exercise as an underused evidence-based intervention in the prevention and treatment of substance use problems.

DISCUSSION QUESTIONS

1. What role might exercise play in primary prevention of substance use disorders among adolescents?
2. How might you use exercise in the treatment of withdrawal, cravings, and relapse prevention in your practice with individuals with substance use disorders?
3. What strategies could you use for overcoming barriers to exercise initiation and continuation in patients with substance use disorders?
4. What are the implications of rising dopamine, endorphin, and endocannabinoid levels in response to exercise? Is substance use a shortcut for the natural rewards of physical activity?
5. Can people get addicted to exercise? What might be some interventions to target this problem?

RECOMMENDED READINGS

Lichtenstein MB, Hinze CJ, Emborg B, et al: Compulsive exercise: links, risks and challenges faced. Psychol Res Behav Manag 10:85–95, 2017

Linke SE, Ussher M: Exercise-based treatments for substance use disorders: evidence, theory, and practicality. Am J Drug Alcohol Abuse 41(1):7–15, 2015

Lynch WJ, Peterson AB, Sanchez V, et al: Exercise as a novel treatment for drug addiction: a neurobiological and stage-dependent hypothesis. Neurosci Biobehav Rev 37(8):1622–1644, 2013

Smith MA, Lynch WJ: Exercise as a potential treatment for drug abuse: evidence from preclinical studies. Front Psychiatry 2:82, 2012

REFERENCES

Adams JM, Miller TW, Kraus RF: Exercise dependence: diagnostic and therapeutic issues for patients in psychotherapy. J Contemp Psychother 33(2):93–107, 2003

American Psychiatric Association: Diagnostic and Statistical Manual of Mental Disorders, 5th Edition. Arlington, VA, American Psychiatric Association, 2013

Brown RA, Abrantes AM, Read JP, et al: A pilot study of aerobic exercise as an adjunctive treatment for drug dependence. Ment Health Phys Act 3(1):27–34, 2010 20582151

Buchowski MS, Meade NN, Charboneau E, et al: Aerobic exercise training reduces cannabis craving and use in non-treatment seeking cannabis-dependent adults. PLoS One 6(3):e17465, 2011 21408154

Chen HI, Kuo YM, Liao CH, et al: Long-term compulsive exercise reduces the rewarding efficacy of 3,4-methylenedioxymethamphetamine. Behav Brain Res 187(1):185–189, 2008 17949827

Cress ME, Buchner DM, Prohaska T, et al: Best practices for physical activity programs and behavior counseling in older adult populations. J Aging Phys Act 13(1):61–74, 2005 15677836

Devaud LL, Walls SA, McCulley WD 3rd, et al: Voluntary wheel running attenuates ethanol withdrawal-induced increases in seizure susceptibility in male and female rats. Pharmacol Biochem Behav 103(1):18–25, 2012 22871538

Ehringer MA, Hoft NR, Zunhammer M: Reduced alcohol consumption in mice with access to a running wheel. Alcohol 43(6):443–452, 2009 19801274

Fontes-Ribeiro CA, Marques E, Pereira FC, et al: May exercise prevent addiction? Curr Neuropharmacol 9(1):45–48, 2011 21886560

Goldstein RZ, Volkow ND: Drug addiction and its underlying neurobiological basis: neuroimaging evidence for the involvement of the frontal cortex. Am J Psychiatry 159(10):1642–1652, 2002 12359667

Hausenblas HA, Downs DS: Exercise dependence: a systematic review. Psychol Sport Exerc 3(2):89–123, 2002

Hosseini M, Alaei HA, Naderi A, et al: Treadmill exercise reduces self-administration of morphine in male rats. Pathophysiology 16(1):3–7, 2009 19131225

Inman RA, da Silva SMG, Bayoumi RR, et al: Cultural value orientations and alcohol consumption in 74 countries: a societal-level analysis. Front Psychol 8:1963, 2017 29209246

Kalivas PW: The glutamate homeostasis hypothesis of addiction. Nat Rev Neurosci 10(8):561–572, 2009 19571793

Korhonen T, Kujala UM, Rose RJ, et al: Physical activity in adolescence as a predictor of alcohol and illicit drug use in early adulthood: a longitudinal population-based twin study. Twin Res Hum Genet 12(3):261–268, 2009 19456218

Landolfi E: Exercise addiction. Sports Med 43(2):111–119, 2013 23329605

Lett BT, Grant VL, Koh MT, et al: Prior experience with wheel running produces cross-tolerance to the rewarding effect of morphine. Pharmacol Biochem Behav 72(1–2):101–105, 2002 11900775

Lichtenstein MB, Hinze CJ, Emborg B, et al: Compulsive exercise: links, risks and challenges faced. Psychol Res Behav Manag 10:85–95, 2017 28435339

Linke SE, Ussher M: Exercise-based treatments for substance use disorders: evidence, theory, and practicality. Am J Drug Alcohol Abuse 41(1):7–15, 2015 25397661

Lynch WJ, Piehl KB, Acosta G, et al: Aerobic exercise attenuates reinstatement of cocaine-seeking behavior and associated neuroadaptations in the prefrontal cortex. Biol Psychiatry 68(8):774–777, 2010 20692647

Lynch WJ, Peterson AB, Sanchez V, et al: Exercise as a novel treatment for drug addiction: a neurobiological and stage-dependent hypothesis. Neurosci Biobehav Rev 37(8):1622–1644, 2013 23806439

Miladi-Gorji H, Rashidy-Pour A, Fathollahi Y: Anxiety profile in morphine-dependent and withdrawn rats: effect of voluntary exercise. Physiol Behav 105(2):195–202, 2012 21871908

Miller ML, Vaillancourt BD, Wright MJ Jr, et al: Reciprocal inhibitory effects of intravenous d-methamphetamine self-administration and wheel activity in rats. Drug Alcohol Depend 121(1–2):90–96, 2012 21899959

Mitchell MS, Goodman JM, Alter DA, et al: Financial incentives for exercise adherence in adults: systematic review and meta-analysis. Am J Prev Med 45(5):658–667, 2013 24139781

Moore MJ, Werch CE: Sport and physical activity participation and substance use among adolescents. J Adolesc Health 36(6):486–493, 2005 15901513

Muller AE, Clausen T: Group exercise to improve quality of life among substance use disorder patients. Scand J Public Health 43(2):146–152, 2015 25527637

Noonan MA, Bulin SE, Fuller DC, et al: Reduction of adult hippocampal neurogenesis confers vulnerability in an animal model of cocaine addiction. J Neurosci 30(1):304–315, 2010 20053911

Peterson AB, Abel JM, Lynch WJ: Dose-dependent effects of wheel running on cocaine-seeking and prefrontal cortex Bdnf exon IV expression in rats. Psychopharmacology (Berl) 231(7):1305–1314, 2014 24173624

Roessler KK: Exercise treatment for drug abuse—a Danish pilot study. Scand J Public Health 38(6):664–669, 2010 20529968

Schmidt HD, Pierce RC: Cocaine-induced neuroadaptations in glutamate transmission: potential therapeutic targets for craving and addiction. Ann N Y Acad Sci 1187:35–75, 2010 20201846

Sigfúsdóttir ID, Thorlindsson T, Kristjánsson AL, et al: Substance use prevention for adolescents: the Icelandic Model. Health Promot Int 24(1):16–25, 2009 19074445

Smith MA, Lynch WJ: Exercise as a potential treatment for drug abuse: evidence from preclinical studies. Front Psychiatry 2:82, 2012 22347866

Smith MA, Pitts EG: Access to a running wheel inhibits the acquisition of cocaine self-administration. Pharmacol Biochem Behav 100(2):237–243, 2011 21924284

Smith MA, Pitts EG: Wheel running decreases the positive reinforcing effects of heroin. Pharmacol Rep 64(4):960–964, 2012 23087148

Smith MA, Pennock MM, Walker KL, et al: Access to a running wheel decreases cocaine-primed and cue-induced reinstatement in male and female rats. Drug Alcohol Depend 121(1–2):54–61, 2012 21885215

Taylor AH, Ussher MH, Faulkner G: The acute effects of exercise on cigarette cravings, withdrawal symptoms, affect and smoking behaviour: a systematic review. Addiction 102(4):534–543, 2007 17286639

Terry-McElrath YM, O'Malley PM: Substance use and exercise participation among young adults: parallel trajectories in a national cohort-sequential study. Addiction 106(10):1855–1865, discussion 1866–1867, 2011 21561496

Thanos PK, Tucci A, Stamos J, et al: Chronic forced exercise during adolescence decreases cocaine conditioned place preference in Lewis rats. Behav Brain Res 215(1):77–82, 2010 20615434

Ussher M, Sampuran AK, Doshi R, et al: Acute effect of a brief bout of exercise on alcohol urges. Addiction 99(12):1542–1547, 2004 15585045

Veliz P, Boyd CJ, McCabe SE: Nonmedical prescription opioid and heroin use among adolescents who engage in sports and exercise. Pediatrics 138(2):e20160677, 2016 27456500

Weinstock J, Farney MR, Elrod NM, et al: Exercise as an adjunctive treatment for substance use disorders: rationale and intervention description. J Subst Abuse Treat 72:40–47, 2017 27666958

Zlebnik NE, Anker JJ, Gliddon LA, et al: Reduction of extinction and reinstatement of cocaine seeking by wheel running in female rats. Psychopharmacology (Berl) 209(1):113–125, 2010 20112008

CHAPTER 9

Physical Exercise in the Management of Attention-Deficit/Hyperactivity Disorder

Erin Schoenfelder, Ph.D.

Tyler Sasser, Ph.D.

Mark A. Stein, Ph.D., ABPP

KEY POINTS

- Physical activity is associated with improved attentional functioning and symptoms of attention-deficit/hyperactivity disorder (ADHD).

- Children with ADHD have lower physical activity than other children, and obesity and cardiovascular disease are common in adults with ADHD, contributing to cumulative health risks.

- Interventions to increase physical activity and reduce sedentary activities for children and adults with ADHD are a promising component of a comprehensive treatment plan.

ATTENTION-DEFICIT/HYPERACTIVITY DISORDER SYMPTOMS, IMPAIRMENTS, AND ASSOCIATED HEALTH RISKS

Attention-deficit/hyperactivity disorder (ADHD) is a prevalent and often chronic disorder that affects 6%–10% of children and adolescents (Polanczyk et al. 2014) and 4% of adults (Kessler et al. 2006). ADHD is characterized by developmentally atypical attention and impulse control that interfere with functioning across numerous domains—including academic/occupational domains, family, and social functioning (McQuade and Hoza 2015). Moreover, ADHD is associated with cumulative health risk behaviors, including increased rates of smoking, substance abuse, unhealthy eating habits, risky sexual behavior, and unsafe driving practices (Schoenfelder and Kollins 2016). Recent evidence indicates that ADHD may also inhibit healthy lifestyle behaviors, such as being physically active, that prevent chronic health problems.

A common misconception is that individuals with ADHD are *more* physically active than those without the disorder. However, individuals with ADHD have been consistently shown to have *lower* rates of activity (Cook et al. 2015; Dalsgaard et al. 2015; Khalife et al. 2014). Together with unhealthy eating (e.g., bingeing), a more sedentary lifestyle contributes to increased risk of metabolic and cardiovascular disease and may help explain decreased life expectancy associated with ADHD (Cortese and Tessari 2017; Dalsgaard et al. 2015). As of yet, little attention has been paid to improving health behaviors and activity levels for this high-risk population. Increasing physical activity may mitigate the negative health outcomes associated with ADHD, and additionally, recent studies indicate that increasing physical activity may improve ADHD symptoms and associated functional impairments (Hoza et al. 2016). In this chapter, we review evidence on the relationship between physical activity and ADHD and highlight future directions in which activity can be used to improve the health, functioning, and perhaps life course of individuals with ADHD.

BENEFITS OF PHYSICAL ACTIVITY IN ATTENTION-DEFICIT/HYPERACTIVITY DISORDER

Executive functions—frontal lobe processes such as response inhibition and working memory involved in monitoring and regulating behavior—are often compromised in ADHD and feature prominently in theories of the disorder (Antshel et al. 2014). The development of executive function skills occurs from infancy into young adulthood, and there has been increased interest in interventions designed to target these skills.

Physical activity has been linked to neurocognitive development and healthy brain functioning, leading some researchers to consider the potential benefits of physical activity for fostering executive function skill development generally (Diamond and Lee 2011) and in individuals with ADHD specifically (Gapin et al. 2011). Indeed, both brief and sustained periods of physical activity are associated with improved executive functions in laboratory-based studies across the lifespan (Verburgh et al. 2013). A meta-analysis found small to medium effects of activity in improving inhibitory control and working memory, the executive functions implicated in ADHD (Tan et al. 2016). Importantly, physical activity is found to additionally benefit mood and overall mental health (Ahn and Fedewa 2011).

The neurocognitive benefits of physical activity perhaps may be even greater for individuals with ADHD than for the general population (Gapin and Etnier 2010). Children with ADHD who participate in moderate to vigorous activity, defined as physical activity ranging from walking at a brisk pace to aerobic exercise, demonstrate improvement on cognitive tasks measuring sustained attention, response inhibition, stimulus processing, and response accuracy (Gapin and Etnier 2010; Halperin and Healey 2011; Pontifex et al. 2013; Verret et al. 2012). A recent meta-analysis of 20 studies indicated that physical activity has moderate to large effects on the symptoms and functioning of children with ADHD as well as on their mood and anxiety symptoms (Cornelius et al. 2017). Another meta-analysis reported an overall medium effect size of physical activity on executive function and motor skills of children with ADHD; effects did not vary by activity intensity but increased with duration (Vysniauske et al. 2016). Additionally, observational studies have documented a link between physical activity and real-world functional outcomes for youth with ADHD, such as classroom behavior or scores on reading and math standardized achievement tests (Hillman et al. 2009b).

The neurobiological mechanisms underlying the relation of physical activity to executive function and ADHD symptoms are underresearched, but there is evidence that physical activity causes brain changes associated with executive function. Children and adults with ADHD have decreased cortical arousal and activation in the frontal cortex compared with peers without ADHD as measured by electroencephalography (Arns et al. 2013). This includes differences on theta- and alpha-wave measurements, which are associated with self-regulation and attentional control, although the strength of the association with ADHD has been debated (Arns et al. 2013). Periods of acute physical activity are associated with enhanced alpha- and theta-wave amplitudes (Hillman et al. 2009a, 2014; Pontifex et al. 2013). One study found that children with ADHD who received an 8-week physical activity intervention exhibited smaller theta wave/alpha wave ratios over the frontal and central brain sites, which was associated with better attentional control, than children with ADHD in the control condition at posttest (Huang et al. 2017). Levels of brain-derived neurotrophic factor (BDNF), a neuroprotein that promotes healthy brain growth and functioning, are also found to differ for individuals with ADHD (Liu et al. 2015). Physical activity enhances BDNF levels (Huang et al. 2014), and this neurobiological change may constitute another mechanism by which exercise increases attention. However, more research is needed to understand the processes by which changes in neurological functioning and associated behavioral improvements occur.

Recently, there have been efforts to design interventions to increase exercise and physical activity in both clinical and nonclinical populations. Family-based physical activity interventions are found to be effective for healthy children ages 5–12 years (Brown et al. 2016), but such interventions have not focused on children with ADHD, who are at higher risk for suboptimal health behaviors and who face unique challenges in increasing their activity levels. In the only large-scale randomized trial of a physical activity intervention for children with ADHD, a 31-minute before-school exercise program improved both parent and teacher ratings of ADHD symptoms and functional outcomes across 12 weeks, indicating lasting effects of the intervention throughout the day (Hoza et al. 2015).

Several smaller pilot studies have explored innovative strategies to increase physical activity for youth with ADHD using real-world strategies integrated into their daily routines. One study provided a 45-minute physical activity lunch program for children with ADHD and found improved fitness, motor skills, and parent and teacher behavioral ratings (Verret et al. 2012). Another recent study provided adolescents with ADHD with wearable health trackers (i.e., a Fitbit band) and a motivational social media group; these interventions were found to be highly satisfying for the youth and increased their active steps taken per day (Schoenfelder et al. 2017).

As of yet, the effects of physical activity have not been systematically studied in adults with ADHD. However as suggested by Archer and Kostrzewa (2012, p. 195), exercise has "beneficial effects against stress, anxiety, depression, negative affect and behavior, poor impulse control, and compulsive behavior concomitant with improved executive functioning, working memory and positive affect, as well as improved conditions for relatives and care-givers." These are common comorbidities as well as impairments associated with persistent ADHD. To our knowledge, there is no published research on interventions to increase physical activity specifically for adults with ADHD.

PHYSICAL ACTIVITY AS ADJUNCTIVE TREATMENT

The most common medical treatment for ADHD throughout the lifespan is stimulant medication. However, adherence is poor, especially for adolescents (Adler and Nierenberg 2010), and stimulant medication is frequently discontinued despite continued impairment (Molina et al. 2009). Adults with ADHD often prefer immediate-release stimulants, which provide decreased and more variable duration of treatment compared with sustained-release and long-acting formulations (Safren et al. 2007).

The evidence that physical activity interventions improve longer-term developmental and ADHD-related functioning suggests that it is likely to be useful as an adjunct to medication and cognitive-behavioral treatments (Halperin and Healey 2011; Molina et al. 2009). Exercise researchers such as psychiatrist John Ratey have suggested that exercise and increased activity "may actually be a replacement for stimulant medication, but, for most, it's complementary—something they should absolutely do, along with taking meds, to help increase attention and improve mood" (ADDitude editors 2019). One study of children with ADHD found that physical activity led to similar improvements on executive function tasks regardless of whether or not the children were taking a stimulant (methylphenidate) (Medina et al. 2010). Physical activity may be appropriate as an alternative to pharmacotherapy in subclinical or mild cases of ADHD or in cases of poor response or tolerability. Just as in diabetes, for which insulin levels are modified on the basis of environmental and lifestyle changes, further research is needed to determine if stimulant dosage or duration may be decreased if supplemented with physical activity.

Because trials of pharmacological and behavioral treatments for ADHD have not evaluated physical activity as an outcome, little is known about the effects of ADHD treatments on individuals' activity levels. Moreover, activity level is not addressed as a target in existing evidence-based behavioral treatments for ADHD, namely, behavior management training (BMT) for parents of children with ADHD or cognitive-behavioral therapy for adults with the disorder. However, the highly effective summer treatment program for youth with ADHD created by William Pelham Jr. (Pelham et al. 2000) uses behavioral strategies to improve sports participation and skills in a summer camp setting, which is likely to increase longer-term physical activity involvement. This intensive program, which is offered at several sites in the United States, includes a point system to motivate and reward active engagement and skill development in sports ranging from soccer to basketball, as well as other behavioral and social skills in youth with ADHD. Despite the robust effectiveness of this program, a component analysis has not yet evaluated the relative benefit of increased physical activity within this complex intervention. It is quite possible that also targeting physical activity would add incrementally to the impact associated with behavioral treatments for ADHD.

OVERCOMING BARRIERS TO PHYSICAL ACTIVITY

Lower rates of physical activity for children with ADHD may be due in part to ADHD, psychiatric comorbidity, and socioeconomic-related barriers to participating in organized activities in their community. For instance, children with ADHD exhibit increased rates of disruptive, noncompliant, and aggressive behavior as well as inconsistent motivation (Spencer et al. 2007). They demonstrate greater rates of oppositional behavior and inconsistent sportsmanship in recreational sports settings, interfering with their engagement and success in sports and thus reducing longer-term physical activity (Johnson and Rosen 2000). Moreover, parents of children with ADHD experience more stress and have high rates of ADHD, depression, and substance use disorders themselves (Roizen et al. 1996). They also tend to use less effective and more negative, punitive, and inconsistent parenting approaches than do parents of youth without ADHD (Johnston and Mash 2001). As such, parents of children with ADHD may have considerable difficulty initiating or encouraging participation in physical activity and/or limiting their own sedentary behaviors, such as media use (Weiss et al. 2011).

Providers working with individuals with ADHD can support the health and functioning of this population by evaluating activity level and supporting family and environmental changes to increase physical activity. Families should be encouraged to identify appropriate organized opportunities in their community and incorporate physical activity into their daily routine. For example, families can make plans to walk a family pet together, play a sport, start the day with yoga, or play physical activity–focused games before homework time, which could benefit mood and focus. Behavioral barriers may be addressed with BMT for parents of children with ADHD. BMT is found to improve rates of compliance and on-task behavior and reduce oppositional behavior (Zwi et al. 2011), which would improve the child's ability to follow a coach's instructions, interact with peers, and learn sports skills. Practitioners working with adults with ADHD should consider incorporating physical activity goals into treatment plans and provide support for patients to schedule, remind themselves about, and track their progress with activity.

Just as behavioral and environmental supports are necessary to encourage on-task behaviors at school and in the workplace, similar principles should be used to encourage exercise within family and school settings to overcome motivational barriers to exercise. These may include strategies to increase novelty, such as varying the exercise or activity, developing a schedule and monitoring system, and identifying social and other rewards, such as exercising in a group or training for a 5K event or hike.

There are a variety of ways to integrate physical activity into a treatment plan for patients for ADHD.

Case Example 1

Michael was an overweight 10-year-old with ADHD. Prior to stimulant treatment, Michael was not able to participate in organized sports because of his disruptive and oppositional behavior. With treatment, he was able to participate in swim lessons and eventually join a swim team. Michael's attention and focus improved during swim practices, as did his appropriate participation and social skills. In middle school, Michael continued on the swim team and maintained friendships he made through this activity. As his social engagement and behavior improved, gains were also observed in his academic functioning.

Physical activity may similarly help adults with ADHD.

Case Example 2

Jane is a 22-year-old patient with ADHD taking community college classes in the evening while working for a clothing retailer during the day. She found it difficult to focus during her classes and stay organized with her materials and deadlines, which led to low grades and jeopardized her graduation. She did not feel the need to take stimulants at work because of low organizational demands, and when she took medication for class in the evenings she experienced insomnia. With her treatment provider, Jane created a schedule to do a 20-minute walk with her roommate's dog before leaving for class in the evening and then to do a 15-minute video workout before beginning to study after class. Jane noticed that her focus was improved following her workouts, and she was able to complete tasks more efficiently and leave extra time to plan her weekly to-do list.

FUTURE DIRECTIONS

Despite promising results from clinic- and school-based interventions targeting physical activity in children with ADHD, exercise is not typically addressed as part of comprehensive ADHD treatment. Interventions to increase physical activity in children and adults with ADHD have the potential to foster executive functioning development, reduce ADHD symptomatology, improve everyday functioning, and promote health, with implications for longer-term well-being. Family-based interventions, which work with caregivers to create lasting lifestyle and behavior changes, may be an appropriate avenue for increasing physical activity in children specifically.

Further research is needed to determine how best to include exercise in a comprehensive treatment plan for ADHD. Important questions remain regarding the relationship of activity and executive functioning with ADHD symptoms. For example, there is limited evidence as to the duration of the cognitive benefits of physical activity and precisely how they occur on a neurobiological level. It is also unclear what intensity and duration of activity are needed to produce meaningful benefits. As yet, we know very little about dose-response effects, maintenance, and generalization. Furthermore, there is almost no current evidence regarding the effects of stimulant medication on physical activity and the role of medication in either augmenting or suppressing the benefits of physical activity to improve cognitive functioning. Finally, there is minimal existing literature on the effects of physical activity for adults with ADHD or on interventions to increase activity in this population specifically.

In summary, individuals with ADHD are at risk for a host of negative outcomes, including obesity and cardiovascular disease, and studies suggest that physical activity is associated with improved ADHD symptoms in children and improved cognitive functioning across the lifespan. Yet little is yet known about how to increase exercise in this population in real-world settings in order to have meaningful outcomes. Assessment of physical activity and a regular exercise schedule should be included as part of a comprehensive evaluation. Despite remaining gaps in the literature in this area, clinicians may improve both the health and attentional functioning of their patients with ADHD by helping them establish a more active lifestyle.

DISCUSSION QUESTIONS

1. What factors may affect the activity level of children and adults with ADHD?
2. What is the incremental benefit of adding exercise to an ADHD treatment plan?
3. How can clinicians help children, adolescents, and adults with ADHD exercise more and increase their activity level?

RECOMMENDED READINGS

Cornelius C, Fedewa AL, Ahn S: The effect of physical activity on children with ADHD: a quantitative review of the literature. Journal of Applied School Psychology 33(2):136–170, 2017

Halperin JM, Healey DM: The influences of environmental enrichment, cognitive enhancement, and physical exercise on brain development: can we alter the developmental trajectory of ADHD? Neurosci Biobehav Rev 35(3):621–634, 2011

Hoza B, Smith AL, Shoulberg EK, et al: A randomized trial examining the effects of aerobic physical activity on attention-deficit/hyperactivity disorder symptoms in young children. J Abnorm Child Psychol 43(4):655–667, 2015

REFERENCES

ADDitude editors: Everything you need to know about ADHD. New York, ADDitude, 2019. Available at: www.additudemag.com/what-is-adhd-symptoms-causes-treatments. Accessed January 11, 2019.

Adler LD, Nierenberg AA: Review of medication adherence in children and adults with ADHD. Postgrad Med 122(1):184–191, 2010 20107302

Ahn S, Fedewa AL: A meta-analysis of the relationship between children's physical activity and mental health. J Pediatr Psychol 36(4):385–397, 2011 21227908

Antshel KM, Hier BO, Barkley RA: Executive functioning theory and ADHD, in Handbook of Executive Functioning. Edited by Goldstein S, Naglieri JA. New York, Springer, 2014, pp 107–120

Archer T, Kostrzewa RM: Physical exercise alleviates ADHD symptoms: regional deficits and development trajectory. Neurotox Res 21(2):195–209, 2012 21850535

Arns M, Conners CK, Kraemer HC: A decade of EEG theta/beta ratio research in ADHD: a meta-analysis. J Atten Disord 17(5):374–383, 2013 23086616

Brown HE, Atkin AJ, Panter J, et al: Family based interventions to increase physical activity in children: a systematic review, meta-analysis and realist synthesis. Obes Rev 17(4):345–360, 2016 26756281

Cook BG, Li D, Heinrich KM: Obesity, physical activity, and sedentary behavior of youth with learning disabilities and ADHD. J Learn Disabil 48(6):563–576, 2015 24449262

Cornelius C, Fedewa AL, Ahn S: The effect of physical activity on children with ADHD: a quantitative review of the literature. Journal of Applied School Psycholgy 33(2):136–170, 2017

Cortese S, Tessari L: Attention-deficit/hyperactivity disorder (ADHD) and obesity: update 2016. Curr Psychiatry Rep 19(1):4, 2017 28102515

Dalsgaard S, Østergaard SD, Leckman JF, et al: Mortality in children, adolescents, and adults with attention deficit hyperactivity disorder: a nationwide cohort study. Lancet 385(9983):2190–2196, 2015 25726514

Diamond A, Lee K: Interventions shown to aid executive function development in children 4 to 12 years old. Science 333(6045):959–964, 2011 21852486

Gapin J, Etnier JL: The relationship between physical activity and executive function performance in children with attention-deficit hyperactivity disorder. J Sport Exerc Psychol 32(6):753–763, 2010 21282836

Gapin JI, Labban JD, Etnier JL: The effects of physical activity on attention deficit hyperactivity disorder symptoms: the evidence. Prev Med 52(suppl 1):S70–S74, 2011 21281664

Halperin JM, Healey DM: The influences of environmental enrichment, cognitive enhancement, and physical exercise on brain development: can we alter the developmental trajectory of ADHD? Neurosci Biobehav Rev 35(3):621–634, 2011 20691725

Hillman CH, Buck SM, Themanson JR, et al: Aerobic fitness and cognitive development: Event-related brain potential and task performance indices of executive control in preadolescent children. Dev Psychol 45(1):114–129, 2009a 19209995

Hillman CH, Pontifex MB, Raine LB, et al: The effect of acute treadmill walking on cognitive control and academic achievement in preadolescent children. Neuroscience 159(3):1044–1054, 2009b 19356688

Hillman CH, Pontifex MB, Castelli DM, et al: Effects of the FITKids randomized controlled trial on executive control and brain function. Pediatrics 134(4):e1063–e1071, 2014 25266425

Hoza B, Smith AL, Shoulberg EK, et al: A randomized trial examining the effects of aerobic physical activity on attention-deficit/hyperactivity disorder symptoms in young children. J Abnorm Child Psychol 43(4):655–667, 2015 25201345

Hoza B, Martin CP, Pirog A, et al: Using physical activity to manage ADHD symptoms: the state of the evidence. Curr Psychiatry Rep 18(12):113, 2016 27807701

Huang CJ, Huang CW, Tsai YJ, et al: A preliminary examination of aerobic exercise effects on resting EEG in children with ADHD. J Atten Disord 21(11):898–903, 2017 25359761

Huang T, Larsen KT, Ried-Larsen M, et al: The effects of physical activity and exercise on brain-derived neurotrophic factor in healthy humans: A review. Scand J Med Sci Sports 24(1):1–10, 2014 23600729

Johnson RC, Rosen LA: Sports behavior of ADHD children. J Atten Disord 4(3):150–160, 2000

Johnston C, Mash EJ: Families of children with attention-deficit/hyperactivity disorder: review and recommendations for future research. Clin Child Fam Psychol Rev 4(3):183–207, 2001 11783738

Kessler RC, Adler L, Barkley R, et al: The prevalence and correlates of adult ADHD in the United States: results from the National Comorbidity Survey Replication. Am J Psychiatry 163(4):716–723, 2006 16585449

Khalife N, Kantomaa M, Glover V, et al: Childhood attention-deficit/hyperactivity disorder symptoms are risk factors for obesity and physical inactivity in adolescence. J Am Acad Child Adolesc Psychiatry 53(4):425–436, 2014 24655652

Liu D-Y, Shen X-M, Yuan F-F, et al: The physiology of BDNF and its relationship with ADHD. Mol Neurobiol 52(3):1467–1476, 2015 25354496

McQuade JD, Hoza B: Peer relationships of children with ADHD, in Attention-Deficit Hyperactivity Disorder: A Handbook for Diagnosis and Treatment. New York, Guilford, 2015, pp 210–222

Medina JA, Netto TL, Muszkat M, et al: Exercise impact on sustained attention of ADHD children, methylphenidate effects. Atten Defic Hyperact Disord 2(1):49–58, 2010 21432590

Molina BS, Hinshaw SP, Swanson JM, et al: The MTA at 8 years: prospective follow-up of children treated for combined-type ADHD in a multisite study. J Am Acad Child Adolesc Psychiatry 48(5):484–500, 2009 19318991

Pelham WE, Gnagy EM, Greiner AR, et al: Behavioral versus behavioral and pharmacological treatment in ADHD children attending a summer treatment program. J Abnorm Child Psychol 28(6):507–525, 2000 11104314

Polanczyk GV, Willcutt EG, Salum GA, et al: ADHD prevalence estimates across three decades: an updated systematic review and meta-regression analysis. Int J Epidemiol 43(2):434–442, 2014 24464188

Pontifex MB, Saliba BJ, Raine LB, et al: Exercise improves behavioral, neurocognitive, and scholastic performance in children with attention-deficit/hyperactivity disorder. J Pediatr 162(3):543–551, 2013 23084704

Roizen NJ, Blondis TA, Irwin M, et al: Psychiatric and developmental disorders in families of children with attention-deficit hyperactivity disorder. Arch Pediatr Adolesc Med 150(2):203–208, 1996 8556127

Safren SA, Duran P, Yovel I, et al: Medication adherence in psychopharmacologically treated adults with ADHD. J Atten Disord 10(3):257–260, 2007 17242421

Schoenfelder EN, Kollins SH: Topical review: ADHD and health-risk behaviors: toward prevention and health promotion. J Pediatr Psychol 41(7):735–740, 2016 26717959

Schoenfelder E, Moreno M, Wilner M, et al: Piloting a mobile health intervention to increase physical activity for adolescents with ADHD. Prev Med Rep 6:210–213, 2017 28373931

Spencer TJ, Biederman J, Mick E: Attention-deficit/hyperactivity disorder: diagnosis, lifespan, comorbidities, and neurobiology. Ambul Pediatr 7(1 suppl):73–81, 2007 17261486

Tan BW, Pooley JA, Speelman CP: A meta-analytic review of the efficacy of physical exercise interventions on cognition in individuals with autism spectrum disorder and ADHD. J Autism Dev Disord 46(9):3126–3143, 2016 27412579

Verburgh L, Königs M, Scherder EJ, et al: Physical exercise and executive functions in preadolescent children, adolescents and young adults: a meta-analysis. Br J Sports Med 48(12):973–979, 2013 23467962

Verret C, Guay MC, Berthiaume C, et al: A physical activity program improves behavior and cognitive functions in children with ADHD: an exploratory study. J Atten Disord 16(1):71–80, 2012 20837978

Vysniauske R, Verburgh L, Oosterlaan J, et al: The effects of physical exercise on functional outcomes in the treatment of ADHD: a meta-analysis. J Atten Disord 2016 26861158Epub ahead of print

Weiss MD, Baer S, Allan BA, et al: The screens culture: impact on ADHD. Atten Defic Hyperact Disord 3(4):327–334, 2011 21948003

Zwi M, Jones H, Thorgaard C, et al: Parent training interventions for attention deficit hyperactivity disorder (ADHD) in children aged 5 to 18 years. Cochrane Database Syst Rev (12):CD003018, 2011 22161373

CHAPTER 10

Physical Exercise in the Management of Autism Spectrum Disorders

Janani Venugopalakrishnan, M.D. M.P.H.

Antonio Hardan, M.D.

KEY POINTS

- People with autism spectrum disorder (ASD) are commonly less active than neurotypical peers.

- Physical exercise is associated with improvements in specific symptoms of ASD and may help with common problems such as anxiety and disruptive behaviors.

- Tailoring physical activity to the individual's interests and engaging family support and participation may help people with ASD achieve sustained, regular exercise in their daily routines.

Autism spectrum disorder (ASD) is a neurodevelopmental disorder specified in the fifth edition of the *Diagnostic and Statistical Manual of Mental Disorders* (DSM-5; American Psychiatric Association 2013) as present during the early developmental period, with deficits in social communication and interaction in addition to restricted, repetitive patterns of behavior, interests, or activities. ASD is a common developmental disability and one of the most common neurological disorders in children. ASD includes the DSM-IV (American Psychiatric Association 1994) diagnoses of autistic disorder, Asperger's disorder, childhood disintegrative disorders, and pervasive developmental disorder not otherwise specified. The symptoms cause significant impairment in social, occupational, and other areas of functioning and are not better explained by developmental delays or intellectual disability. There can be associated intellectual disability, language impairments, neurodevelopmental disorders, and genetic and medical conditions. Severity levels are often defined by the levels of support that are required in the context of deficits in social communication and repetitive restricted behaviors. The causes for ASD are heterogeneous and multifactorial and include drug and toxin exposures, prematurity, infections, pregnancy or birth complications, gene deletions, mutations, chromosomal anomalies, and advanced paternal age.

Social deficits in ASD include poor socioemotional reciprocity, reduced sharing of interests, and deficits in verbal and nonverbal communication causing difficulties in developing, maintaining, and understanding relationships. Restricted and repetitive patterns of behaviors include stereotypic behaviors, insistence on sameness, and restricted or fixated interests. Stereotypic behaviors allude to repetitive use of objects; verbal or motor movements such as rocking, jumping, hand flapping, spinning, pacing, tapping, and gazing; and vocalizations. Sensory problems include hyporeactivity or hyperreactivity to sensory stimuli along with challenges in regulating auditory, visual, and tactile inputs in the environment. These behaviors can be distracting, and because they interfere with attention to tasks, acquisition of skills, mastery of simple tasks, and positive social behaviors, they disrupt learning as well (Kern et al. 1982). In addition, there is an increased occurrence of mood and behavioral challenges in ASD, such as aggression, outbursts, impulsivity, hyperactivity, anxiety, depression, and self-injurious behaviors, making it hard for the individual to function in social settings and respond positively to the environment.

There are no available treatments that will cure symptoms of autism, but there are several interventions that aim at decreasing maladaptive behaviors and improving social communication deficits and restricted, repetitive behaviors. These include behaviorally based interventions (early intensive behavioral interventions); speech, physical, and occupational therapy; sensory integration therapies; pharmacotherapies; auditory and visual interventions; and several naturalistic behavioral interventions such as the Early Start Denver Model (Dawson et al. 2010), applied behavioral analysis, and pivotal response treatment. Interestingly, there have been numerous investigations examining the effects of physical exercise on decreasing the frequency and intensity of some of the core deficits and associated behaviors, with reports from some special education teachers providing preliminary evidence of improved cooperation and attention span after physical activities, gym class, and field trips (Burns and Ault 2009).

Mounting evidence suggests that physical exercise plays an important role in promoting mental and physical health, and it is gaining attention related to improved behaviors, cognitive functioning, and academic performance both in neurotypical children and in children with ASD. This area of research in individuals with ASD was facilitated by the combination of an overall increase in interest in exercise in the general population and the recent trends of prevalence rates of ASD. According to the Centers for Disease Control and Prevention's 2014 Autism and Developmental Disabilities Monitoring Network, prevalence of ASD is 1 in 59 children age 8 years (16.8 per 1,000; Baio et al. 2018). Different types of physical activities ranging from aerobic exercises to jogging, aquatics, martial arts, basketball, mind-body-based programs, horseback riding, yoga, stationary biking, and fencing have been studied in detail (Bahrami et al. 2012; Chan et al. 2015; Pan 2011; Schmitz Olin et al. 2017). Findings from these investigations indicate that physical activity may improve attention, cognitive functioning, and socioemotional reciprocity in individuals with ASD (Koehne et al. 2016; Neely et al. 2015). Reduction of outbursts and stereotypic behaviors are some of the other noted benefits of exercise (Bremer et al. 2016). Improvements in the social communication domain and reduction in self-stimulatory behaviors have also been observed

(Neely et al. 2015; Rafie et al. 2017). Individual case reports from clinical practice are also notable for mild cognitive and behavioral improvements post-exercise (Chan et al. 2015; Lang et al. 2010).

NEED FOR EXERCISE IN AUTISM SPECTRUM DISORDERS

The cognitive, motor, and social limitations experienced by people with ASD are barriers to accessing physical activity on a regular basis. This leads to a higher need in this group because of the increased prevalence of metabolic issues such as obesity and other associated medical comorbidities. Individuals with ASD have lower fitness scores and are less fit because sedentary behaviors are more commonly seen in this population compared with typically developing peers (McCoy et al. 2016; Tyler et al. 2014).

Decreasing activity levels are noted as children with ASD age; elementary-age children with ASD are more active than older children (Pan and Frey 2006). Moreover, restricted interests limited to technology—overuse of media, specifically, video games and television—can cause a highly sedentary lifestyle, leading to weight gain. When compared with their peers, children with ASD demonstrate a lower likelihood of being actively involved in a sport or club activity in the previous year (McCoy et al. 2016). The greater the severity of autism, the higher the chances of decreased physical activity and sports and club participations (McCoy et al. 2016).

Individuals with ASD tend to focus comparatively less on exercise and spend less time doing moderate to vigorous physical activity, necessitating more targeted programs aiding in physical interventions (Stanish et al. 2017). There is evidence suggesting that adolescents with ASD are less active overall than their typically developing peers, with higher chances of obesity, higher body mass index, and higher chances of increased weight or obesity (Srinivasan et al. 2014). Prevalence of obesity is 30.4% in the ASD group compared with 23.6% in youth without ASDs (Must et al. 2014). Higher rates of feeding and gastrointestinal problems in this population are also contributory factors to obesity. Obesity leads to other significant health consequences, such as diabetes, cardiovascular disease, hypertension, and stroke.

Psychopharmacological treatments such as atypical antipsychotics and disordered eating are also contributory factors to obesity. Weight gain, metabolic syndrome, and cardiac problems are some of the side effects secondary to medications commonly used in this population, making it all the more crucial for patients to have healthy physical activity levels. Bone mineral density is another studied physical parameter that is found to be lower in boys with ASD when compared with neurotypical prepubertal control subjects, indicating further low physical activity levels (Neumeyer et al. 2013). As a result, increased risks of fractures are seen in children and adults with ASD.

Children with ASD isolate themselves and prefer focusing on their own interests, which is a contributory factor to reduced activity levels; exercising is crucial for minimizing the impact of this lifestyle. Finally, physical activity might lead to a decrease in stereotypic behaviors and maladaptive behaviors such as aggression, outbursts, and self-injurious behaviors, thus leading to an improvement in quality of life.

CHALLENGES FOR PEOPLE WITH AUTISM SPECTRUM DISORDER

Compared with peers or typically developing children, individuals with autism do not exercise as regularly (McCoy et al. 2016). As mentioned in the previous section, the specific challenges in this group related to behavioral, physical, and cognitive deficits limit interest and access to physical activity. Society's perception of behavioral problems in the ASD group is higher than the actual levels of impairment, which is a social constraint leading to restricted access (Llewellyn and Hogan 2010).

Difficulties exist in individuals with ASD with regard to social interactions, turn taking, and understanding social cues and explicit instructions during activities. Therefore, participation in group physical activities is limited, and exercising is at times restricted to solitary sports, which are less entertaining than team sports. Segregation of activities based on skill level of the person and decreased accessibility to some of the more competitive games are other barriers in accessing opportunities for physical exercise (Pan and Frey 2006).

Reduced motor skill levels compared with peers can also be a deterrent factor that results in youth choosing something easier, such as watching media or playing online games, rather than physical activity. Delayed motor development, reduced lower body flexibility, less motor proficiency, and limited endurance are seen in children with ASD. Physical challenges also exist in the form of reduced visuospatial and visuomotor skills in ASD, leading to poor coordination and balance. Motor difficulties lead to frequent falls and accidents, limiting access to certain activities. There are limited choices when it comes to activities in this group, and the level of competition in addition to advanced skill set requirements for some exercise regimens reduce opportunities for children with ASD to engage in physical activity.

Behavioral problems such as aggression, agitation, and other comorbid mental health issues (e.g., anxiety, hyperactivity, impulsivity) are frequently observed in individuals with ASD, which by itself limits consistent involvement in physical activities and following through on expectations. It also makes it more challenging to sustain any activity, especially exercise. Disruptions in routine because of illnesses or other physical factors can also cause a setback in exercise regimens. Maladaptive fear and anxiety related to injuries and accidents during exercise can also lead to exercise avoidance in certain children.

Sensory problems, especially hyperstimulation from noises and crowded areas on a field or in the gymnasium, can cause maladaptive behavior and anxiety. Sleep disturbances and a disrupted circadian rhythm are common in this population, causing lethargy and irritability along with an increase in behavioral disturbances. This leads to increased daytime tiredness and disruption, which makes adherence to a regular exercise routine difficult. However, many of these problems are likely to improve in response to physical exercise, which reduces barriers to continued participation and is key to optimizing behavioral and socioemotional outcomes.

EVIDENCE-BASED RESEARCH AND ANECDOTAL EXPERIENCES

Exercise studies have been completed in individuals with ASD across different age groups varying from preschoolers to adults. Improvements in social and motor skills were noted in both children and adults who underwent individual exercise interventions (Sowa and Meulenbroek 2012). No changes in communication were noted. A crossover study of a 14-week aquatic program showed improvements in aquatic skills and physical fitness in children with ASD and their siblings ages 7–12 years. In certain peer- or sibling-assisted exercise programs, children with ASD showed more improvement than typically developing peers in social and physical interaction (Chu and Pan 2012). A metanalytic review studied exercise in individuals with ASD ranging in age from 3 to 41 years, and a variety of exercises including walking, aquatics, biking, jogging, and weight training were analyzed. The authors found that exercise led to a reduction of stereotypic behaviors and aggression. Participants also showed a reduction in off-task behaviors (Lang et al. 2010). Martial arts training was shown to produce sustained benefits in reduction of stereotypic behaviors up to 30 days after the intervention. Improvements in motor proficiency, academic responses, and on-task behaviors were also noted (Neely et al. 2015; Rafie et al. 2017). Fatigue was not considered to be the reason for decreased disruptive behaviors, especially because academic function-ing, motor functioning, and on-task behaviors after the physical activity showed improvement (Elliott et al. 1994).

The mechanisms underlying the effect of exercise on behaviors in ASD are not clear, but, as outlined in Chapter 2, "Physical Exercise and the Brain," neurogenesis, angiogenesis, and neuromodulation may be implicated.

Case Example 1

John is a 16-year-old male adolescent who stopped attending special day school secondary to severe anxiety, impulsivity, and disruptive behaviors. He has been homeschooled for the past 3 years. He presented with a long-standing history of extreme hypersensitivity to loud noises; aggression; diffi-culty transitioning, especially from media-related activities; and anxiety. He was enrolled in an unstructured fitness program and given access to gym equipment with a parent twice a week for 1 hour each time. After 3 months, John's parents reported decreased aggression and outbursts following these activities. John was also receiving psychotropic medication, but no changes were made during the 3 months of exercise participation.

Case Example 2

Sam is a 14-year-old male adolescent with behavioral difficulties such as aggression in addition to having attention-deficit/hyperactivity disorder (ADHD), combined type. He also has comorbid medical problems and underwent staged orthopedic surgeries over a period of 3 years, necessi-tating physical therapy and exercise. He was in an intensive physical ther-apy treatment program at home that included walking, stretching, and weightlifting with therapists and a trainer. Sam's parents noted improve-ments in his attitude, decreased anxiety, and better emotion regulation and redirectability when Sam was involved in physical activity. Discontin-uation of activities led to an increase in maladaptive behaviors and poor adjustment both at home and in the school setting, and the exercises sub-sequently were reinstated.

Intensive exercises such as jogging and horseback riding have a better effect than milder forms such as walking. Inviting people to choose their own preferred activities rather than having the activities imposed on them improves compliance and motivation. Greater participation is seen when there are shorter bouts of moderate- to vigorous-intensity exercises when compared with longer bouts. Individuals with ASD tend to do better with frequent reinforcement and goal setting (LaLonde et al. 2014). They also tend to do better when there are fewer demands to socialize in the specific activities. Moreover, having a peer buddy in the exercise programs pro-vides support, improved social interactions, and motivation to stick to the regimen.

Studies of physical exercise have found benefits for motor skills, body mass index, and mood. Improvements were noted in perceptual motor skills in adolescents with autism in a group setting after a 10-week intervention of exercises that included ball games, motor activities, and sports (Rafie et al. 2017). A 9-month treadmill-walking program in adolescents with severe autism showed increased treadmill-walking behaviors and reduction in body mass index (Pitetti et al. 2007). Brand et al. (2015) noted an improvement in mood and sleep after regular aerobic exercise and motor skills training.

Case Example 3

Dave is a 17-year-old adolescent with ASD and ADHD, combined type who struggles with severe impulsivity and hyperactivity that affect his daily functioning. Simple exercise techniques of running in the backyard and doing a few push-ups were noted to calm him down in the late evenings, making bedtime routines and transitions easier.

COGNITION

Antecedent physical activity prior to educational sessions is known to improve academic engagement as well as decrease stereotyping during instruction among individuals with ASD. Chan et al. (2015) studied groups receiving the Chinese martial art known as nei gong, progressive muscle relaxation, or no intervention. After 1 month, improved memory skills were seen in the nei gong (exercise) group when they were given a computerized visual memory task, as noted by increased electroencephalographic theta coherence between the frontal and posterior brain regions. This was not observed in the progressive muscle relaxation and control groups with no intervention. The program was considered to improve memory processing by regulating neural functional connectivity through the mind-body exercise, thus enhancing memory functioning in individuals with autism (Chan et al. 2015).

Oriel et al. (2011) found that aerobic exercises performed prior to classroom activities increased academic engagement. This was shown by significant differences in correct responses in the exercise group compared with a control group after 15 minutes of jogging or running. Stereotypic behaviors, number of correct versus incorrect responses, and percentage of on-task behaviors were measured (Oriel et al. 2011). In a different study, a dance/movement intervention strategy was shown to improve inference of emotions in adults with ASD. In this study, better academic performance was noted after exercise of mild intensity (Koehne et al. 2016). In a study of individuals with ASD and ADHD (Tan et al. 2016),

61.75% showed better cognitive performance after exercise as shown by improved on-task behaviors and performance on simple learning tasks. The results showed small to medium benefits in the exercise group for enhancing cognition. In a 10-week comparative study of a therapeutic horse-riding program (Gabriels et al. 2012), individuals with ASD showed improvements in postcondition assessments in the realm of self-regulation behaviors, stereotypies, motor skills, and expressive language. Benefits to mood and decreased lethargy and irritability were also noted.

Another study noted improved communication skills, responding, and expression in a 12-week study with 24 sessions of structured exercise activities (Zhao and Chen 2018). Incorporating the principles of the Treatment and Education of Autistic and Related Communication-Handicapped Children (TEACCH) model and the Program for the Education and Enrichment of Relational Skills (PEERS) into the exercise regimen helped achieve improvements in social skills. The PEERS model is a 14-week evidence-based social skills intervention to help teenagers with ASD make friends. Parental assessments showed that parents identified benefits of this 12-week structured exercise program in increasing social interaction and communication skills in children with ASD.

Several additional studies highlight the importance of physical activity in improving social skills and executive functioning. Incorporating a reward system promotes motivation to participate, as reported by Zhao and Chen (2018). Active video game play that includes augmented reality technology was tested as a simulation for physical activity but was inconsistent in improving social skills outcomes (Chung et al. 2015). A water exercise swimming program improved aquatic skills in addition to social improvements (Pan 2010). Benefits in executive functioning and motor skills proficiency were noted after a 12-week table tennis intervention (Pan et al. 2017).

EFFECT OF EXERCISE ON STEREOTYPIC BEHAVIORS

Schmitz Olin et al. (2017) examined the effect of physical activity on stereotypic behaviors in ASD. Exercise does not seem to eliminate stereotypic behaviors but might help in their reduction and might increase their functionality. Schmitz Olin et al. (2017) studied the effects of different intensities of aerobic exercises on stereotypic behaviors such as hand flapping, body rocking, and echolalia. Exercise was delivered in either a mild- to moderate-intensity format or a high-intensity format, and the frequency of stereotypies was measured 1 hour before and after exercising. Mild- to moderate-intensity aerobic exercise proved to be beneficial in decreasing stereotypic behaviors, whereas high-intensity exercise worsened these behaviors (Schmitz Olin et al. (2017).

Liu et al. (2015) found that 15 minutes of moderate to vigorous exercise decreased stereotypic behaviors up to 2 hours later. The reduction in stereotypies was noted regardless of age, gender, and disorder. In another study, reduction in stereotypic activities for small intervals was specifically noted after a short-term exercise intervention only with no other confounding variables (Petrus et al. 2008). Bahrami et al. (2012) examined the effectiveness of a 14-week program of kata techniques (a form of martial arts) in reducing stereotypies. The exercise group was found to have benefited in reduced behaviors even 1 month after training.

In another study, Tse et al. (2018) suggested that matching the type of exercise to the stereotypy could produce a beneficial effect. This was evidenced by decreased hand flapping after 15 minutes of a ball-tapping exercise intervention, whereas a body-rocking group did not respond significantly to the same ball-tapping exercise. This research suggested that matching the biomechanics of stereotypies to a particular exercise intervention can be more beneficial in targeting the specific repetitive behavior. Lowest levels of self-stimulatory behaviors were observed after exercise and not after activities such as regular academics or television watching. This was demonstrated by studying boys with ASD in language training sessions that followed either physical exercise, television watching, or regular academic work (Watters and Watters 1980). In a study of adults with autism and moderate to severe intellectual disability, a 65% improvement in stereotypies and 57% reduction in maladaptive behaviors (e.g., aggression, loud vocalizations, self-injurious behaviors) were observed after vigorous aerobic exercises (Elliott et al. 1994). Additionally, this study also proved the importance of exercise intensity by comparing exercise with regular motor activities.

Case Example 4

Landon is a 22-year-old male adolescent with ASD and moderate intellectual disability who also has obsessive-compulsive disorder, severe anxiety, and aggression. He presented to the clinic with hypersensitivities to loud noises and also had stereotypic behaviors of rocking and pacing, which greatly limited his social and environmental interactions and led to increases in his anxiety. He was in a year-long aquatic program, attending swim lessons two times per week and accessing a gym with a parent. His behaviors, especially aggression, were noted to be better on days when he exercised. Landon's parents also noted a decrease in self-stimulatory behaviors after exercise, attributing it to the anxiety-reduction benefits of physical activity.

Of note, the patients in these case examples were receiving medications for comorbid conditions and behavioral problems, but the improvements in behaviors following an exercise program were specifically brought to the attention of the treating provider by the patients' parents without any modifications to the concomitant medications.

LIMITATIONS

The literature described here should be interpreted with caution. Generalizability of the investigated exercise conditions is limited because of restricted availability of structured settings with accommodations for ASD and specialized equipment to meet motor and sensory needs. Nonstandardized measurement parameters in some of these studies are also limiting factors. Generalization and replicability are limited by the wide spectrum of behaviors and deficits displayed in ASD, which causes individual differences in response to the interventions. Small sample size, lack of randomization, and restricted time-based interventions are other factors that hinder the generalizability of these studies.

Most investigations focused on male subjects, and there are inadequate data on female subjects. Much of the research also focuses on high-functioning individuals with ASD and is not inclusive of children with more severe, intellectually disabling forms of ASD. In addition, there is a dearth of literature in the early childhood age group. The varied types of exercise modalities studied, with differences in intensities and duration, and the varied presentations of ASDs make it difficult to identify optimal exercise recommendations for targeted behaviors. There were many studies on the effects of exercise on stereotypic behaviors but very few studies evaluating cognitive and executive function outcomes.

FUTURE DIRECTIONS

Further research is warranted in both individual and group settings to replicate the preliminary findings of exercise improving skills in individuals with ASD. Large randomized controlled trials are needed to provide more conclusive answers on the effectiveness of different types of physical activities on core features of ASD as well as associated behaviors. Specific research into the neurobiological mechanisms of the effects of physical exercise in animal models and individuals with ASD is also needed. Longitudinal follow-up studies are needed to see if the benefits of physical activity are maintained over a period of years. Recent studies focused mostly on high-functioning individuals with ASD, and more research that includes individuals with intellectual disability and severe levels of autism is warranted.

Special instructors who are experienced with the challenges and needs of children with ASD can be helpful in decreasing anxiety surrounding choosing the type of exercise and following instructions. Occupational and physical therapy evaluations can be helpful when choosing the specific type of exercise for certain families and children. Individualized activities that take into account the particular individual's difficulties in both motor and sensory areas can be helpful to address the child's needs. Special gym areas with sensory activities aligned to visuospatial and motor needs and other considerations such as noise reduction strategies can be helpful in addressing difficulties arising from sensory overstimulation for individuals with ASD. However, advocating for more inclusive play areas, activities, and games for people with ASD rather than providing limited segregated facilities is advantageous in increasing access and social opportunities. Technology designed to encourage movement, such as apps and games that reward physical activity, may also haver promise for children and adults with ASD.

CONCLUSION

A broad range of research and clinical evidence suggests that incorporating exercise into the daily routines of individuals with ASD may lead to benefits in social, cognitive, behavioral, and physical well-being. Motor skill interventions have also been shown to improve communication skills and academic performance. Physical activity is less costly and less time consuming than other interventions and hence is more affordable to a majority of the population. It is also easy to implement at home, in the park, and at school in the child's natural environment, making it one of the most accessible ways to manage maladaptive behaviors. Most investigators conclude that fatigue is unlikely to explain the observed improvements in outbursts or other maladaptive behaviors, suggesting that the direct effects of exercise on brain health and plasticity are contributing to these benefits. Involving supports from family and peers has been shown to improve social interactions and provide sustained motivation to participate in physical activity.

DISCUSSION QUESTIONS

1. In your practice, does physical activity produce long-term benefits in reduction of maladaptive behaviors and coping with the sensory needs of children with ASD?
2. What types of exercise might you expect to have the greatest benefits for cognition, aggression, stereotypic behaviors, hyperactivity, impulsivity, or anxiety in patients with ASD?

3. How might you help a family to overcome the initial hurdle of engaging their child in a sustained physical activity?

RECOMMENDED READINGS

Elliott RO Jr, Dobbin AR, Rose GD, et al: Vigorous, aerobic exercise versus general motor training activities: effects on maladaptive and stereotypic behaviors of adults with both autism and mental retardation. J Autism Dev Disord 24(5):565–576, 1994

Petrus C, Adamson SR, Block L, et al: Effects of exercise interventions on stereotypic behaviours in children with autism spectrum disorder. Physiother Can 60(2):134–145, 2008

Sorensen C, Zarrett N: Benefits of physical activity for adolescents with autism spectrum disorders: a comprehensive review. Review Journal of Autism and Developmental Disorders 1(4):344–353, 2014

REFERENCES

American Psychiatric Association: Diagnostic and Statistical Manual of Mental Disorders, 4th Edition. Washington, DC, American Psychiatric Association, 1994

American Psychiatric Association: Diagnostic and Statistical Manual of Mental Disorders, 5th Edition. Arlington, VA, American Psychiatric Association, 2013

Bahrami F, Movahedi A, Marandi SM, et al: Kata techniques training consistently decreases stereotypy in children with autism spectrum disorder. Res Dev Disabil 33(4):1183–1193, 2012 22502844

Baio J, Wiggins L, Christensen DL, et al: Prevalence of autism spectrum disorder among children aged 8 Years—Autism and Developmental Disabilities Monitoring Network, 11 sites, United States, 2014. MMWR Surveill 67(6):1–23, 2018 29701730

Brand S, Jossen S, Holsboer-Trachsler E, et al: Impact of aerobic exercise on sleep and motor skills in children with autism spectrum disorders—a pilot study. Neuropsychiatr Dis Treat 11:1911–1920, 2015 26346856

Bremer E, Crozier M, Lloyd M: A systematic review of the behavioural outcomes following exercise interventions for children and youth with autism spectrum disorder. Autism 20(8):899–915, 2016 26823546

Burns BT, Ault R: Exercise and autism symptoms: a case study. Psi Chi Journal of Undergraduate Research 14(2):43–51, 2009

Chan AS, Han YM, Sze SL, et al: Neuroenhancement of memory for children with autism by a mind-body exercise. Front Psychol 6:1893, 2015 26696946

Chu CH, Pan CY: The effect of peer- and sibling-assisted aquatic program on interaction behaviors and aquatic skills of children with autism spectrum disorders and their peers/siblings. Res Autism Spectr Disord 6(3):1211–1223, 2012

Chung PJ, Vanderbilt DL, Soares NS: Social behaviors and active videogame play in children with autism spectrum disorder. Games Health J 4(3):225–234, 2015 26182068

Dawson G, Rogers S, Munson J, et al: Randomized, controlled trial of an intervention for toddlers with autism: the Early Start Denver Model. Pediatrics 125:e17–e23, 2010 19948568

Elliott RO Jr, Dobbin AR, Rose GD, et al: Vigorous, aerobic exercise versus general motor training activities: effects on maladaptive and stereotypic behaviors of adults with both autism and mental retardation. J Autism Dev Disord 24(5):565–576, 1994 7814306

Gabriels RL, Agnew JA, Holt KD, et al: Pilot study measuring the effects of therapeutic horseback riding on school-age children and adolescents with autism spectrum disorders. Res Autism Spectr Disord 6(2):578–588, 2012

Kern L, Koegel RL, Dyer K, et al: The effects of physical exercise on self-stimulation and appropriate responding in autistic children. J Autism Dev Disord 12(4):399–419, 1982 7161239

Koehne S, Behrends A, Fairhurst MT, et al: Fostering social cognition through an imitation- and synchronization-based dance/movement intervention in adults with autism spectrum disorder: a controlled proof-of-concept study. Psychother Psychosom 85(1):27–35, 2016 26609704

LaLonde KB, MacNeill BR, Wolfe Eversole L, et al: Increasing physical activity in young adults with autism spectrum disorders. Res Autism Spectr Disord 8(12):1679–1683, 2014

Lang R, Koegel KL, Ashbaugh K, et al: Physical exercise and individuals with autism spectrum disorders: a systematic review. Res Autism Spectr Disord 4(4):565–576, 2010

Liu T, Fedak AT, Hamilton M: Effect of physical activity on the stereotypic behaviors of children with autism spectrum disorder. International Journal of School Health 3(1):e28674, 2015

Llewellyn A, Hogan K: The use and abuse of models of disability. Disabil Soc 15(1):157–165, 2010

McCoy SM, Jakicic JM, Gibbs BB: Comparison of obesity, physical activity, and sedentary behaviors between adolescents with autism spectrum disorders and without. J Autism Dev Disord 46(7):2317–2326, 2016 26936162

Must A, Phillips SM, Curtin C, et al: Comparison of sedentary behaviors between children with autism spectrum disorders and typically developing children. Autism 18(4):376–384, 2014 24113339

Neely L, Rispoli M, Gerow S, et al: Effects of antecedent exercise on academic engagement and stereotypy during instruction. Behav Modif 39(1):98–116, 2015 25271070

Neumeyer AM, Gates A, Ferrone C, et al: Bone density in peripubertal boys with autism spectrum disorders. J Autism Dev Disord 43(7):1623–1629, 2013 23124396

Oriel KN, George CL, Peckus R, et al: The effects of aerobic exercise on academic engagement in young children with autism spectrum disorder. Pediatr Phys Ther 23(2):187–193, 2011 21552085

Pan CY: Effects of water exercise swimming program on aquatic skills and social behaviors in children with autism spectrum disorders. Autism 14(1):9–28, 2010 20124502

Pan CY: The efficacy of an aquatic program on physical fitness and aquatic skills in children with and without autism spectrum disorders. Res Autism Spectr Disord 5(1):657–665, 2011

Pan CY, Frey GC: Physical activity patterns in youth with autism spectrum disorders. J Autism Dev Disord 36(5):597–606, 2006 16652237

Pan CY, Chu CH, Tsai CL, et al: The impacts of physical activity intervention on physical and cognitive outcomes in children with autism spectrum disorder. Autism 21(2):190–202, 2017 27056845

Petrus C, Adamson SR, Block L, et al: Effects of exercise interventions on stereotypic behaviours in children with autism spectrum disorder. Physiother Can 60(2):134–145, 2008 20145777

Pitetti KH, Rendoff AD, Grover T, et al: The efficacy of a 9-month treadmill walking program on the exercise capacity and weight reduction for adolescents with severe autism. J Autism Dev Disord 37(6):997–1006, 2007 17151799

Rafie F, Ghasemi A, Zamani Jam A, et al: Effect of exercise intervention on the perceptual-motor skills in adolescents with autism. J Sports Med Phys Fitness 57(1–2):53–59, 2017 27028719

Schmitz Olin S, McFadden BA, Golem DL, et al: The effects of exercise dose on stereotypic behavior in children with autism. Med Sci Sports Exerc 49(5):983–990, 2017 28060033

Sowa M, Meulenbroek R: Effects of physical exercise on autism spectrum disorders: a meta-analysis. Res Autism Spectr Disord 6(1):46–57, 2012

Srinivasan SM, Pescatello LS, Bhat AN: Current perspectives on physical activity and exercise recommendations for children and adolescents with autism spectrum disorders. Phys Ther 94(6):875–889, 2014 24525861

Stanish HI, Curtin C, Must A, et al: Physical activity levels, frequency, and type among adolescents with and without autism spectrum disorder. J Autism Dev Disord 47(3):785–794, 2017 28066867

Tan BWZ, Pooley JA, Speelman CP: A meta-analytic review of the efficacy of physical exercise interventions on cognition in individuals with autism spectrum disorder and ADHD. J Autism Dev Disord 46(9):3126–3143, 2016 27412579

Tse CYA, Pang CL, Lee PH: Choosing an appropriate physical exercise to reduce stereotypic behavior in children with autism spectrum disorders: a non-randomized crossover study. J Autism Dev Disord 48(5):1666–1672, 2018 29196864

Tyler K, MacDonald M, Menear K: Physical activity and physical fitness of school-aged children and youth with autism spectrum disorders. Autism Res Treat 2014:312163, 2014 25309753

Watters RG, Watters WE: Decreasing self-stimulatory behavior with physical exercise in a group of autistic boys. J Autism Dev Disord 10(4):379–387, 1980 6927742

Zhao M, Chen S: The effects of structured physical activity program on social interaction and communication for children with autism. BioMed Res Int 2018:1825046, 2018 29568743

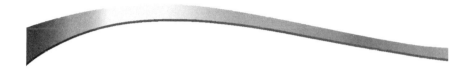

PART III

Healthy Body, Healthy Mind

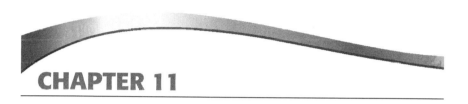

CHAPTER 11

Yoga and Tai Chi for People With Psychiatric Disorders

Michelle Guo, B.A.

Michael E. Thase, M.D.

Anup Sharma, M.D., Ph.D.

KEY POINTS

- The percentage of people in the United States who are using yoga and tai chi is increasing, suggesting increased interest in these mind-body approaches in the general population and accessibility for those with psychiatric disorders.
- Yoga and tai chi can significantly reduce psychiatric symptoms in diverse clinical populations.
- Studies of mind-body practices have demonstrated that yoga and tai chi interventions, in comparison with control interventions, can alter pathophysiological processes and change the structure and function of key brain regions.

Pharmacotherapy and psychotherapy are effective first-line treatments for psychiatric disorders such as major depressive disorder (MDD), anxiety disorders, schizophrenia, and sleep disorders. Although these therapies can make significant improvements in the lives of people with psychiatric disorders, the responses to these treatments can be inconsistent. Additionally, some patients may be discouraged about using pharmacological and psychotherapy interventions because of concerns regarding tolerability, side effects, cost, and access. As a result, effective and tolerable adjunctive therapies are needed for patients who do not respond to pharmacological monotherapy or for those who prefer evidence-based lifestyle approaches to treat their psychiatric conditions.

Mind-body practices constitute a large and diverse group of lifestyle practices that can substantially affect neurophysiology in both healthy individuals and people with psychiatric disorders (Sharma and Newberg 2015). The National Health Interview Survey suggested that the use of yoga, tai chi, and qi gong has increased linearly over time, from 5.8% in 2002 to 6.7% in 2007 to 10.1% in 2012 (Clarke et al. 2015). Notably, the increase in yoga accounts for 80% of the prevalence and occurs in all age groups ages 18 and older. Mind-body practices such as yoga and tai chi appear to be favorable for individuals across a wide range of ages and experience levels, suggesting the potential for therapeutic impact across the life span. Among the active areas of investigation is the use of mind-body approaches for people living with mental health conditions.

YOGA INTERVENTIONS FOR PSYCHIATRIC DISORDERS

Yoga is a multicomponent system that includes breathing exercises (pranayama), posture sequences (asanas), and meditation practices (Balaji et al. 2012). Each of these components can impact neurobiological functioning. Yoga combines the effects of physical postures, which have been linked to mood changes (Phillips et al. 2003), and meditation, which increases levels of brain-derived neurotrophic factor (Xiong and Doraiswamy 2009). Yoga breathing practices also result in physiological effects such as parasympathetic activation, reduction in stress responses, and modulation of thalamic activity (Brown and Gerberg 2005).

Sharma et al. (2017) performed a randomized pilot study to evaluate the feasibility, efficacy, and tolerability of Sudarshan Kriya yoga (SKY) as an adjunctive treatment in patients with MDD and incomplete response to antidepressant treatment. SKY is a breathing-based meditation technique that brings practitioners into a restful, meditative state (Sharma et al. 2017). Initial research has demonstrated that SKY has a well-tolerated antidepressant effect in patients with depression due to alcohol dependence (Vedamurthachar et al. 2006) and inpatients with MDD (Janakiramaiah et al. 2000). Furthermore, SKY reduces cortisol, increases prolactin, and improves antioxidant status in practitioners (Janakiramaiah et al. 1998; Sharma et al. 2003).

On the basis of this research, Sharma et al. (2017) developed a randomized pilot study of SKY for outpatients who were diagnosed with MDD according to DSM-IV-TR (American Psychiatric Association 2000) criteria and were taking stable doses of antidepressant medication. Patients were recruited on the basis of total scores on the 17-item Hamilton Depression Rating Scale (HDRS-17) at screening and baseline visits. At baseline, the mean HDRS-17 total score was 20.4, indicating moderate depression despite medication therapy.

The randomized, rater-blind, waitlist-controlled study consisted of 25 participants, including 13 participants in the active group (SKY intervention) and 12 participants in the waitlist control group (Sharma et al. 2017). All participants were required to continue their antidepressant medications, without dosage changes, for the entire study duration. The yoga intervention consisted of two phases of a manual-based group program. During the first phase, participants completed a six-session SKY program, which included SKY breathing, yoga postures, sitting meditation, and stress education, for 3.5 hours per day. During the second phase, participants attended weekly SKY follow-up sessions (1.5 hours per session) and completed a home practice version of SKY (20–25 minutes per day).

The SKY intent-to-treat (ITT) sample demonstrated a greater improvement from baseline to 2 months in HDRS-17 total score compared with the waitlist control (mean difference –10.27; $P=0.0032$) (Sharma et al. 2017). For both the ITT and completer samples, SKY showed greater improvement compared with the waitlist control in secondary efficacy measures, including the Beck Depression Inventory (ITT mean difference –15.48, completer mean difference –18.61; $P=0.0043$) and Beck Anxiety Inventory (ITT mean difference –5.19, completer mean difference –6.23; $P=0.0005$). These results support the efficacy and tolerability of SKY as an adjunctive treatment for MDD outpatients with inadequate response to antidepressant medications. Additionally, this study identifies the response of adjunctive SKY treatment in comparison to continuing the participants' current medication regimen. Although this study did not include an active control group, the degree and duration of improvement observed following SKY suggests its potential as an effective adjunctive treatment for a people living with significant depressive symptoms.

SKY has also been evaluated in the treatment of patients with generalized anxiety disorder (GAD). Katzman et al. (2012) performed a pilot trial to study the efficacy and tolerability of SKY as an adjunctive treatment for outpatients with GAD who had not achieved remission after at least 8 weeks of traditional anxiolytic therapy and had received previous treatments with cognitive-behavioral therapy and/or mindfulness-based stress reduction. Pharmacological treatments for GAD have side effects, such as nausea and weight gain (Kennedy et al. 2001). These side effects, combined with variable efficacy, can make long-term remission difficult to achieve (Katzman et al. 2008).

Patients in this study had a primary diagnosis of GAD with a Hamilton Anxiety Rating Scale (HAM-A) total score of 20 or greater and a Clinical Global Impression–Severity of Illness (CGI-S) score of 5–7. The 5-day, 22-hour SKY course was taught by a psychiatrist who was also an experienced yoga teacher certified to teach the SKY course. Patients were taught breathing techniques, yoga stretches, and guided meditation. They also engaged in discussion of cognitive coping and stressor evaluation throughout the course.

This study revealed that 4 weeks after completing the course, HAM-A total score was significantly reduced compared with preintervention scores in the 29 patients who completed the HAM-A in the ITT sample ($t=4.59$; $P<0.01$) (Katzman et al. 2012). The response rate was 73% (decrease of at least 50% on the HAM-A), and remission rate was 41% (HAM-A score of ≤7), which compare favorably with other studies of psychotherapy and pharmacotherapy (Nimatoudis et al. 2004). There were no significant changes on the Intolerance to Uncertainty Scale or the Multidimensional Perfectionism Scale, which measure self-oriented, other-oriented, and socially prescribed perfectionism, suggesting that intolerance to uncertainty and perfectionism are unlikely to account for the reduction in anxiety associated with taking the SKY course. Instead, this study indicates that a significant improvement in emotion-oriented coping ($t=-3.45$; $P<0.02$) may mediate the effect of SKY on anxiety. Katzman et al.'s (2012) study suggested that SKY may have potential in the treatment of unremitted GAD through improved emotional regulation.

Van der Kolk et al. (2014) conducted a clinical trial to evaluate the use of yoga therapy for women experiencing posttraumatic stress disorder (PTSD) symptoms. Because of the rates of incomplete response for exposure therapy in the treatment of PTSD (Bradley et al. 2005), identification of effective adjunctive therapies is critical. The authors identified yoga therapy as a potential option for these patients. Yoga therapy combines the effects of meditation and breathing exercises on the modulation of arousal (Breslau et al. 1995). In addition, yoga therapy fosters emotion regulation through observing fear rather than initiating avoidance (Hölzel et al. 2011). The physical postures of hatha yoga help practitioners develop flexibility and body awareness for the physiological aspects of physical sensations, which is important for recognizing triggered emotional responses (Wilamowska et al. 2010).

The principal investigators collaborated with certified yoga professionals with master's and doctorate degrees in psychology to develop a 10-week, trauma-informed weekly yoga program (Van der Kolk et al. (2014). This program specifically focused on the treatment of women 18–58 years old with chronic, treatment-nonresponsive PTSD, defined as having at least 3 years of prior therapy for the treatment of PTSD without significant improvement in symptoms. The yoga intervention included breathing, postures, and meditation. The program encouraged self-inquiry and openness about sensations in the body, with the instructor using invitational phrases to demonstrate sensitivity. The control intervention was a 10-week weekly women's health education class that focused on active participation and support and did not discuss issues related to trauma. Thirty-two women were randomly assigned to each group, and each group met for 1 hour per week.

The results of this study suggested that yoga therapy offers effective education in body awareness for emotion regulation (Van der Kolk et al. (2014). Body awareness offers participants an opportunity to gain a sense of control and tolerance over their own physical responses to environmental stimuli. Although both groups demonstrated significant decreases on the Clinician-Administered PTSD Scale, the decrease had a greater effect size for the yoga group ($d=1.07$ compared with $d=0.66$; $P<0.05$). Both groups exhibited significant decreases in the Davidson Trauma Scale during the first half of treatment (after 5 weeks), but these improvements were maintained only in the yoga group and not in the control group at the conclusion of the 10-week program. The effect sizes observed in the yoga group were comparable to those of standard psychotherapeutic and pharmacological treatments. Both the yoga group and the control group offered social aspects, but only the yoga group had a focus on the physical body and interoception. Thus, the yoga physical aspects appear to be the elements of the yoga intervention responsible for reducing PTSD symptoms. The results of this study offer the possibility of posttrauma recovery through yoga therapy approaches.

Duraiswamy et al. (2007) performed a randomized controlled trial of yoga therapy for moderately ill patients with schizophrenia compared with an active physical exercise control group. Sixty-one patients with a confirmed diagnosis of schizophrenia and a CGI-S score of 4 or more were enrolled in the study. A therapist trained to teach both yoga therapy and physical exercise therapy taught the programs for each group. The yoga treatment included breathing exercises, relaxation techniques, and asanas to build physical strength and stability. Some specific asanas included Bhujangasana (cobra posture) and Dandasana (staff posture). The physical exercise group practiced brisk walking, jogging, and relaxation. The subjects in both groups received training 1 hour a day for 15 days, 5 days a week. Both groups were evaluated using the Positive and Negative Syndrome Scale for Schizophrenia (PANSS).

Four months after the beginning of the study, the patients randomly assigned to the yoga therapy group had a significant difference in mean total PANSS compared with the active control group (effect size 0.74; $P=0.03$) (Duraiswamy et al. 2007). The change in PANSS was largely due to reductions in negative symptoms, depression, and anergia scores. The results of this single-blind randomized controlled trial of yoga therapy suggest that yoga can be effective as an adjunct treatment for people with schizophrenia.

Not only has yoga been effective in the treatment of adult psychiatric disorders; it has also been shown to have benefits in the treatment of children ages 6–11 with attention-deficit/hyperactivity disorder (ADHD). A recent Indian study analyzed the impact of a 6-week yoga intervention for 55 children with ADHD screened using the Initial Teacher Vanderbilt Assessment (Mehta et al. 2012). Twice-weekly morning sessions consisted of 25 minutes of yoga and meditation, 30 minutes of play therapy, and 5 minutes of discussion and feedback from the children. Baseline, 6-week, and 1-year assessments on the Vanderbilt ADHD questionnaire were completed by teachers and parents.

The teachers' Vanderbilt scores for children in the program demonstrated significant decreases from the baseline to both the 6-week and the 1-year assessment time points (median score 13 at baseline, 4.0 at 6 weeks, and 0.5 at 1 year; $P<0.0001$ for each comparison to baseline). Similarly, parents' Vanderbilt scores also demonstrated an improvement, with median score 9.0 at baseline, 6.0 at 6 weeks, and 5.0 at 1 year ($P<0.001$ for each comparison to baseline). In both teacher and parent assessment, however, there was no significant improvement between the scores at 6 weeks and 1 year. Despite this, after 1 year of participating in the program, 91.9% of the children had ADHD symptoms that had improved from baseline on the basis of parent reports. Additional studies on the child and adolescent population are warranted to develop a fuller picture of the potential for yoga to treat mental health conditions across the life span.

Case Example 1

Brian is a 30-year-old young professional with a history of depression and anxiety beginning in adolescence. He recently learned that he would be laid off from his job at a startup company. He was devastated by the news because he had moved across the country to join this company. Since learning of his unemployment, Brian had developed significant return of depression and anxiety consistent with a major depressive episode, despite being compliant with the antidepressant medication he had been taking regularly for a number of years. Attempts to increase his medication were not met with further improvement. Given that Brian had previously received a number of medications since a young age, he was resistant to trying a new medication at this time. Because Brian had previously expressed a strong interest in yoga and meditation techniques, his psychiatrist provided him information about an upcoming SKY program in his area. He was instructed to continue his medication while completing an 8-week trial period with the SKY program. Brian enrolled in the course and learned the SKY practice. He continued attending weekly SKY group sessions and maintained his home SKY practice regularly (five times per week) for 8 weeks. At the end of the trial, Brian reported significant improvements in mood, interest, sleep, and anxiety. He felt more capable and decided to begin the process of searching for another job.

TAI CHI INTERVENTIONS FOR PSYCHIATRIC DISORDERS

Tai chi is a mind-body exercise with origins in China. It is founded on slow, intentional movements coordinated with breathing that aim to relax and strengthen the body and mind and improve health (Wayne and Kaptchuk 2008). Tai chi interventions for psychiatric disorders are designed to focus on the combination of aerobic exercise, stress reduction, and mindfulness meditation. Tai chi has been shown to promote relaxation and reduce sympathetic nervous system stimulation (Irwin et al. 2008; Reid-Arndt et al. 2012). Electroencephalogram (EEG) studies of participants undergoing tai chi exercise have found increased frontal EEG alpha, beta, and theta wave activity, suggesting increased relaxation and attentiveness (Liu et al. 2003; Pan et al. 1994). Moreover, compared with other forms of aerobic exercise, tai chi can be more readily implemented among older adults with physical limitations due to chronic illness or poor balance (Blumenthal et al. 1999).

Lavretsky et al. (2011) performed a randomized controlled trial to evaluate the efficacy of a tai chi adjunct treatment compared with a health education control for geriatric patients with depression. All 112 participants (age 60 and older) were treated with the drug escitalopram for 6 weeks, after which any patients who did not achieve remission were randomly assigned to either tai chi or health education. At randomization, subjects had a mean HDRS-24 score of 16 or higher. Throughout the study, all participants continued escitalopram treatment. Both the tai chi and health education interventions were held for 2 hours once a week for 10 weeks. The tai chi intervention emphasized control over arousal-related responsiveness through the practice of repetitious, low-intensity, and slow-paced movement. The health education intervention offered an active control for nonspecific elements of treatment such as social support. Participants received didactic lectures on key topics about depression, stress, sleep, and health-related issues and participated in group discussions.

The results of this study suggested that the use of tai chi as a complementary treatment for geriatric depression was more effective than health education. Although both intervention groups demonstrated reduced severity of depression, greater reductions in severity were observed in those participating in tai chi compared with those participating in health education (group × time interaction: $F_{[5,285]}=2.26$; $P<0.05$). In the tai chi group, 94% of the subjects achieved depression response, defined as HDRS-17 scores of 10 or lower, and 65% achieved remission, defined as HDRS scores of 6 or lower (Lavretsky et al. 2011). Only 77% of the health education participants achieved depression response, and 51% achieved remission ($P<0.06$). Moreover, tai chi and escitalopram compared with health education and escitalopram yielded greater improvements in physical functioning (group × time interaction: $F_{[1,66]}=5.73$; $P=0.02$) and cognition (group × time interaction: $F_{[1,65]}=5.29$; $P<0.05$) and greater reductions in the inflammatory marker C-reactive protein (time effect: $F_{[2,78]}=3.14$; $P<0.05$). These results are suggestive of the potential of tai chi to reduce depression symptoms in a geriatric population with MDD.

Yeung et al. (2012) proposed a tai chi intervention to reduce depressive symptoms among Chinese Americans. In a randomized controlled trial, middle-aged Chinese immigrants with MDD were randomly assigned to either a tai chi intervention group or a waitlist control group. Participants in the tai chi intervention attended 1-hour group classes held twice weekly for 12 weeks. Compared with the waitlist control group, the tai chi intervention group demonstrated improved response rates, defined as a decrease of 50% or more on the HDRS-17 (24% vs. 0%) and remission rates, defined as an HDRS-17 score of 7 or lower (19% vs. 0%). However, these differences did not reach statistical significance. This pilot study identified tai chi as a promising intervention for treating MDD in Chinese immigrant populations, especially where access to and knowledge of mental health resources is limited.

Case Example 2

Theresa is a 65-year-old woman who lives with her children. Over the course of the past 6 months, her family noted that she had been more withdrawn and isolative. Her son took her to see her primary care physician, who believed that Theresa might be experiencing symptoms of depression. Her physician also noted that Theresa had been demonstrating some deterioration in her physical health, including increased weight gain and poor posture. Given that Theresa did not exercise and was not interested in psychiatric medication at this time, her primary physician suggested she take a tai chi program at a local medical health center. She instructed Theresa to attend at least twice weekly. Theresa found the classes to be light and engaging. She continued attending the classes regularly for several weeks. At her 3-month follow-up appointment, Theresa appeared to be doing better. Her mood was improved; she was more engaged and had started attending more social events. Altogether, her overall lifestyle had improved.

RISKS ASSOCIATED WITH YOGA AND TAI CHI

In considering whether to recommend yoga and tai chi as a therapeutic option to patients, providers should weigh the benefits and risks. Relatively few adverse events have been reported in healthy individuals. Adverse events have been associated with forceful breathing and particular postures, such as headstand (Cramer et al. 2013). Yoga interventions designed for individuals with psychiatric disorders should be tailored to limit these adverse events and be maximally inclusive by instead incorporating gentle breathing and postures. The use of the squat movement in tai chi has led to knee pain or knee injury (Chen et al. 2011). Thus, patients with severe medical conditions are advised to work with therapists who have experience working with medical populations. To protect the knee joint, interventions should be designed to avoid repetitive use of the squat. With both yoga and tai chi, instructors should also be advised to offer reminders to patients to practice at their own level and slowly increase intensity to avoid injury.

LIMITATIONS OF STUDIES

Although these studies offer promising insights into the mechanisms of yoga and tai chi in the treatment of psychiatric disorders, the strength of their conclusions is limited by several factors. Most of these studies are open label and unblinded; therefore, demand characteristics may have affected outcome measures (Katzman et al. 2012). Comparing the efficacy of different interventions is difficult because of differences in patient populations, baseline illness status, control group treatment (active vs. wait-list), aspects of interventions (such as quality of instructors and length of intervention), and methodological rigor of study.

Available data in these studies often were limited because of participant dropout. Reasons for participant dropout included disinterest, physical injury not resulting from intervention, or conflict with work schedule. Even with ITT analysis, the results are limited by lack of data for participants who were lost to follow-up.

Finally, mind-body interventions may offer patients suffering from social isolation a source of social support. Although some studies have specifically identified that the intervention was significantly more efficacious than the control condition when social interaction was controlled for, Cho (2008) identified that effects of a tai chi intervention on a group of older Chinese patients with depression disappeared when changes in social support were controlled for. Therefore, the effects of social support must be carefully analyzed in studies of mind-body interventions conducted in group sessions.

SUGGESTIONS FOR FUTURE RESEARCH

As with all clinical studies on populations of patients with psychiatric illnesses, small sample sizes limit statistical power. To improve our understanding of the potential of yoga and tai chi to reduce symptoms of psychiatric illness, larger sample sizes are necessary. More studies on patients with clinically diagnosed conditions will help elucidate the effects of these mind-body exercises on patients with more severe degrees of psychiatric illness. Last, more studies on young adults and adolescents with psychiatric disorders will contribute to our ability to provide long-lasting therapeutic options for patients earlier in their illness course.

FACILITATING PARTICIPATION

Clinical practitioners interested in suggesting mind-body interventions for their patients need to be able to communicate key aspects of the interventions, especially for patients who have not experienced them. A discussion around the nature of the intervention is essential for understanding how patients conceptualize the intervention, gauging interest level, and assessing feasibility of implementation. Drawing from clinical practitioners' own personal experiences to describe intervention specifics will greatly assist patients considering a mind-body intervention. Practitioners should also be able to offer basic information regarding how a given mind-body intervention may impact psychiatric symptoms. With regard to implementation, practitioners who are able to offer specific suggestions with regard to teachers, classes, or workshops will further help direct patients to suitable community resources. Practitioners may suggest that patients consider a trial period to determine the suitability of the intervention. Following the trial period, practitioners can subsequently communicate specifics regarding frequency and duration of practice shown to impact clinical symptoms. Practitioners may suggest that patients complete paper or digital logs to keep track of their compliance with a mind-body intervention. A number of mind-body phone applications are available that can help patients stay connected to the intervention.

CONCLUSION

In this chapter, we have summarized several important clinical findings from studies of yoga and/or tai chi in the treatment of psychiatric conditions. These findings demonstrate to providers how these mind-body exercises can be used in conjunction with conventional modalities to help patients achieve improved therapeutic responses and ultimately remission.

DISCUSSION QUESTIONS

1. How do yoga and tai chi differ from current psychiatric treatments (medication and psychotherapy)?
2. When considering complementary approaches for the treatment of psychiatric disorders, when would a provider recommend yoga or tai chi? What are the benefits and risks to consider?
3. What kind of patient would be well suited for yoga or tai chi in the treatment of a psychiatric disorder? What kind of patient would be less well suited?

RECOMMENDED READINGS

Sharma A, Newberg AB: Mind-body practices and the adolescent brain: clinical neuroimaging studies. Adolesc Psychiatry (Hilversum) 5(2):116–124, 2015

Sharma A, Barrett MS, Cucchiara AJ, et al: A breathing-based meditation intervention for patients with major depressive disorder following inadequate response to antidepressants: a randomized pilot study. J Clin Psychiatry 78(1):e59–e63, 2017

REFERENCES

American Psychiatric Association: Diagnostic and Statistical Manual of Mental Disorders, 4th Edition, Text Revision. Washington, DC, American Psychiatric Association, 2000

Balaji PA, Varne SR, Ali SS: Physiological effects of yogic practices and transcendental meditation in health and disease. N Am J Med Sci 4(10):442–448, 2012 23112963

Blumenthal JA, Babyak MA, Moore KA, et al: Effects of exercise training on older patients with major depression. Arch Intern Med 159(19):2349–2356, 1999 10547175

Bradley R, Greene J, Russ E, et al: A multidimensional meta-analysis of psychotherapy for PTSD. Am J Psychiatry 162(2):214–227, 2005 15677582

Breslau N, Davis GC, Andreski P: Risk factors for PTSD-related traumatic events: a prospective analysis. Am J Psychiatry 152(4):529–535, 1995 7694900

Brown RP, Gerbarg PL: Sudarshan Kriya yogic breathing in the treatment of stress, anxiety, and depression: part I-neurophysiologic model. J Altern Complement Med 11(1):189–201, 2005 15750381

Chen HL, Liu K, You QS: Attention should be paid to preventing knee injury in tai chi exercise. Inj Prev 17(4):286–287, 2011 21788230

Cho KL: Effect of tai chi on depressive symptoms amongst Chinese older patients with major depression: the role of social support. Med Sport Sci 52:146–154, 2008 18487894

Clarke TC, Black LI, Stussman BJ, et al: Trends in the use of complementary health approaches among adults: United States, 2002–2012. Natl Health Stat Rep (79):1–16, 2015 25671660

Cramer H, Krucoff C, Dobos G: Adverse events associated with yoga: a systematic review of published case reports and case series. PLoS One 8(10):e75515, 2013 24146758

Duraiswamy G, Thirthalli J, Nagendra HR, et al: Yoga therapy as an add-on treatment in the management of patients with schizophrenia—a randomized controlled trial. Acta Psychiatr Scand 116(3):226–232, 2007 17655565

Hölzel BK, Lazar SW, Gard T, et al: How does mindfulness meditation work? Proposing mechanisms of action from a conceptual and neural perspective. Perspect Psychol Sci 6(6):537–559, 2011 26168376

Irwin MR, Olmstead R, Motivala SJ: Improving sleep quality in older adults with moderate sleep complaints: a randomized controlled trial of tai chi chih. Sleep 31(7):1001–1008, 2008 18652095

Janakiramaiah N, Gangadhar B, Murthy PJNV, et al: Therapeutic efficacy of Sudarshan Kriya yoga (SKY) in dysthymic disorder. NIMHANS J 17:21–28, 1998

Janakiramaiah N, Gangadhar BN, Naga Venkatesha Murthy PJ, et al: Antidepressant efficacy of Sudarshan Kriya yoga (SKY) in melancholia: a randomized comparison with electroconvulsive therapy (ECT) and imipramine. J Affect Disord 57(1–3):255–259, 2000 10708840

Katzman MA, Vermani M, Jacobs L, et al: Quetiapine as an adjunctive pharmaco-therapy for the treatment of non-remitting generalized anxiety disorder: a flexible-dose, open-label pilot trial. J Anxiety Disord 22(8):1480–1486, 2008 18455360

Katzman MA, Vermani M, Gerbarg PL, et al: A multicomponent yoga-based, breath intervention program as an adjunctive treatment in patients suffering from generalized anxiety disorder with or without comorbidities. Int J Yoga 5(1):57–65, 2012 22346068

Kennedy SH, Eisfeld BS, Cooke RG: Quality of life: an important dimension in assessing the treatment of depression? J Psychiatry Neurosci 26(suppl):S23–S28, 2001 11590966

Lavretsky H, Alstein LL, Olmstead RE, et al: Complementary use of tai chi chih augments escitalopram treatment of geriatric depression: a randomized controlled trial. Am J Geriatr Psychiatry 19(10):839–850, 2011 21358389

Liu Y, Mimura K, Wang L, et al: Physiological benefits of 24-style Taijiquan exercise in middle-aged women. J Physiol Anthropol Appl Human Sci 22(5):219–225, 2003 14519910

Mehta S, Shah D, Shah K, et al: Peer-mediated multimodal intervention program for the treatment of children with ADHD in India: one-year followup. ISRN Pediatr 2012:419168, 2012 23316384

Nimatoudis I, Zissis NP, Kogeorgos J, et al: Remission rates with venlafaxine extended release in Greek outpatients with generalized anxiety disorder: a double-blind, randomized, placebo controlled study. Int Clin Psychopharmacol 19(6):331–336, 2004 15486518

Pan W, Zhang L, Xia Y: The difference in EEG theta waves between concentrative and non-concentrative qigong states—a power spectrum and topographic mapping study. J Tradit Chin Med 14(3):212–218, 1994 7799657

Phillips WT, Kiernan M, King AC: Physical activity as a nonpharmacological treatment for depression: a review. J Evid Based Integr Med 8(2):139–152, 2003

Reid-Arndt SA, Matsuda S, Cox CR: Tai chi effects on neuropsychological, emotional, and physical functioning following cancer treatment: a pilot study. Complement Ther Clin Pract 18(1):26–30, 2012 22196570

Sharma A, Newberg AB: Mind-body practices and the adolescent brain: clinical neuroimaging studies. Adolesc Psychiatry (Hilversum) 5(2):116–124, 2015 27347478

Sharma A, Barrett MS, Cucchiara AJ, et al: A breathing-based meditation intervention for patients with major depressive disorder following inadequate response to antidepressants: a randomized pilot study. J Clin Psychiatry 78(1):e59–e63, 2017 27898207

Sharma H, Sen S, Singh A, et al: Sudarshan Kriya practitioners exhibit better antioxidant status and lower blood lactate levels. Biol Psychol 63(3):281–291, 2003 12853172

van der Kolk BA, Stone L, West J, et al: Yoga as an adjunctive treatment for posttraumatic stress disorder: a randomized controlled trial. J Clin Psychiatry 75(6):e559–e565, 2014 25004196

Vedamurthachar A, Janakiramaiah N, Hegde JM, et al: Antidepressant efficacy and hormonal effects of Sudarshana Kriya yoga (SKY) in alcohol dependent individuals. J Affect Disord 94(1–3):249–253, 2006 16740317

Wayne PM, Kaptchuk TJ: Challenges inherent to t'ai chi research: part I—t'ai chi as a complex multicomponent intervention. J Altern Complement Med 14(1):95–102, 2008 18199021

Wilamowska ZA, Thompson-Hollands J, Fairholme CP, et al: Conceptual background, development, and preliminary data from the unified protocol for transdiagnostic treatment of emotional disorders. Depress Anxiety 27(10):882–890, 2010 20886609

Xiong GL, Doraiswamy PM: Does meditation enhance cognition and brain plasticity? Ann N Y Acad Sci 1172:63–69, 2009 19743551

Yeung A, Lepoutre V, Wayne P, et al: Tai chi treatment for depression in Chinese Americans: a pilot study. Am J Phys Med Rehabil 91(10):863–870, 2012 22790795

CHAPTER 12

Mindfulness and Meditation in the Management of Psychiatric Disorders

Lynn Yudofsky, M.D.

David Spiegel, M.D.

KEY POINTS

- Mindfulness meditation is becoming widely used in mainstream medicine, and a growing amount of research indicates that it can be effective in the treatment of a number of psychiatric disorders.
- Several studies now show that mindfulness meditation can lead to structural and functional neurobiological changes.
- Mindfulness has been demonstrated to benefit clinicians who use it and also can help reduce burnout in medicine.

Meditation is "the act of giving your attention to only one thing, either as a religious activity or as a way of becoming calm and relaxed" (*Cambridge English Dictionary*, https://dictionary.cambridge.org/us/dictionary/english/meditation). The use of meditation began thousands of years ago, predominantly in religious contexts. A form of meditation, mindfulness, is the focus of this chapter. For millennia, meditation has been used in various religious contexts. Two of the best-known religions in which meditation has played an integral role are Buddhism and Hinduism, but meditation has also been a part of Islamic, Jewish, and Christian religions (Trousselard et al. 2014).

Jon Kabat-Zinn (1994), who is credited as introducing mindfulness to Western culture, conceptualized mindfulness as "paying attention in a particular way: on purpose, in the present moment, and nonjudgmentally" (p. 4). At the University of Massachusetts in 1997, Kabat-Zinn helped to secularize and even medicalize mindfulness meditation by developing mindfulness-based stress reduction (MBSR) techniques and by founding the Stress Reduction Clinic and the Center for Mindfulness in Medicine, Health Care, and Society. He delineated seven factors of mindfulness: "non-judging, patience, beginner's mind, trust, non-striving, acceptance, and letting go" (Kabat-Zinn 1990, p. 33). Through Kabat-Zinn's pioneering work, what was once a religious practice was transformed into a scientific methodology that began to be used to help individuals with both medical and psychiatric disorders as well as those who suffer from general stress.

In addition to MBSR, there are many other types of mindfulness programs that have been developed over the years. For the purpose of this chapter, however, we focus primarily on MBSR and mindfulness-based cognitive therapy (MBCT) as well as mindfulness-based relapse prevention (MBRP) programs. MBCT, which combines mindfulness techniques with cognitive-behavioral therapy, was originally developed as a treatment for depression and has been expanded as a treatment for other psychiatric disorders in addition to depression (Hofmann and Gómez 2017).

MBRP is a program developed at the University of Washington Addictive Behaviors Research Center that uses mindfulness skills to help people with addictions (Bowen et al. 2009).

From the primary care outpatient clinic to the surgical operating room to the psychiatry psychotherapeutic office, mindfulness and other forms of meditation are rapidly gaining popularity in mainstream medicine. Additionally, mindfulness meditation is being increasingly used in the business sector, in schools at all levels, and even in prisons. Currently, there are multiple mindfulness apps, YouTube videos, and even a magazine called *Mindful*. Research measuring the benefits of meditation for specific disorders—both medical and psychiatric—is growing. In addition to alleviating *symptoms* of a number of medical and psychiatric conditions, research has shown that mindfulness meditation improves specific *disorders,* including anxiety and mood disorders, attention-deficit/hyperactivity disorder, eating and sleep disorders, substance use disorders, and psychotic disorders. Although mindfulness has been used to treat a full range of psychiatric disorders, for the purpose of this chapter, we discuss the most common psychiatric illnesses and those that have been studied most intensively: anxiety, depression, and addiction disorders.

We have divided this chapter into three main sections. The first section reviews research studies based on the benefits of mindfulness for various commonly occurring psychiatric disorders, including anxiety, mood, and addictive disorders. In the second section, we consider published research on the neurological mechanisms involved in mindfulness. In the third section, we discuss benefits of mindfulness for the clinician and demonstrate how mindfulness may be implemented in clinical practice. Because of the vast and growing number of research studies of mindfulness interventions for psychiatric disorders, the majority of the studies presented in this chapter are meta-analyses.

MINDFULNESS AS A TREATMENT FOR PSYCHIATRIC ILLNESS

Numerous studies have supported the benefits of mindfulness in helping individuals cope with physical illnesses, from the common cold to epilepsy. Representative examples include a narrative review of the evidence of mindfulness-based treatments for physical conditions by Linda E. Carlson (2012) that reviewed the literature on mindfulness interventions for patients with diabetes, chronic pain, irritable bowel syndrome, arthritis, fibromyalgia, back pain, cardiovascular disease, and HIV/AIDS. Her analysis revealed that mindfulness was effective in varying degrees in the treatment of these conditions. In this review, she concluded that individuals receive benefits from mindfulness across different conditions, given that the symptoms of all these conditions (and others) can be worsened by stress. In her studies of mindfulness for people with cancer (Carlson and Garland 2005; Carlson et al. 2004, 2013, 2015), she demonstrated both psychological and physiological benefits, including normalization of cortisol patterns and prevention of telomere shortening. Mindfulness can help individuals learn ways of coping with their symptoms—and consequent stress—in more accepting, compassionate, and relaxed ways that lead to symptom relief.

Just as mindfulness helps alleviate physical symptoms, a number of studies have shown that it can also help reduce cognitive and emotional symptoms. In a systematic review and meta-analysis of mindfulness for psychiatric disorders, Goldberg et al. (2018) evaluated 142 randomized controlled trials to determine the efficacy of mindfulness-based treatment on clinical symptoms of psychiatric illnesses. At posttreatment, mindfulness was shown to be superior to no treatment ($d=0.55$), minimal treatment ($d=0.37$), nonspecific active controls ($d=0.35$), and specific active controls ($d=0.23$). At follow-up, mindfulness-based interventions were superior to no-treatment conditions ($d=0.50$), nonspecific active controls ($d=0.52$), and specific active controls ($d=0.29$). Mindfulness conditions did not differ from minimal treatment conditions ($d=0.38$) and evidence-based treatments ($d=0.09$). According to the study, the effects of mindfulness were most consistently supported in major depression and tobacco and other specific substance use disorders.

Although many studies corroborate that mindfulness is an effective treatment for certain commonly occurring psychiatric disorders, how exactly does mindfulness help improve psychiatric symptoms? This question was addressed by Gu et al. (2015) in a systematic review and meta-analysis of 20 meditation studies. This team of researchers studied how MBSR and MBCT improve mental health and well-being. They investigated the mechanisms of the effects of MBCT and MBSR by measuring capacities for mindfulness, self-compassion, emotional reactivity, cognitive reactivity, repetitive negative thinking (rumination, worry, and concerns), psychological flexibility, and autobiographical memory specificity (the ability to retrieve memories of specific personal events). This study reported evidence that mindfulness affects mental health outcomes by increasing one's capacity for awareness and acceptance and by decreasing ruminations and worries.

Mindfulness Meditation for People With Anxiety and Depression

Given the emphasis on nonjudgment, relaxation, letting go, and acceptance, it is not surprising that mindfulness is becoming a widely recognized treatment for anxiety disorders and major depression. Serpa et al. (2014) conducted a prospective study of 79 veterans with various psychiatric diagnoses who participated in a 9-week MBSR course. Participants had acute and active psychiatric conditions, including psychosis, substance use, and personality disorders, and 24% of them had active suicidal ideation (Serpa et al. 2014). The only exclusion criterion was advanced dementia. By analyzing data collected in pre-MBSR and post-MBSR questionnaires, the researchers determined that the veterans had significant reductions in anxiety, depression, and suicidal ideation.

In a meta-analysis of mindfulness-based therapy, Khoury et al. (2013) examined 209 studies to evaluate the efficacy of mindfulness for the symptoms of a varied range of psychiatric conditions. This study showed that mindfulness was particularly helpful for reducing depression, anxiety, and stress and that mindfulness was more effective than several other types of interventions, including psychological education (Hedges' $g=0.61$; 95% confidence interval [CI] 0.27–0.96), supportive therapy (Hedges' $g=0.37$; 95% CI 0.17–0.57; $I^2=64\%$), relaxation procedures (Hedges' $g=0.19$; 95% CI 0.03–0.35), and imagery or suppression techniques (Hedges' $g=0.26$; 95% CI 0.10–0.53). Effect-size estimates suggested that mindfulness is moderately effective in pre and post comparisons ($n=72$ studies; Hedges' $g=0.55$) with waitlist control subjects ($n=67$; Hedges' $g=0.53$) and when compared with other active treatments ($n=68$; Hedges' $g=0.33$), including other psychological treatments ($n=35$; Hedges' $g=0.22$). In this study of clinical effectiveness, mindfulness did not differ significantly from cognitive-behavioral therapy, behavioral therapies, or pharmacological treatment.

In a randomized controlled trial for generalized anxiety disorder (GAD), 93 individuals with GAD were randomly assigned to either an 8-week group intervention with MBSR or to the control, a stress-management education program (Hoge et al. 2013). Anxiety symptoms were measured with the Hamilton Anxiety Rating Scale (HAM-A; primary outcome measure), the Clinical Global Impression–Severity of Illness and Clinical Global Impression–Improvement scales (CGI-S and CGI-I), and the Beck Anxiety Inventory (BAI). Participants who received MBSR had a significantly larger reduction in anxiety according to CGI-S, CGI-I, and BAI. Participants who received MBSR also had increased positive statements about themselves. Both interventions had significant reductions in HAM-A scores; the difference was not significant.

Mindfulness has also been shown to be effective when delivered in person or via the Internet. This is important because many people do not have time to attend a mindfulness session each week, do not have access to treatment, cannot afford treatment, are concerned about stigma, or are reluctant to leave their homes because of the nature of their illness. Digital health care and convenience medicine are growing trends with the general public. In one study, 91 participants diagnosed with GAD, panic disorder, social anxiety disorder, or anxiety disorder not otherwise specified were randomly assigned to an Internet-based mindfulness treatment group or to an online discussion forum control group (Boettcher et al. 2014). Participants in the mindfulness treatment group showed a larger decrease of symptoms of anxiety, depression, and insomnia and a moderate improvement in quality of life compared with the control group.

Six randomized controlled trials were included in a systematic review and meta-analysis of the effect of MBCT for prevention of relapse in recurrent major depressive disorder (Piet and Hougaard 2011). MBCT significantly reduced the risk of relapse or recurrence, with a risk ratio of 0.66 for MBCT compared with treatment as usual or placebo controls, corresponding to a relative risk reduction of 34%. In a preplanned subgroup analysis, the relative risk reduction was 43% for participants with three or more previous episodes, whereas no risk reduction was found for participants with only two episodes. In two studies, MBCT was at least as effective as maintenance antidepressant medication. This suggests that mindfulness could be an effective treatment for preventing relapse of depression in individuals who have had three or more previous episodes. In those patients with depression who have significant side effects from or are unable to tolerate psychiatric medications, MBCT may be considered as a potential alternative.

Case Example 1

Rose is a 60-year-old woman with chronic pain and GAD. Prior to psychiatric assessment and treatment, Rose regularly overused narcotics and benzodiazepines to help control pain and anxiety. After her psychiatrist took a thorough history of the quality and course of her psychiatric and medical symptoms, Rose was offered the option of trying mindfulness. Although skeptical of how this treatment could help her symptoms, Rose was amenable to learning mindfulness techniques. Her psychiatrist began by introducing her to the practice of mindfulness through a discussion of its history, followed by a brief overview of research findings on mindfulness and an explanation of how the practice is conducted. The psychiatrist next taught Rose mindfulness exercises, including mindful breathing and body scans, and led her in a 5- to 10-minute mindfulness exercise at the end of each weekly session. The body scan involved focusing attention toward sensations in one's body, with the goal of helping to increase awareness and relieve stress and tension. Rose's psychiatrist asked her to rate her pain and anxiety separately, each on a scale of 1–10 (10 being the highest) before and after each mindfulness session. At first Rose noticed that her mind was wandering a lot during these exercises, and her psychiatrist reminded her that the mind naturally wanders. When she noticed her attention drifting, she learned to gently bring her attention back to her breathing.

Over the course of several sessions, Rose's doctor slowly began to increase the length of the exercises until Rose was able to easily engage in a 20-minute mindfulness exercise. After each session, Rose consistently rated her pain and anxiety as decreased. She then began using these exercises on her own outside the appointments but initially noticed that she had trouble remembering to do them. Her consistency progressively improved with each trial. She and her psychiatrist then agreed on a regular practice schedule comprising approximately 15–20 minutes daily of mindfulness exercises. She chose to do the exercises in the morning because this was when the levels of her pain and anxiety were at their highest. She came to believe that her mindfulness exercises "set up a positive tone for the rest of my day." Gradually, over the course of 2 months, Rose noticed that her anxiety and pain levels decreased, as did her use of benzodiazepines and narcotic pain medication. She observed that she felt more in control of her symptoms and found that, on many days, she did not need pain and anxiety medications.

Mindfulness Meditation for People With Addictions

Mindfulness has also been demonstrated to be effective in helping people with addiction disorders—including individuals with addictions to substances as well as those who struggle with so-called behavioral addictions such as binge eating and gambling. Mindfulness has been shown to both help reduce cravings and help prevent relapse. In a randomized controlled trial of 168 participants with substance use disorders, MBRP was compared with treatment as usual (Bowen et al. 2009). Participants who received MBRP had significantly lower rates of relapse during the 4-month postintervention period compared with those who received treatment as usual. The study also suggested that, compared with individuals receiving treatment as usual, those in the MBRP group had fewer cravings, acted with increased awareness, and had increased acceptance of negative experiences.

Bowen et al. (2014) conducted a study of the long-term efficacy of MBRP in individuals who successfully completed a substance use program for drug and ethyl alcohol use. They compared MBRP with relapse prevention or psychoeducation and 12-step programs (treatment as usual) by randomly assigning 286 participants to MBRP, relapse prevention, or treatment as usual and monitoring them for 12 months. Both relapse prevention and MBRP produced a significant reduction in risk of relapse to drug use and heavy drinking. At 6-month follow-up, relapse prevention delayed time to first substance use, and MBRP and relapse prevention participants reported significantly fewer heavy drinking days compared with treatment-as-usual participants. At 12-month follow-up, compared with relapse prevention and treatment as usual, individuals who received

MBRP reported significantly decreased heavy drinking and significantly fewer days of substance use. This study suggests that MBRP may be an effective long-term approach to help mitigate drug and alcohol relapse.

In a recent systematic review and meta-analysis of 42 studies of mindfulness and addiction, Li et al. (2017) documented significant effects of mindfulness treatments in reducing the severity and frequency of substance use, the intensity of craving for psychoactive substances, and severity of stress. Of note, in cigarette smokers, mindfulness increased rates of posttreatment abstinence compared with alternative treatments, and participants were 76% more likely to achieve abstinence (Li et al. 2017).

An abundance of research supports the benefit of mindfulness for tobacco users. In a systematic literature review of this topic, de Souza et al. (2015) reviewed 198 articles and reported that mindfulness prevented relapse, reduced the number of cigarettes smoked, decreased cravings, and improved coping skills. Their findings are highly relevant given that tobacco remains the leading cause of preventable death in the world (Centers for Disease Control and Prevention 2017b). The researchers did note, however, that further carefully designed studies are needed in this area to support or disprove their findings (de Souza et al. 2015).

Several studies examine the effectiveness of mindfulness in treating people with binge-eating disorders and obesity. In a literature review of mindfulness-based interventions for obesity, O'Reilly et al. (2014) found that of the 21 studies included in the review, 18 showed that mindfulness improved obesity-related eating behaviors—especially binge eating, external eating (which occurs when one is exposed to cues to eat such as sights and smells), and emotional eating. These findings have broad importance given that persons with obesity have greater risk of developing several chronic illnesses, including, but not limited to, heart disease, type II diabetes, stroke, and even some forms of cancer (Centers for Disease Control and Prevention 2017a). In addition, most individuals who are obese try multiple treatment modalities to help them lose weight, many of which are expensive, are ineffective in producing long-term results, or have high risk, such as extreme dieting, diet pills, or even surgery. Although further research is needed in this area, there are data to suggest that mindfulness may be more effective, safer, and a more economical treatment for obesity-related eating disorders than many other more commonly used interventions.

Case Example 2

Harold is a 40-year-old male patient with obesity and type II diabetes who tends to binge eat "junk food" when he experiences stress. His psychiatrist discussed with him the fundamental concepts of mindfulness and how it could be used to help him reduce stress and combat binge eating. In Harold's mindfulness exercises, he learned how to relax; slow down; enjoy his food more; notice when he feels full; and not engage in other activities during eating, such as watching television or surfing the Web on his cell phone. Harold began to notice that he was more attuned to his level of hunger and to noticing when he was full. He began eating less overall and slowly started losing weight. His psychiatrist also discussed how to increase exercise by going on "mindful walks" in which Harold would pay close attention to his sensations and surroundings while walking (i.e., the feeling of his feet against the ground, the breeze against his skin, the smell of the flowers, the sounds of wildlife, and trying to notice different details of his surroundings). He found these daily walks enjoyable and relaxing and noticed that his level of stress began to decrease. Over a few months of engaging in mindful eating and walking, Harold's weight continued to drop—as did his fasting glucose levels. Like Rose, Harold progressively felt in more control of his medical and psychiatric symptoms.

MINDFULNESS AND THE BRAIN

A recent area of research inquiry is the neurobiological changes that occur in the practice of meditation and mindfulness. Fox et al. (2014) conducted a systematic review and meta-analysis to determine if there are structural brain changes associated with meditation. They evaluated 123 differences in brain structure from 21 neuroimaging studies involving approximately 300 meditators. The study used anatomical likelihood estimation meta-analysis and found eight brain regions that were consistently changed in meditators: frontopolar cortex or Brodmann area 10 (meta-awareness), hippocampus (memory consolidation and reconsolidation), anterior cingulate and midcingulate (self-regulation), orbitofrontal cortex (emotion regulation), sensory cortices and insula (exteroceptive and interoceptive body awareness), superior longitudinal fasciculus (intrahemispheric communication), and corpus callosum (interhemispheric communication). However, the authors noted some limitations, including methodological limitations and publication bias among the studies they evaluated.

In another meta-analysis, Boccia et al. (2015) investigated magnetic resonance imaging (MRI) studies that included 37 individual functional MRI (fMRI) experimental studies on functional activations during meditation tasks (642 participants), 63 fMRI experimental studies on functional changes ascribable to meditation (1,652 participants, including both meditators and control subjects), and 10 experimental structural MRI studies of structural changes ascribable to meditation (581 participants). The meta-analysis used activation likelihood estimation analysis, which indicated that meditation practice causes functional and structural brain changes in areas involved in attention, memory formation, and executive functioning as well as self-referential processes, including self-awareness and self-regulation. One widely cited study found changes in activity in the default mode network, which processes self-reflection, particularly reduced activity in the posterior cingulate cortex (Brewer et al. 2011). These researchers suggested that their results could provide further evidence of the benefit of mindfulness in the prevention of age-related cognitive decline and the treatment of mood, anxiety, and addiction disorders. Several studies revealed that mindfulness meditation leads to changes in white and gray matter in the brain. Hölzel et al. (2011) proposed that mindfulness increases gray matter density, and Doll et al. (2015) concluded that mindfulness is associated with intrinsic functional connectivity (i.e., synchronized ongoing activity) between the default mode network and the salience network. Tang et al. (2010) found that even short courses of meditation (4 weeks or 11 hours) can produce white matter changes involving the anterior cingulate cortex (involved in self-regulation) in the brain.

Mindfulness has also been studied in the context of immune response. Tang et al. (2007) showed that a short course of meditation (5 days) can result in decreased cortisol levels and increased immunoreactivity. These studies and others indicate that short courses of meditation can not only produce significant effects in one's subjective experience but also can lead to objective changes at the cellular, genetic, and neuronal level. In a systematic review of randomized controlled trials, Black and Slavich (2016) studied the effects of mindfulness meditation on immune system parameters, with a focus on five outcomes: 1) circulating and stimulated inflammatory proteins, 2) cellular transcription factors and gene expression, 3) immune cell count, 4) immune cell aging, and 5) antibody response. The findings suggested possible effects of mindfulness meditation on specific markers of inflammation, cell-mediated immunity, and biological aging. The researchers, however, noted that further studies are necessary, and the study was limited by the large differences in study design, assay procedures, and patient populations.

MINDFULNESS FOR THE MENTAL HEALTH PROVIDER

Benefits of Mindfulness for Clinicians

Mindfulness has been shown to benefit not only the patient but also the clinician by helping to prevent physician burnout. In a review of eight studies involving mindfulness training for health care providers and teachers, Luken and Sammons (2016) found that six studies showed significant reduction in job burnout after participants received mindfulness training.

In fact, mindfulness can also decrease stress for staff in high-intensity medical settings such as the emergency department. In one study of 50 emergency department nurses, mindfulness was shown to decrease anxiety, depression, and burnout (Westphal et al. 2015).

Mindfulness can also help physicians deliver higher quality of care. In an observational study of 45 clinicians treating patients with HIV, it was found that patient visits with high-mindfulness clinicians or physicians who rated themselves as more mindful were more likely to be characterized by a patient-centered pattern of communication (adjusted odds ratio of a patient-centered visit was 4.14; 95% CI 1.58–10.86), in which both patients and clinicians engaged in more rapport building and discussion of psychosocial issues (Beach et al. 2013). Clinicians with high mindfulness scores also displayed more positive emotional tone with patients (adjusted β=1.17; 95% CI 0.46–1.9). Patients were more likely to give high ratings on clinician communication (adjusted prevalence ratio [APR]=1.48; 95% CI 1.17–1.86) and to report high overall satisfaction (APR=1.45; 95 CI 1.15–1.84) with high-mindfulness clinicians.

Incorporating Mindfulness Into Clinical Practice

Physicians who practice mindfulness may be more effective at teaching mindfulness to their patients (see Chapter 18, "Physician Lifestyle and Health-Promoting Behavior"). Christiane Wolf and J. Greg Serpa, in their book *A Clinician's Guide to Teaching Mindfulness*, recommended that clinicians incorporate mindfulness into their practices because both patients and clinicians derive significant benefit therefrom (Wolf and Serpa 2015). There is not a single template to incorporate mindfulness into clinical practice. In a narrative review of mindfulness in health care systems, Demarzo et al. (2015) concluded that mindfulness-based interventions are "complex interventions" that require innovative and creative approaches and delivery models in order to implement them in a cost-effective and accessible way. In other words, there is no one-size-fits-all approach.

First, clinicians should seek out appropriate training. Perhaps the clinician can find a mentor to help guide him or her in learning mindfulness treatments or can take a course at an academic institution or in the community. Excellent online training programs and tools and many illuminating books on mindfulness may be used. Second, when bringing mindfulness into treatment, the clinician must take into account the fact that every patient and patient problem and need is unique. Taking a comprehensive medical and neuropsychiatric history is essential because there are elements in the history that will help inform which type of mindfulness intervention to choose. There are insufficient syndrome-specific outcome data in the literature to definitively recommend one mindfulness approach over another for specific conditions. Therefore, there is room for judicious, respectful, and safe modification of standard mindfulness approaches based on the specific needs and personal proclivities of the individual patient. For example, when treating patients for tobacco cessation, we may have them use mindfulness techniques to cope with uncomfortable sensations that arise when they are having cravings or urges to smoke. Specifically, this is called *urge surfing*, a technique developed by Alan Marlatt (Bowen and Marlatt 2009). One way of beginning is for clinicians to conduct session-by-session mindfulness trainings with their patients, as delineated by Wolf and Serpa (2015).

A clinician who is beginning to introduce mindfulness treatments in his or her practice might initiate and/or end each patient session with a 5-minute mindfulness exercise, such as a body scan (a mindfulness relaxation exercise involving awareness of sensations in one's body in the present moment), and encourage the patient to practice the same regimen at home daily. Remind your patients that, just like exercise, 5–10 minutes of mindfulness daily is better than no minutes and can have psychological, physiological, and neurological benefits. For more in-depth practice, depending on the patient and the disorder being treated, you can perhaps encourage your patient to enroll in an 8-week MBSR program.

CONCLUSION

There is now a significant body of evidence that shows the effectiveness of mindfulness meditation for patients with psychiatric disorders. Mindfulness meditation produces documented neurobiological changes in individuals who practice it. For patients with severe psychiatric illness, mindfulness may be best used in conjunction with other treatments, but for other patients, mindfulness may offer some benefits over medications, given that it has a lower side-effect profile than many medications, is cost-effective (there are multiple free apps and online videos), has lasting benefit, and is convenient because the patient can practice anywhere. Finally, mindfulness meditation has been shown to deliver significant benefit to those clinicians who use it.

DISCUSSION QUESTIONS

1. Given that mindfulness has been shown to be effective in the treatment of psychiatric disorders, how can we incorporate mindfulness into sessions with patients? What is the best way to train clinicians who would like to incorporate mindfulness into their practice?

2. How can we motivate and encourage our patients to practice mindfulness on their own, outside of office visits?
3. How can we best integrate mindfulness into the workplace for health care providers to help prevent burnout and reduce stress?

RECOMMENDED READINGS

Lake JA, Spiegel D: Complementary and Alternative Treatments in Mental Health Care. Washington, DC, American Psychiatric Publishing, 2007

Wolf C, Serpa JG: A Clinician's Guide to Teaching Mindfulness: The Comprehensive Session-by-Session Program for Mental Health Professionals and Health Care Providers. Oakland, CA, New Harbinger, 2015

Zerbo E, Schlechter A, Desai S, et al: Becoming Mindful: Integrating Mindfulness Into Your Psychiatric Practice. Arlington, VA, American Psychiatric Association Publishing, 2017

REFERENCES

Beach MC, Roter D, Korthuis PT, et al: A multicenter study of physician mindfulness and health care quality. Ann Fam Med 11(5):421–428, 2013 24019273

Black DS, Slavich GM: Mindfulness meditation and the immune system: a systematic review of randomized controlled trials. Ann N Y Acad Sci 1373(1):13–24, 2016 26799456

Boccia M, Piccardi L, Guariglia P: The meditative mind: a comprehensive meta-analysis of MRI studies. BioMed Res Int 2015:419808, 2015 26146618

Boettcher J, Aström V, Påhlsson D, et al: Internet-based mindfulness treatment for anxiety disorders: a randomized controlled trial. Behav Ther 45(2):241–253, 2014 24491199

Bowen S, Marlatt A: Surfing the urge: brief mindfulness-based intervention for college student smokers. Psychol Addict Behav 23(4):666–671, 2009 20025372

Bowen S, Chawla N, Collins SE, et al: Mindfulness-based relapse prevention for substance use disorders: a pilot efficacy trial. Subst Abus 30(4):295–305, 2009 19904665

Bowen S, Witkiewitz K, Clifasefi SL, et al: Relative efficacy of mindfulness-based relapse prevention, standard relapse prevention, and treatment as usual for substance use disorders: a randomized clinical trial. JAMA Psychiatry 71(5):547–556, 2014 24647726

Brewer JA, Worhunsky PD, Gray JR, et al: Meditation experience is associated with differences in default mode network activity and connectivity. Proc Natl Acad Sci USA 108(50):20254–20259, 2011 22114193

Carlson LE: Mindfulness-based interventions for physical conditions: a narrative review evaluating levels of evidence. ISRN Psychiatry 2012:651583, 2012

Carlson LE, Garland SN: Impact of mindfulness-based stress reduction (MBSR) on sleep, mood, stress and fatigue symptoms in cancer outpatients. Int J Behav Med 12(4):278–285, 2005 16262547

Carlson LE, Speca M, Patel KD, et al: Mindfulness-based stress reduction in relation to quality of life, mood, symptoms of stress and levels of cortisol, dehydroepiandrosterone sulfate (DHEAS) and melatonin in breast and prostate cancer outpatients. Psychoneuroendocrinology 29(4):448–474, 2004 14749092

Carlson LE, Doll R, Stephen J, et al: Randomized controlled trial of mindfulness-based cancer recovery versus supportive expressive group therapy for distressed survivors of breast cancer. J Clin Oncol 31(25):3119–3126, 2013 23918953

Carlson LE, Beattie TL, Giese-Davis J, et al: Mindfulness-based cancer recovery and supportive-expressive therapy maintain telomere length relative to controls in distressed breast cancer survivors. Cancer 121(3):476–484, 2015 25367403

Centers for Disease Control and Prevention: Overweight and Obesity: Adult Obesity Facts. Atlanta, GA, Centers for Disease Control and Prevention, 2017a. Available at: www.cdc.gov/obesity/data/adult.html. Accessed January 13, 2018.

Centers for Disease Control and Prevention: Smoking and Tobacco Use, Fast Facts: Diseases and Death. Atlanta, GA, Centers for Disease Control and Prevention, 2017b. Available at: www.cdc.gov/tobacco/data_statistics/fact_sheets/fast_facts/index.htm. Accessed January 7, 2018.

Demarzo MMP, Cebolla A, Garcia-Campayo J: The implementation of mindfulness in healthcare systems: a theoretical analysis. Gen Hosp Psychiatry 37(2):166–171, 2015 25660344

de Souza IC, de Barros VV, Gomide HP, et al: Mindfulness-based interventions for the treatment of smoking: a systematic literature review. J Altern Complement Med 21(3):129–140, 2015 25710798

Doll A, Hölzel BK, Boucard CC, et al: Mindfulness is associated with intrinsic functional connectivity between default mode and salience networks. Front Hum Neurosci 9:461, 2015 26379526

Fox KC, Nijeboer S, Dixon ML, et al: Is meditation associated with altered brain structure? A systematic review and meta-analysis of morphometric neuroimaging in meditation practitioners. Neurosci Biobehav Rev 43:48–73, 2014 24705269

Goldberg SB, Tucker RP, Greene PA, et al: Mindfulness-based interventions for psychiatric disorders: a systematic review and meta-analysis. Clin Psychol Rev 59:52–60, 2018 29126747

Gu J, Strauss C, Bond R, et al: How do mindfulness-based cognitive therapy and mindfulness-based stress reduction improve mental health and wellbeing? A systematic review and meta-analysis of mediation studies. Clin Psychol Rev 37:1–12, 2015 25689576

Hofmann SG, Gómez AF: Mindfulness-based interventions for anxiety and depression. Psychiatr Clin North Am 40(4):739–749, 2017 29080597

Hoge EA, Bui E, Marques L, et al: Randomized controlled trial of mindfulness meditation for generalized anxiety disorder: effects on anxiety and stress reactivity. J Clin Psychiatry 74(8):786–792, 2013 23541163

Hölzel BK, Carmody J, Vangel M, et al: Mindfulness practice leads to increases in regional brain gray matter density. Psychiatry Res 191(1):36–43, 2011 21071182

Kabat-Zinn J: Full Catastrophe Living: Using the Wisdom of Your Body and Mind to Face Stress, Pain, and Illness. New York, Delacourt, 1990

Kabat-Zinn J: Wherever You Go, There You Are: Mindfulness Meditation in Everyday Life. New York, Hyperion, 1994

Khoury B, Lecomte T, Fortin G, et al: Mindfulness-based therapy: a comprehensive meta-analysis. Clin Psychol Rev 33(6):763–771, 2013 23796855

Li W, Howard MO, Garland EL, et al: Mindfulness treatment for substance misuse: a systematic review and meta-analysis. J Subst Abuse Treat 75:62–96, 2017 28153483

Luken M, Sammons A: Systematic review of mindfulness practice for reducing job burnout. Am J Occup Ther 70(2):7002250020p1-7002250020p10, 2016 26943107

O'Reilly GA, Cook L, Spruijt-Metz D, et al: Mindfulness-based interventions for obesity-related eating behaviours: a literature review. Obes Rev 15(6):453–461, 2014 24636206

Piet J, Hougaard E: The effect of mindfulness-based cognitive therapy for prevention of relapse in recurrent major depressive disorder: a systematic review and meta-analysis. Clin Psychol Rev 31(6):1032–1040, 2011 21802618

Serpa GJ, Taylor S, Tillisch K: Mindfulness-based stress reduction (MBSR) reduces anxiety, depression, and suicidal ideation in veterans. Med Care 52(12 suppl 5):S19–S24, 2014 25397818

Tang Y-Y, Ma Y, Wang J, et al: Short-term meditation training improves attention and self-regulation. Proc Natl Acad Sci U S A 104(43):17152–17156, 2007 17940025

Tang Y-Y, Lu Q, Geng X, et al: Short-term meditation induces white matter changes in the anterior cingulate. Proc Natl Acad Sci USA 107(35):15649–15652, 2010 20713717

Trousselard M, Steiler D, Claverie D et al: The history of mindfulness put to the test of current scientific data: unresolved questions [in French]. Enceephale 40(6):474–480, 2014 25194754

Westphal M, Bingisser MB, Feng T, et al: Protective benefits of mindfulness in emergency room personnel. J Affect Disord 175(April):79–85, 2015 25597793

Wolf C, Serpa JG: A Clinician's Guide to Teaching Mindfulness. Oakland, CA, New Harbinger, 2015

CHAPTER 13

Diet and Nutrition in the Prevention and Adjuvant Treatment of Psychiatric Disorders

Jonathan Burgess, M.D.

> Emerging and compelling evidence for nutrition as a crucial factor in the high prevalence and incidence of mental disorders suggests that diet is as important to psychiatry as it is to cardiology, endocrinology, and gastroenterology.
>
> *Sarris et al. 2015*

KEY POINTS

- Diet and nutrition can impact risk for and symptoms of many psychiatric disorders.
- Mechanisms include impact of diet on neuroinflammation and oxidative stress.
- Specific nutrient deficiencies also may contribute to onset and severity of psychiatric disorders.

The nascent field of lifestyle psychiatry has significant evidence that in addition to mindfulness, sleep, and exercise, diet is a foundational component in the prevention and treatment of neurological and psychiatric illnesses. Indeed, the Royal Australian and New Zealand College of Psychiatrists Clinical Practice Guidelines for Mood Disorders (Malhi et al. 2015) now recommend addressing diet as part of standard of care for mood disorders. Dietary psychiatry research has steadily matured from observational studies to double-blind randomized controlled trials regarding microbiome interventions, nutrient and supplement interventions, and comprehensive dietary interventions that have demonstrated efficacy in treating psychiatric disorders. These results suggest that research into dietary interventions for psychiatric conditions will likely bear fruit for generations to come in our efforts to maximize health and minimize harm of the human mind through modifiable lifestyle habits.

There are three basic mechanisms through which diet impacts mental health: 1) the microbiome, 2) neuroinflammation and oxidative stress, and 3) individual nutrients. The microbiome is discussed in Chapter 14, "The Gut-Brain Axis and Microbiome in Psychiatric Disorders." Neuroinflammation and oxidative stress are discussed throughout this chapter. Last, individual nutrients are necessary cofactors in the production of neurotransmitters. For example, serotonin production begins with the amino acid tryptophan and requires cofactors of iron, calcium, magnesium, zinc, folate, vitamin B_6, and vitamin C. Dopamine and norepinephrine begin with tyrosine and require iron, copper, magnesium, folate, vitamin B_6, and vitamin C. Nutrient insufficiencies in any of these minerals and vitamins may decrease levels of these basic neurotransmitters and may be factors in the development of psychiatric disorders. Additionally, if there is insufficiency or deficiency, these nutrients may be factors in cases of psychiatric disorders that remain treatment-resistant despite pharmacological treatment.

MOOD DISORDERS

Unipolar Depressive Disorders

Observational Studies of Diet and Depressive Disorders

In one of the first prospective cohort studies that examined whole foods—rather than individual nutrients—in relation to depression, Akbaraly et al. (2009) discovered that individuals consuming the highest tertile versus the lowest tertile of *whole foods* (e.g., vegetables, fruits, fish) were 26% less likely to develop depression over a 5-year period. Additionally, those eating the highest tertile versus the lowest tertile of processed foods (e.g., refined carbs, processed meats, fried foods) had a 58% increased risk of developing depression. The results were significant after accounting for sociodemographics, smoking and physical activity, and medical illnesses.

Researchers have studied the Mediterranean diet, which consists primarily of plant-based foods: vegetables, legumes, whole grains, nuts, seeds, fruits, and olive oil with some fish and moderate consumption of meat and poultry. Psaltopoulou et al. (2013) completed a meta-analysis of nine case-control, cross-sectional cohort studies that evaluated adherence to the Mediterranean diet and neurological and psychiatric conditions. In a dose-dependent response, moderate adherence to the Mediterranean diet significantly reduced the risk of depression by 27%, whereas high adherence significantly reduced risk of depression by 32%.

Nanri et al. (2013) examined the relationship of diet and suicide through the Japanese Public Health Center–based Prospective Study. A total of 89,037 enrollees from 1995 to 1998 were evaluated during a 20-year follow-up period. Compared with the lowest quartile, the highest quartile of adherence to a "prudent" diet that emphasized vegetables, fruits, soy products, mushrooms, seaweeds, and fish was associated with a 54% reduced risk of suicide, with high statistical significance after accounting for sociodemographics, health behaviors, and medical illnesses.

Mechanisms of Diet, Oxidative Damage, and Neuroinflammation in Depressive Disorders

Diet, activity level, and genetic factors contribute to neuro-oxidative stress, which activates immune-inflammatory pathways through multiple feedback loops, resulting in neuronal damage. Oxidation damages neurons by producing epitopes that increase immunoglobulin G and immunoglobulin M autoantibodies that bind to neuronal signaling proteins, impairing downstream signaling pathways that affect cell survival, neuroplasticity, and neurotransmission. Additionally, there is direct oxidative damage to neuronal membranes, leading to aberrant cell functioning, apoptosis, and decreased neurogenesis.

Although there are genetic predispositions for inflammation that increase the risk for depression and decrease responsiveness to antidepressants, several modifiable factors can affect oxidative immune-inflammatory pathways. In an obese state, adipocytes are enlarged and release leptin and tumor necrosis factor alpha (TNF-α), which are pro-inflammatory compounds that contribute to the low-grade inflammatory state of obesity. Additionally, serum and tissue levels of reactive oxygen species are impacted by dietary choices. Vegetables, nuts, fruits, and olive oil contain potent antioxidants that increase neuronal antioxidant capacity, thereby reducing neuronal damage and the neuroinflammatory state that contributes to depressive symptoms. Plant polyphenols enhance neuroplasticity and modulate neurotrophic factors such as brain-derived neurotrophic factor (BDNF). Additionally, specific nutrients are implicated in psychiatric health.

Nutrient Studies and Depressive Disorders

Omega-3 Essential fatty acids are precursors to eicosanoids, which are hormone-like substances that function in nearly every tissue in the body. Remarkably, omega-3 and omega-6 fatty acids produce eicosanoids that have opposing effects in nearly every facet. For instance, omega-3 produces eicosanoids that are anti-inflammatory and anticoagulant to platelets, whereas omega-6 eicosanoids are pro-inflammatory and procoagulant to platelets. Additionally, omega-3 fatty acids versus omega-6 fatty acids are competitive inhibitors of each other because they compete for the same enzymes that transform omega-3 and omega-6 fatty acids into their biologically active compounds. Therefore, if the body has a significant imbalance of omega-3 or omega-6, one fatty acid can substantially impair the pathways of the other.

Regarding psychiatric health, essential fatty acids constitute up to 20% of the dry weight of the brain and modulate norepinephrine, dopamine, serotonin, neuroinflammation, apoptosis, neurogenesis, and BDNF levels. Sarris et al. (2016) completed a meta-analysis of eight double-blind randomized controlled trials that used adjuvant omega-3 fatty acids for depression, finding significant improvement in psychiatric symptoms, with an effect size of 0.61 ($P=0.009$). When the analysis was restricted to supplemental eicosapentaenoic acid (EPA) rather than combined EPA plus docosahexaenoic acid (DHA) omega-3 supplements, the effect size became larger (0.69; $P=0.007$), suggesting that EPA may be the dominant therapeutic agent for depression. Of note, EPA is more specific as an anti-inflammatory agent, whereas DHA is a primary constituent of structural brain volume. DHA is discussed later in the sections on schizophrenia and cognitive disorders.

Zinc Zinc is an essential mineral that impacts pathways of cell growth, apoptosis, immunity, and neuronal functions and is a reducing agent in neuro-oxidation reactions. Serum zinc levels are lower in people with depression, and the severity of depression is related to the severity of zinc deficiency. Sarris et al. (2016) reviewed two double-blind randomized controlled trials for zinc as adjuvant treatment in depression and found that zinc significantly improved depressive symptoms in one trial and significantly improved depressive symptoms in treatment-resistant cases of depression.

L-Methylfolate L-Methylfolate is a reduced form of folate and the only form of folate that crosses the blood-brain barrier. Papakostas et al. (2012) published the results from two double-blind randomized controlled trials ($n=148$; $n=75$) using L-methylfolate as adjuvant treatment to selective serotonin reuptake inhibitors (SSRIs). A dose of 7.5 mg of L-methylfolate did not improve depression. However, 15 mg of L-methylfolate more than doubled the response rate of SSRIs alone (32.3% vs. 14.6%), marked by a reduction of 50% or more on the Hamilton Depression Rating Scale. L-Methylfolate is U.S. Food and Drug Administration (FDA) approved for suboptimal folate levels in depressed patients. Other forms of folate have produced inconclusive results in double-blind randomized controlled trials.

Other nutrients Selenium, magnesium, and vitamin D also have wide-ranging effects on neuronal health, redox reactions, and neurotransmission. Although deficiencies in these nutrients have been associated with depression in epidemiological data, the evidence for these single-nutrient supplements as treatment for clinical symptoms of depression remains inconclusive.

Dietary Interventions and Unipolar Depressive Disorders

Brinkworth and colleagues (2009) completed a randomized controlled trial ($N=106$) for individuals with a body mass index (BMI) of 25 or greater who had no evidence of clinical depression. Individuals were randomly assigned to eat either a high-fat, very low carbohydrate diet or a high-plant, high-carbohydrate diet for 1 year. Calories and weight loss were equal for each group. At 52-week follow-up, the high-plant, high-carbohydrate group demonstrated significantly improved mood, with medium to large effect sizes as measured by the total Profile of Mood States scale, with particular improvements in anger-hostility, confusion-bewilderment, depression-dejection, and total mood disturbance.

Brinkworth and colleagues repeated the trial in 2016 ($N=115$) and found no difference in mood between the high-fat versus high-carbohydrate groups (Brinkworth et al. 2016). However, the investigators changed the methodology of the study to include exercise, which has known mood-enhancing effects. The investigators also changed the types of fats used in the study, replacing saturated fats with polyunsaturated fats, which may also have impacted mood.

In a previous small double-blind randomized controlled crossover trial ($N=12$) that tested the impact of saturated versus unsaturated fatty acids on mood, Kien et al. (2013) supplied individuals with premade foods, altering only the proportion of long-chain saturated versus unsaturated fat in the recipes. After 3 weeks of intervention, the individuals who consumed higher polyunsaturated fats had significantly lower anger-hostility and trend-level improvements in total mood disturbance and depression-dejection. The findings of these trials are interesting, and replication in larger trials is needed.

Regarding prevention of clinical depression, Stahl et al. (2014) published an interesting study on the impact of dietary coaching in the prevention of depression in older adults with subsyndromal depressive symptoms. The study randomly assigned 247 patients to an intervention group of problem-solving therapy versus a dietary coaching control group. Subsyndromal depression progressed to clinical depression in 20%–25% of those without intervention. Only 10.5% of patients in both trial arms progressed to depression, which was consistent with previous randomized controlled trials for interventions for the prevention of depression (Stahl et al. 2014). The interventions also reduced symptom burden of depressive symptoms by 40%, as measured by the Beck Depression Inventory. Of note, the total intervention time was 5.5 hours over 2 years, demonstrating remarkable efficiency in therapeutic value for dietary coaching in the prevention of clinical depression in older adults.

In the treatment of clinical depression, Jacka et al. (2017) completed a landmark trial demonstrating the efficacy of diet as adjuvant treatment in moderate to severe depression. In addition to standard of care, 67 patients with clinical depression were randomly assigned to 7 hours of instruction on the Mediterranean diet versus a control group with 7 hours of social support. Inclusion criteria for the trial was a "poor" diet as measured by a diet screening tool. The dietary intervention group achieved increased remission from depression at a fourfold rate compared with the control group (32% vs. 8%) and significant improvement in depressive symptoms compared with the control group ($P \le 0.03$). The effect size of the dietary intervention was very large, at 1.16. Although this intervention will need to be reexamined in larger trials, these results suggest that dietary improvement as adjuvant treatment to psychotherapy and psychopharmacology may be a powerful treatment in patients with depression who have poor baseline dietary status.

Bipolar Spectrum Disorders

Observational Studies of Diet and Bipolar Spectrum Disorders

There are few epidemiological studies related to dietary practices and bipolar disorder. In 2003, Noaghiul and Hibbeln conducted a cross-national comparison of seafood consumption and rates of bipolar disorders and schizophrenia. The association of fish consumption and schizophrenia did not reach significance in this study, although other studies have shown association. However, lower consumption of seafood was exponentially associated with increased rates of bipolar disorders, with high statistical significance ($P<0.0001$) and high level of correlation ($r=0.85$) (Noaghiul and Hibbeln 2003). Specific types of seafood were not calculated, which is of increasing importance with regard to the balance of the benefits of omega-3 fatty acids versus the neurological detriments of mercury. For example, a single serving of albacore tuna exceeds the recommended allowance of mercury for a full week of food.

In 2011, Jacka and colleagues completed a rigorous cross-sectional analysis evaluating the relationship between diet and bipolar disease in women (Jacka et al. 2011a). Structured clinical interviews were conducted with 1,046 women. Their diets were categorized as "traditional," which emphasized whole grains, vegetables, fruit, fish, lamb, and beef; "Western," which emphasized processed foods; and "modern," which emphasized fruits, salads, fish, tofu, beans, nuts, yogurt, and red wine. Each standard deviation increase of the Western and modern diets was associated with an 88% and 72% increased risk of having a diagnosis of bipolar disorder, respectively. Each standard deviation increase of the traditional diet was associated with a 47% decreased risk of bipolar disorder. The cross-sectional design of the study does not allow for causation analysis. However, Western diets have been associated with increased risk of unipolar depression that was not explained by reverse causality analysis. Interestingly, the modern diet association with bipolar disorder appears to be an outlier in the data. The modern diet would be considered nutrient-dense and anti-inflammatory, which could be expected to reduce symptoms of bipolar disorder. However, the cross-sectional association could possibly be explained by dietary changes secondary to the diagnosis of bipolar disorder. Future studies will have to examine these speculations in a prospective fashion.

Mechanisms of Oxidative Damage and Inflammation in Bipolar Spectrum Disorder

Bipolar disorder shares many similar oxidative damage and immune-inflammatory processes that are active in depression, with several key distinguishing features. In bipolar disorder, inflammatory markers cycle with bouts of mania and depression. During manic episodes, TNF-α, interleukin (IL)-2, IL-6, IL-8, and interferon-γ are elevated. As mania resolves, most inflammatory markers decrease to baseline levels. However, TNF-α continues to be elevated. During depressive episodes, IL-6 increases before returning to baseline during remission of episodes. Bipolar patients with a history of suicidal behavior have chronically high IL-6. It must also be noted that the cyclic nature of bipolar illness, which may have differential effects on nutrient metabolism during states of illness and euthymia, adds complexity regarding nutrition research in bipolar disorder.

The cycles of inflammation in bipolar episodes contribute to *allostatic load*, which is defined as the "wear and tear" that the body endures with each distressing episode of increased inflammatory and oxidative markers. Inflammatory cytokines reduce sensitivity of glucocorticoid and insulin receptors, provoking hypercortisolemia and insulin resistance. In bipolar disorder, this metabolic dysregulation combined with increased platelet and endothelial aggregation and autonomic disturbance contributes to cardiovascular disease being the primary cause of mortality in bipolar patients. In fact, severity of bipolar disease, evidenced by psychotic features, predicts higher levels of cardiovascular disease. Regardless of how nutrition may impact core symptoms of bipolar disorder, comprehensive dietary improvement is warranted for cardiovascular benefit.

Nutrient Studies and Bipolar Spectrum Disorders

Omega-3   Sarris et al. (2012) conducted a systematic review and meta-analysis of double-blind randomized controlled trials that evaluated the use of omega-3 in patients with bipolar disorder. EPA/DHA supplementation demonstrated significant improvement in bipolar depression, with a modest effect size of 0.34. The most successful double-blind randomized controlled trial ($N=44$) used high doses of 6.2 g of EPA and 3.4 g of DHA. The intervention group demonstrated such marked improvement that the trial was ended early so that the control group could achieve similar clinical benefits. Of the six trials for bipolar mania, none achieved clinical significance. However, meta-analysis found trend-level improvement ($P \leq 0.15$), suggesting possible benefit.

N-acetylcysteine and glutathione   N-acetylcysteine (NAC) is both an over-the-counter supplement and a pharmaceutical drug. NAC is simply a highly bioavailable form of the amino acid cysteine. Cysteine is the rate-limiting ingredient in the production of glutathione, the main antioxidant of the central nervous system. In psychiatry, glutathione deficiency is relevant in depression, bipolar disorder, and schizophrenia. Regarding bipolar disorder, Berk et al. (2008a) demonstrated the efficacy of 2 g NAC daily in the treatment of bipolar depression. A sample of 75 patients with bipolar I disorder or bipolar II disorder and a recent manic or depressive episode (within the past 6 months) were randomly assigned to NAC or placebo. At 24 weeks, there were significant improvements in the NAC group regarding depressive symptoms, with medium to large effect sizes. Of note, the benefits progressed over time, with some symptom categories requiring the length of the study to demonstrate significance. At study completion, the removal of NAC from the intervention group for 4 weeks caused depressive symptoms to return to baseline, suggesting that NAC was the key ingredient in symptom improvement. However, a follow-up trial by Berk for bipolar maintenance (Berk et al. 2012) did not show significant results with NAC. More trials are under way (Ellengaard et al. 2018).

It is noteworthy that several nutrients and foods help preserve glutathione levels. Cysteine is found in cruciferous vegetables, yogurt, and oats. Antioxidant vitamins C and E help to replenish oxidized glutathione to its own active antioxidant state. Selenium is an essential cofactor for glutathione production. In fact, for clinical trials evaluating NAC, consumption of 500 IU of vitamin E or 200 µg of selenium supplementation per day is typically exclusionary. Interestingly, an individual can meet 200 µg of selenium per day with two to four Brazil nuts. Although it is too soon to recommend Brazil nuts as a dietary treatment for psychiatric disorders, one could contemplate intentionally adding this food as an ingredient in an otherwise healthful anti-inflammatory diet for future dietary psychiatry randomized controlled trials. However, selenium is a mineral that, like lithium, does have toxicity levels, so if these dietary trials come to fruition, therapeutic levels of selenium will require attention.

Branched-chain amino acids Branched-chain amino acids (BCAAs) (e.g., valine, isoleucine, leucine) competitively inhibit the entry of tyrosine through the blood-brain barrier, attenuating dopamine and catecholamine production in the central nervous system. Scarna et al. (2003) tested the administration of BCAAs as adjuvant treatment for acute mania. This study was based on a previous clinical trial that demonstrated that BCAAs could blunt the effects of methamphetamine in healthy volunteers. In the Scarna et al. (2003) double-blind randomized controlled trial, 25 patients experiencing acute mania were provided with a drink containing 60 g of BCAAs versus placebo for 7 days as adjuvant treatment to standard of care. The intervention significantly decreased manic symptoms within 6 hours, with a large effect size. After the 7-day intervention, the participants were followed for an additional 7 days and demonstrated significantly fewer manic symptoms than the control group during the follow-up period. Of note, BCAAs can cause liver toxicity at high doses, so patients taking valproate were excluded from the trial.

Broad-spectrum micronutrient formulas It is worth a cautionary mention that there have been reports of bipolar symptom reduction due to broad-spectrum micronutrient formulas (sold as EMPower Plus and Daily Essential Nutrients). The formulas consist of 16 minerals, 14 vitamins, 3 antioxidants, and 3 amino acids. The reports began in 2001, when Kaplan et al. (2001) published the results of an open-label clinical trial for 11 bipolar patients who achieved a 55% reduction in symptoms and 50% reduction in need for medications. However, the one unpublished double-blind randomized controlled trial (N=40) that tested this formula for use in bipolar patients demonstrated no improvement of symptoms compared with placebo (Kaplan 2012). Micronutrient formulas are discussed further in the section on attention-deficit hyperactivity disorder (ADHD).

Ketogenic Diet and Bipolar Spectrum Disorders

The rationale for using a ketogenic diet in bipolar disorder is logical and remains hypothetical. Seizure disorder medications have been successful in treating bipolar disorder, and ketogenic diets have been successfully used for seizure disorders; therefore, perhaps ketogenic diets will impact bipolar disorder. Indeed, there have been case reports of symptom reduction in people with bipolar disorder and schizoaffective disorder with the use of a ketogenic diet (Palmer 2017). However, randomized clinical trials will be required to discover whether this approach is applicable to a broader population of patients with bipolar disorder or whether there are ways to predict when a ketogenic diet might be suitable for a subset of bipolar patients.

SCHIZOPHRENIA SPECTRUM DISORDERS

Observational Studies of Diet and Schizophrenia Spectrum Disorders

In 2004, psychiatrist Malcolm Peet completed an ecological study that evaluated 2-year outcomes for people with schizophrenia in relation to diet (Peet 2004a, 2004b). Peet based his hypothesis that diet impacts schizophrenia on prior observational studies that found the following: 1) outcomes for people with schizophrenia spectrum disorders were better in some developing nations (e.g., Nigeria, India) than in developed nations (e.g., United Kingdom, United States), 2) the improvement of schizophrenia outcomes in developing nations mirrored lower levels of cardiometabolic disorders in those nations, 3) patients with schizophrenia have increased cardiometabolic disorders independent of the side effect profile of antipsychotics, and 4) cardiometabolic disease biomarkers are present at illness onset in drug-naïve patients with psychosis. Indeed, the finding of prediabetic biomarkers in drug-naïve patients with first-episode psychosis has recently been confirmed in a systematic review and meta-analysis, demonstrating a 5.44-fold increase of impaired glucose tolerance compared with matched control subjects (Perry et al. 2016).

With these observational studies in mind, Peet posited that psychiatric disorders and cardiometabolic disease may share common etiologies and that the foods that were beneficial for cardiometabolic health would be also be beneficial for psychiatric disorders. Peet's ecological study discovered that consumption of red meat, dairy, and refined sugar significantly worsened 2-year outcomes of patients with schizophrenia, whereas consumption of beans and fish significantly improved outcomes (Peet 2004a, 2004b). Peet's study was one of the first epidemiological studies that established the field of nutritional psychiatry.

Mechanisms for Diet, Brain Volume, and Schizophrenia Spectrum Disorders

Mechanisms in schizophrenia spectrum disorders are similar to those in major depression and bipolar disorders regarding the themes of oxidative stress provoking inflammatory-immune reactions that significantly alter neuronal connectivity and dendritic spines and lead to reductions in supportive glial cells. However, the neuronal damage is more severe in schizophrenia than in mood disorders, such that there are notable changes in brain volume, particularly in the prefrontal cortex and hippocampal-parahippocampal areas, which are areas that relate to executive function, memory, and cognition. Attenuation of loss—and even regrowth—of these brain areas is partially impacted by neurotrophic factors such as BDNF, and BDNF levels have been inversely correlated with symptom severity in schizophrenia.

Previous research established that high-fat, high-sugar diets decreased BDNF levels in the central nervous system (Peet 2004a). In the 5-year, 7,447-person Prevención con Dieta Mediterránea (PREDIMED) trial, Sánchez-Villegas et al. (2011) furthered this finding by demonstrating that a Mediterranean diet that includes walnuts can reduce the risk of low BDNF levels. Within this randomized controlled study comparing the Mediterranean diet with a low-fat diet similar to the one recommended by the American Heart Association (Table 13–1), 234 patients were selected for evaluation of BDNF levels. Compared with the low-fat diet control group, individuals in the Mediterranean diet plus nut group demonstrated 78% reduced odds of having low BDNF levels over a 3-year period ($P<0.05$). Interestingly, the Mediterranean diet plus olive oil did not ap-

TABLE 13–1. Dietary intake questionnaire

Mediterranean diet assessment questionnaire used in the PREDIMED trials	0 points	1 point
1. Do you use extra virgin olive oil as your *main* culinary fat?	No	Yes
2. How much extra virgin olive oil do you consume in a given day (including oil used for frying, salads, out-of-house meals, etc.)?	<4 tbsp	≥4 tbsp
3. How many *vegetable* servings do you consume per day (1 serving=7 oz; consider side dishes as half a serving)?	<2	≥2
4. How many *fruit* units (including natural fruit juices) do you consume per day?	<3	≥3
5. How many servings of *red meat, hamburger,* or *meat products* (e.g., ham, sausage) do you consume per day (1 serving=3.5–5 oz)?	≥1	<1
6. How many servings of *butter, margarine,* or *cream* do you consume per day (1 serving=1 tbsp)	≥1	<1
7. How many *sweet* or *carbonated beverages* do you drink per day?	≥1	<1
8. How much *wine* do you drink per week?	<7 glasses	≥7 glasses
9. How many servings of *legumes* (i.e., beans, peas, lentils) do you consume per week (1 serving=5 oz)?	<3	≥3
10. How many servings of *fish* or *shellfish* do you consume (1 serving=3–5 oz of fish or 7 oz of shellfish)?	<3	≥3
11. How many times per week do you consume of *commercial sweets* or *pastries* (not homemade), such as cakes, cookies, biscuits, or custard?	≥3	<2
12. How many servings of *nuts* (including peanuts) do you consume per week (1 serving=30 g)?	<3	≥3
13. Do you *preferentially* consume *chicken, turkey,* or rabbit meat instead of veal, pork, hamburger, or sausage?	No	Yes or vegetarian
14. How many times per week do you consume vegetables, pasta, rice, or other dishes seasoned with *sofrito* (sauce made with tomato and onion, leek, or garlic and simmered in olive oil)?	<2	≥2

TABLE 13–1. Dietary intake questionnaire *(continued)*

Additional questions for dietary psychiatry (not part of PREDIMED)

	<75%	≥75%
15. What percentage of your grain products are 100% whole grain?	<75%	≥75%
16. Do you consume cruciferous vegetables (broccoli, kale, cabbage, cauliflower, brussels sprouts, bok choy) daily?	No	Yes
17. Do you consume flavanol-rich foods daily (raw cacao, dark chocolate, berries, freshly made green tea)?	No	Yes
18. Do you consume probiotics or fermented foods daily (probiotic supplement, additive-free plain yogurt, kimchi, raw sauerkraut, kombucha)?	No	Yes
19. Do you consume artificial colors, flavors, or preservatives?	Yes	No
20. Do you have abundant exposure to sunshine or consume ≥2,000 IU cholecalciferol daily?	No	Yes

Suggested modifications to the above questionnaire for psychiatry

Questions 1 and 2: Change olive oil to extra virgin olive oil, as per the PREDIMED methodology.

Question 8: Alcohol is not necessary and should be limited to ≤7 drinks per week for women and ≤14 drinks per week for men. Provide 1 point for remaining within these limits.

Question 10: Limit high-mercury fish (e.g., tuna, swordfish) or fish with high omega-6 (e.g., tilapia).

Question 14: Tomato and onion, leek, or garlic may be changed to any vegetables.

Note. The dietary intake questionnaire consists of the free validated 14-item Mediterranean diet assessment questionnaire used in the PREDIMED trials plus 6 additional questions. Scoring for the questionnaire is simple: the more points the better The questionnaire may be used for evaluation and guidance as people assess and improve their diets for optimal cardiometabolic and psychiatric health.

Abbreviations. oz=ounces; PREDIMED= Prevención con Dieta Mediterránea: tbsp =tablespoon(s).
Source. www.predimed.es; Martínez-González et al. 2012; Schröder et al. 2011.

pear to influence BDNF levels (Sánchez-Villegas et al. 2011). These results suggest that specific ingredients in otherwise healthful diets may
have important effects for neurological and psychiatric health.

Nutrient Studies and Schizophrenia Spectrum Disorders

Trace Minerals

Several mineral deficiencies and excesses have been related to neurological and psychiatric disorders, including schizophrenia. Liu et al. (2015)
completed a case-control study comparing serum levels of minerals in
124 people with schizophrenia and serum levels in 124 matched control
subjects without psychiatric disorders. After a multivariate analysis, having schizophrenia was associated with significantly decreased selenium
and copper.

Reports of both increased and decreased copper levels are associated
with having schizophrenia. Copper is a mineral integral to several antioxidant enzymes, and copper deficiency may lead to increased oxidative
damage in the nervous system. However, copper-containing enzymes are
also necessary for the production of dopamine and norepinephrine, allowing for the possibility that copper excess may also alter dopamine production.

Selenium is a necessary cofactor in the production of glutathione,
which is the major antioxidant enzyme in the central nervous system. Do
et al. (2000) found glutathione levels to be 27% lower in the cerebrospinal
fluid and 52% lower in the medial prefrontal cortex in people with schizophrenia versus matched control subjects. Low serum levels of selenium
decrease glutathione production and thereby increase neuro-oxidative
stress. Conversely, higher serum levels of selenium are associated with
lowered risk of schizophrenia and other psychiatric disorders (Liu et al.
2015). However, selenium toxicity is possible, and the tolerable upper
limit is 400 µg per day (one Brazil nut contains 68–91 µg).

N-Acetylcysteine and Glutathione

Berk et al. (2008b) completed a 28-week double-blind randomized controlled trial (N=140) of patients with schizophrenia. Compared with placebo, NAC significantly improved Clinical Global Impression (CGI) and
Positive and Negative Syndrome Scale (PANSS) total, general, and negative
symptoms ($P \leq 0.05$), with moderate effect sizes. After 4 weeks of discontinuing NAC, the improvements in the intervention group returned to baseline
levels of dysfunction. These findings were confirmed in a second double-
blind randomized controlled trial several years later (Farokhnia et al. 2013).

Cholecalciferol (Vitamin D₃)

"Vitamin D" is a misnomer. Cholecalciferol, the substance usually referred to as Vitamin D, is a steroid hormone that affects the expression of hundreds of genes, developmentally and throughout life. As a neurohormone, cholecalciferol impacts differentiation of neurons, interneuronal connectivity, and the development of the dopamine system.

Kinney et al. (2009) completed a systematic review and meta-analysis of 49 studies that examined variations in rates of schizophrenia and possible contributing factors to the disorder. They posited the cholecalciferol hypothesis with evidence that latitude and cold weather correlated with schizophrenia rates more strongly than any other factor measured. Regional areas in high latitudes have 10 times higher rates of schizophrenia than areas near the equator, despite northern regions having greater wealth and better health care systems. Within high-latitude regions, individuals with dark skin (which inhibits cholecalciferol production) or regions where residents ate the least amount of fish (which provides cholecalciferol plus DHA/EPA) had the highest rates of schizophrenia. Conversely, in high-latitude regions where residents consumed 23 kg of fish per person or more per year, the rates of schizophrenia where equal to rates in equatorial regions, suggesting that diet may be a powerful tool in the prevention of schizophrenia spectrum disorders.

Omega-3

Amminger et al. (2010, 2015) conducted a double-blind randomized controlled trial with 81 young people at ultra high risk for developing psychosis. The intervention group was given DHA-EPA supplementation for 3 months, versus a control group that was given a placebo. At 1-year follow-up, 2 patients in the omega-3 group versus 11 patients in the placebo group had developed a psychotic disorder ($P<0.05$). At 6.7-year follow-up, 4 patients in the omega-3 group versus 16 patients in the placebo group had developed a psychotic disorder ($P<0.05$). However, a larger double-blind randomized controlled trial ($N=304$) with similar methodology that additionally included CBT in both treatment arms was unable to confirm that omega-3 provided significant benefit compared with placebo (McGorry et al. 2017). This discrepancy of results most likely represents the multifactorial nature of this neurodevelopmental disorder, which requires comprehensive and personalized interventions rather than a single nutrient supplementation to decrease conversion from ultra high-risk states to clinical psychosis.

Although the evidence of using omega-3 to prevent ultra high risk youth from developing a psychotic disorder remains inconclusive, DHA-EPA supplementation appears to have some benefit regarding symptoms of schizophrenia in those with an established diagnosis. Bozzatello et al.

(2016) completed a systematic review of omega-3 supplementation in schizophrenia. Eight of the 11 double-blind randomized controlled trials reviewed demonstrated significant improvements for psychiatric symptoms in people with nonacute schizophrenia spectrum disorders. However, the one trial that examined omega-3 in acute psychosis demonstrated worsening of psychotic symptoms.

In depression studies, EPA appears to be the most active ingredient because of its anti-inflammatory mechanism, whereas with schizophrenia studies, DHA may be an important component (Hallahan et al. 2016; Pawełczyk et al. 2016). This difference may be accounted for by the need to maintain brain volume in people with schizophrenia spectrum disorders. Essential fatty acids account for up to 20% of the dry mass of the brain, with DHA being the omega-3 constituent. If a consistent source of affordable, low-mercury fish (which provides EPA and DHA plus additional ingredients) is not available for patients, omega-3 supplementation may be warranted.

Folate and L-Methylfolate

Low folate or B_{12} levels can produce chronic inflammation by raising homocysteine, an inflammatory compound linked to both cardiovascular disease and psychiatric disorders. For example, elevated homocysteine levels are associated with higher risk of schizophrenia as well as higher risk for myocardial infarction in the general population. In schizophrenia, folate deficiency may be due to decreased consumption of folate or may be functional, caused by genetic polymorphisms that lead to aberrant folate metabolism. Even with a U.S. Department of Agriculture–recommended intake of dietary folate, functional folate deficiency may still occur and may require supplementation.

Levine and colleagues (2006) completed a 6-month double-blind randomized crossover trial ($N=42$) with folate, B_{12}, and B_6 for patients with elevated homocysteine levels. Compared with placebo, the intervention group experienced significant improvements in PANSS total symptoms and trend-level improvements in positive, negative, and general symptoms ($P=0.02–0.08$). Roffman and colleagues (2018) published a 12-week double-blind randomized controlled trial ($N=55$) using L-methylfolate, the fully reduced bioactive form of folate. Compared with placebo, L-methlylfolate significantly improved PANSS negative symptoms, independent of genetic phenotypes, and improved PANSS total, negative, and general symptoms when accounting for genetic phenotypes. L-Methylfolate also increased cortical thickness on magnetic resonance imaging evaluation (Roffman et al. 2018). Of note, L-methylfolate is FDA approved for hyperhomocysteinemia in people with schizophrenia.

Dietary Interventions and Schizophrenia Spectrum Disorders

The study of the gut-brain axis in schizophrenia includes investigations into food antigens crossing the intestinal epithelium and leading to auto-immunity that may be implicated in the pathology of schizophrenia. Of these food antigens, wheat gluten has received the most attention. Patients with schizophrenia are three to four times more likely to have celiac disease and have higher levels of antigliadin antibody levels than those of the general public. The antigliadin antibodies in patients with schizophrenia can have different specificity than those found in celiac disease, such that their autoimmunogenic activities may be directed to the central nervous system. There have been case reports of improvement or remission from psychosis with a gluten-free diet (Delichatsios et al. 2016).

In the 1960s and 1970s, Dohan and Grasberger (1973) initiated two double-blind randomized controlled trials for inpatients with schizophrenia spectrum disorders ($N=103$ and $N=105$) that investigated standard of care versus standard of care plus a gluten- and milk-free diet. The intervention group demonstrated significant improvement in symptoms, earlier stepdown from locked to open wards, and earlier discharges. Since that time, additional double-blind randomized controlled trials have been repeated, with some studies demonstrating significant benefits of a gluten-free diet for schizophrenia (Singh and Kay 1976) and other studies finding no benefit (Potkin et al. 1981). There is preliminary evidence that there may be a genetic subset of or specific biomarkers in patients with schizophrenia that would help predict who would benefit from gluten-free diets. Trials addressing these factors are currently under way (Kelly 2017, 2018).

Raine et al. (2003) completed a childhood intervention in order to see if a multifactorial approach that included dietary changes could prevent the development of schizotypal personality disorder. A group of 3-year-olds from an underserved community ($N=83$) received an intervention that included a daily healthful meal, increased physical activity, and so-cial-cognitive education. The intervention group was compared with matched control subjects ($N=355$) who received standard education for that community. The multifactorial intervention lasted for 2 years, from the time the children were 3 years old until they were 5 years old. On follow-up assessment at ages 17 and 23 years, the intervention group demonstrated significantly lower schizotypal and disorganization scores. Of note, the children who had signs of malnutrition at age 3 accounted for the thrust of those significant improvements.

DEVELOPMENTAL AND PEDIATRIC PSYCHIATRIC DISORDERS

Observational Studies and Pediatric Onset of Psychiatric Disorders

Jacka et al. (2013) completed the first prospective cohort study (N=23,020 mothers with children) on the pattern of maternal and postnatal diets and its potential impact on internalizing and externalizing behaviors, which are validated predictors of developing psychiatric disorders. Gestational and childhood diet patterns were characterized as "healthy"—consisting of high intakes of vegetables, fruit, whole grains, vegetable oils, eggs, and fish—or "unhealthy," consisting of processed foods.

Jacka and colleagues were able to distinguish the independent effects of maternal diet versus postnatal diet in the development of internalizing and externalizing behaviors. Increased intake of unhealthy foods and decreased intake of healthy foods during early childhood each independently predicted internalizing and externalizing behaviors in children ages 18 months through 5 years, after accounting for sociodemographic and mental health factors, including parental age, gestational age, maternal mental health, and maternal diet during pregnancy. Increased intake of unhealthy foods during pregnancy also predicted increased rates of externalizing behaviors in children independent of the effect of childhood diet. Impressively, the effect of maternal diet and childhood diet was as strong a predictor of psychiatric disorders in childhood as maternal depression, which is an established risk factor for psychiatric disorders in offspring (Jacka et al. 2013).

Observational Studies and Adolescent Mental Health

Given that 75% of mental illnesses first manifest in adolescence and young adulthood, Jacka et al. (2011b) completed a cross-sectional, 2-year prospective study (N=3,040) of adolescents, relating dietary patterns to pediatric mental health. "Healthy" diet scores were based on Harvard School of Public Health's Alternative Healthy Eating Index and the Mediterranean Index, and "unhealthy" diet scores were derived from quantifying amounts of highly processed foods.

Consistent with findings in adult literature, there was a linear dose-response pattern of healthy diets and better mental health and unhealthy diets and worse mental health (P<0.001). Baseline diets also predicted mental health status at 2-year follow-up. Importantly, changes in diet over the 2-year period mirrored changes in mental health status. Increasing healthful foods was associated with improved mental health status, and increasing unhealthful foods was associated with worsened mental health status, after accounting for sociodemographic factors, baseline mental health scores, and baseline diet scores. The authors also found that baseline poor mental health did not predict dietary choices over the 2-year follow-up period, suggesting that reverse causality was unlikely. These data inspire some intriguing theories. Diet is correlated with the development of mental illness at the time of illness onset, and diet may be a modifiable factor to prevent and partially treat mental illness over time (Jacka et al. 2011b). It has yet to be determined whether this is causal or correlated with other factors.

ATTENTION-DEFICIT/HYPERACTIVITY DISORDER

Observational Studies of Diet and Attention-Deficit/Hyperactivity Disorder

There has been international consistency in relating diet quality with the development of ADHD. Howard and colleagues (2011) published a prospective study ($N=2,868$) that followed individuals from gestation to age 14 years in order to determine which factors may increase the risk of developing ADHD. A "Western" dietary pattern, consisting of high consumption of processed foods, was associated with a doubling of the odds of being diagnosed with ADHD by age 14 years after accounting for sociodemographic factors, major stress events during gestational pregnancy, and child physical activity and screen time. Woo et al. (2014) published a case-control study ($N=192$) from Korea that demonstrated a significant inverse dose-response between ADHD and a "traditional healthy" diet, consisting of vegetables, kimchi, whole grains, and fatty fish and low intakes of processed foods, dairy, and meat. The highest versus lowest tertiles of the traditional healthy diet demonstrated a threefold difference in ADHD diagnosis after accounting for sociodemographic factors. Ríos-Hernández et al. (2017) published a case-control study ($N=120$) that found significant inverse associations with a Mediterranean diet and ADHD. The highest versus lowest tertiles of adherence to a Mediterranean diet were associated with sevenfold decreased odds of having ADHD after accounting for sociodemographic factors, tobacco use by family, and child physical activity.

Mechanisms of Diet and Attention-Deficit/ Hyperactivity Disorder: Artificial Food Additives

In addition to nutrient deficiencies, oxidative stress, and inflammation, which appear to be implicated in many psychiatric disorders, there are proposed environmental risk factors implicated in ADHD, including heavy metals, organophosphates, chlorines, and phthalates. One of the most scientifically established chemical exposures related to hyperactivity in children is artificial food additives.

McCann et al. (2007) published a 6-week double-blind randomized crossover trial of 3-year-olds ($n=153$) and 8- to 9-year-olds ($n=144$) to test the effects of artificial food additives on attention and hyperactivity in otherwise healthy children. Prior research was used to determine the mixtures of artificial colors plus the preservative sodium benzoate in order to mimic the types and quantities of artificial colors eaten by children on a daily basis. In nearly every statistical evaluation model, artificial colors and sodium benzoate caused significant or trend-level increases in hyperactivity compared with placebo. The average effect size was 0.18 in this nonclinical population. In clinical populations of patients with ADHD, an effect size of 0.2 equates to about 10% of the observed hyperactive behaviors (McCann et al. 2007).

With regard to the effects of artificial additives on patients who meet diagnostic criteria for ADHD, Sonuga-Barke et al. (2013) published a meta-analysis of eight randomized controlled trials. They separately analyzed rating scales of parents and teachers who were considered insufficiently blinded versus medical providers who were considered "probably blinded." Removing artificial colors from the diets of children with ADHD significantly improved symptoms when evaluated by either parents and teachers or medical providers, with effect sizes of 0.32 ($P=0.02$) and 0.42 ($P=0.004$), respectively. The medical providers reported greater effects with higher significance than did the parents and teachers.

Broad-Spectrum Micronutrient Studies and Attention-Deficit/Hyperactivity Disorder

In 2014, Rucklidge and colleagues published results of the first double-blind randomized controlled trial of broad-spectrum micronutrients for ADHD. In this study, 80 adults with a diagnosis of ADHD were given a broad-spectrum micronutrient formula containing 36 minerals, vitamins, antioxidants, and amino acids. From baseline to 8 weeks, there were significant improvements, with moderate effect sizes (0.46–0.67) in self-reported and observer Conners' Adult ADHD Rating Scales and clinician-rated CGI-Improvement-ADHD and CGI-Improvement-Overall scores (Rucklidge et al. 2014). Subgroup analysis for patients with moderate to severe depression (*n*=22) demonstrated significant improvements in mood, and there were trend-level improvements in mood for all patients in the micronutrient group. At study completion, more than double the patients in the micronutrient group were "much" to "very much" improved on the CGI-Improvement scale (*P*<0.013; Rucklidge et al. 2014).

Rucklidge et al. (2018) published a 10-week double-blind randomized controlled trial (*N*=93) using broad-spectrum micronutrients with children ages 7–12 years diagnosed with ADHD. Using intention-to-treat analysis, micronutrients demonstrated significant improvements on 6 of 16 ADHD scales and subscales compared with placebo, with moderate effect sizes (0.46–0.66), and trend-level improvements on six additional scales and subscales (*P*≤0.10), with small to moderate effect sizes (0.35–0.47). Specifically, broad-spectrum micronutrients improved symptoms of inattention, aggression, and mood dysregulation, but the symptoms of hyperactivity and impulsivity did not improve. Of note, patients using pharmacological treatment for ADHD were excluded from this trial, and the broad-spectrum micronutrient formula was used as a stand-alone nutriceutical treatment (Rucklidge et al. 2018).

Dietary Interventions and Attention-Deficit/Hyperactivity Disorder

Pelsser and colleagues (2011) published the largest trial to date (*N*=100) that examined the effects of a 5-week "restricted elimination" diet on the symptoms of ADHD and oppositional defiant disorder. A restricted elimination diet is a way to simplify a diet to only a few ingredients and then add or remove foods on the basis of symptomatic response. Foods that demonstrated an increase in symptoms were eliminated. For this study, the diet included rice, turkey, lamb, vegetables (e.g., lettuce, carrots, cauliflower, cabbage, beets), pears, and water. These foods were supplemented by potatoes, fruits, corn, and wheat eaten on prescheduled days and in predetermined doses. The diet was designed to maintain sufficient daily nutrient intakes.

ADHD symptoms were established by blinded physicians with the ADHD Rating Scale (ARS) and unblinded parents and teachers with the Abbreviated Conners' Scale (ACS). On the ARS, out of a total score of 54, the elimination diet group improved 23.7 points more than the control group (*P*<0.0001). On the ACS, out of a total score of 30, the elimination diet group improved 11.8 more points than the control group (*P*<0.0001). Of the 50 children in the elimination diet group, 32 were clinical responders, defined as having a 40% or greater reduction of ADHD symptoms. Symptoms of oppositional defiant disorder were reduced by equal magnitude. The effect size of the intervention was 1.6. Whether or not these effects, or the diet, would or could be sustained for extended periods of time remains a topic for future research (Pelsser et al. 2011).

In 2013, Sonuga-Barke and colleagues published a meta-analysis of eight randomized controlled trials that evaluated restricted elimination diets on the symptoms of ADHD. Given that it is difficult to blind the parents and teachers to a comprehensive dietary intervention, parent and teacher ratings may be biased. Indeed, the researchers found that unblinded evaluators reported significant reduction in ADHD symptoms, with an effect size of 1.48 (P=0.01), whereas blinded evaluators reported trend-level reduction in ADHD symptoms, with an effect size of 0.51 (P=0.06; Sonuga-Barke et al. 2013).

AUTISM SPECTRUM DISORDER

Observational Studies of Diet and Autism and Attention-Deficit/Hyperactivity Disorder

In 2018, Sanchez and colleagues published a systematic review and meta-analysis of 32 publications evaluating 684,775 children from 36 cohort and case-control studies in eight countries. The study used dose-response to compare children born to mothers of healthy prepregnancy weight and children born to mothers with prepregnancy overweight and obesity. Prepregnancy overweight increased the odds of any neurodevelopmental disorder by 1.17, and obesity increased the odds by 1.51 (P<0.001). The odds of specific disorders increased as follows: ADHD 1.30 and 1.62 (P≤0.01), autism spectrum disorder (ASD) 1.1 and 1.36 (P≤0.026), intellectual delay 1.19 and 1.58 (P≤0.003), and any emotional or behavioral problems 1.14 (P=0.16) and 1.42 (P≤0.001), respectively (Sanchez et al. 2018). Overweight- and obesity-specific mechanisms include inflammatory milieu during pregnancy leading to a cascade of events that affect brain development, including aberrant cytokine and microglial function. However, weight is a single biometric that may also be a proxy for an otherwise unhealthful diet containing nutritional deficiencies; hyperprocessed, high–glycemic index foods; food additives; heavy metals; pesticides; and endocrine disruptors harmful to neurological health (Sanchez et al. 2018).

Cholecalciferol and Autism Spectrum Disorder

Cholecalciferol is a neurosteroid that alters brain morphology, genes related to neuronal survival, speech and language development, and dopamine synthesis. Cholecalciferol also exhibits anti-inflammatory and antiautoimmune properties, protects mitochondria, upregulates glutathione levels, scavenges oxidative by-products, and chelates heavy metals.

Vinkhuyzen et al. (2018) published a prospective cohort study (N=4,229) that demonstrated significant association between persistent gestational cholecalciferol deficiency and autism traits according to the Social Responsiveness Scale (SRS). By analyzing cholecalciferol levels from maternal serum at 21 weeks' gestation and from infant cord blood, the researchers determined that individuals with persistent gestational cholecalciferol deficiency had significantly more autism traits at age 6 years (P<0.001). By using a dichotomous cutoff SRS score, it was determined that individuals with cholecalciferol deficiency midgestation were 3.8 times more likely to be positive for autism than were individuals with sufficient cholecalciferol at midgestation, after accounting for sociodemographic factors and pregnancy and birth complications (Vinkhuyzen et al. 2018).

Wu et al. (2018) published a case-control study (N=1,550) evaluating the effects of prenatal cholecalciferol on the development of ASD. Neonatal blood was measured for cholecalciferol levels and compared with ASD diagnosis by age 3 years. After adjusting for sociodemographic factors, pregnancy and birth complications, and family history of ASD, with the highest quartile of cholecalciferol as reference, the three lower quartiles were associated with 1.9 (P=0.082), 2.5 (P=0.024), and 3.6 (P<0.001) increased odds of developing ASD. When dividing neonatal cholecalciferol levels into quintiles, a j-shaped curve fit significantly better than a straight linear association (P=0.032), with the lowest risk of ASD at 49.1 nmol/L, occurring at the 76th percentile in the distribution of this cohort (Wu et al. 2018). Interestingly, a nearly identical j-shaped curve has been reported for neonatal cholecalciferol and risk of schizophrenia (McGrath et al. 2010).

Cholecalciferol deficiency in autism appears to extend into childhood. Wang et al. (2016) completed a meta-analysis of 11 studies evaluating cholecalciferol levels in individuals with autism (n=870) versus healthy control subjects (n=782) that found significantly lower levels of cholecalciferol in patients with autism (P=0.0002), with no evidence of publication bias.

Although supplementation with cholecalciferol is appropriate for individuals with insufficient levels, double-blind randomized controlled trials using cholecalciferol for ASD have produced inconsistent results regarding improvement of core ASD symptoms. Further studies are needed to distinguish whether dose, age of supplementation, or genetic differences account for the differential study results.

Sulforaphane, Broccoli, Broccoli Sprouts, and Autism Spectrum Disorders

Singh and colleagues (2014) published an 18-week double-blind randomized controlled trial ($N=44$) testing the effects of a broccoli compound, sulforaphane, in children with ASD. The basis of the study arose from an observation that 35% of patients with ASD have core symptom improvement during a febrile illness. Additionally, the antioxidant capacity of ASD patients is significantly lower than that of individuals without the disorder. Sulforaphane activates the same heat-shock proteins that are activated in febrile illnesses and stimulates transcription of master antioxidant response element genes that increase antioxidant production systemically.

Compared with placebo, the sulforaphane group experienced a significant decrease in symptoms on the Aberrant Behavior Checklist (ABC; $P<0.001$), all the subscales of the ABC ($P \leq 0.05$), and the SRS ($P=0.017$), with significant improvement in the subscales of awareness, communication, motivation, and mannerism. Sixty percent of the sulforaphane group versus 20% of the placebo group were clinical responders on the ABC, and 35% of the sulforaphane group versus 0% of placebo were clinical responders on the SRS ($P=0.036$) Additionally, the sulforaphane group compared with the placebo group was "much" or "very much" improved on CGI-Improvement subscales for social interaction (46.2% vs. 0%; $P=0.007$), abnormal behavior (53.8% vs. 9%; $P=0.014$), and verbal communication (42.3% vs. 0%; $P=0.015$). Importantly, beneficial results were reversed after discontinuing treatment for 4 weeks (Singh et al. 2014).

However, the intervention currently has limits in practicality. The sulforaphane compound used in the trial was pharmaceutical grade, whereas commonly available sulforaphane supplements are unregulated, and prior studies on these products have demonstrated no measurable sulforaphane levels in the serum of those who ingest them. Regarding the 50–150 μmol of sulforaphane used in this trial, 50 μmol sulforaphane is found in 1 tablespoon of broccoli sprouts and 1 cup of broccoli. Last, two of the sulforaphane group experienced a seizure during the intervention. Both patients had prior seizures, and neither was taking antiseizure medication at the time of the seizure during the clinical trial. However, given that sulforaphane activates heat-shock proteins, and seizures can be induced by fever, this is an adverse event and mechanism that warrants close attention (Singh et al. 2014).

Dietary Interventions and Autism Spectrum Disorders

There has been interest in gluten- and casein-free diets for people with autism, which demonstrated benefit in ASD core symptoms in single-blind studies (Knivsberg et al. 2002; Whiteley et al. 2010). However, the one double-blind study (*N*=14) did not demonstrate improvements (Hyman et al. 2016). It may be worth completing a larger double-blind randomized controlled trial in the future, but currently, there is no convincing evidence that these diets improve ASD, and there is some evidence that children who follow these diets have lower bone density. Parents who choose these diets should find adequate sources of calcium (Sathe et al. 2017).

COGNITIVE FUNCTION AND COGNITIVE DISORDERS

Observational Studies of Diet and Cognitive Function and Cognitive Disorders

In 2013, Psaltopoulou and colleagues published a meta-analysis of nine case-control, cross-sectional, and cohort studies that assessed adherence to a Mediterranean diet and the risk of cognitive impairment. In a dose-dependent response, moderate and high adherence to a Mediterranean diet was significantly associated with a 21% and 40% reduced risk of mild cognitive impairment as well as dementia and Alzheimer's disease, without evidence for publication bias (Psaltopoulou et al. 2013).

McEvoy et al. (2017) published a large cross-sectional evaluation (*N*=5,907, average age 67.8 years) evaluating global cognitive function in relation to adherence to the Mediterranean diet and the MIND diet, a hybrid of the Mediterranean diet and Dietary Approaches to Stop Hypertension (DASH). After accounting for sociodemographic factors, health habits, and comorbid illnesses, moderate and high adherence to the Mediterranean diet were associated with 15% (*P*=0.08) and 35% (*P*<0.001) reduced odds of cognitive impairment, respectively. Likewise, moderate and high adherence to the MIND diet were associated with 15% (*P*=0.10) and 30% (*P*=0.001) reduced odds of cognitive impairment, respectively.

Anastasiou et al. (2017) published a cross-sectional study (*N*=1,865, average age 73 years) of the association between cognitive function and rates of dementia and adherence to the Mediterranean diet. The study included a battery of neurologist-administered tests for cognitive performance and dementia. After adjusting for sociodemographic factors, caloric intake, comorbid neurological illnesses, and apolipoprotein E genotype (*APOE*) status, participants' food consumption scores (0–55 points) based on detailed records resulted in 10% reduced odds for dementia for each point greater adherence to the Mediterranean diet (*P*≤0.05). The highest- versus lowest-quartile scores reduced the odds of dementia by 65% ($P \leq 0.05$). Every 2-point and 4-point reduction of the score equaled the same risk as 1 year of aging for diagnosis of dementia and cognitive performance, respectively ($P \leq 0.05$).

Imaging Studies Regarding Diet, Brain Volume, and Cognitive Function

Volumetric loss and loss of interneural connectivity detected by brain imaging are hallmark signs of cognitive impairment and dementia. There have been several high-quality imaging studies evaluating the relationship between diet and weight and the maintenance of brain volume through the aging process. Janowitz et al. (2015) completed two cross-sectional volumetric brain imaging studies ($N=758$, average age 50 years and $N=1,586$, average age 46 years) evaluating the relationship between waist circumference and gray matter. Waist circumference demonstrated a significant inverse relationship to the volume of gray matter in frontal and temporal lobes, limbic system, and hippocampal regions functionally involved with behavioral control, reward, and cognition.

Gu et al. (2015) evaluated brain volume in relation to diet by completing a cross-sectional study of 674 elderly individuals without evidence of dementia. Individuals adherent to a Mediterranean diet had a 5-year difference in brain age, with significantly larger gray matter, white matter, and total brain volumes, with effects particularly noted in the frontal and temporal lobes. Higher proportions of fish and lower proportions of red meat were some of the strongest correlates to improved brain volume. Luciano et al. (2017) completed a longitudinal prospective study ($N=401$) that measured brain volume over time in relation to diet. After adjusting for sex, cardiometabolic risk factors, and cognitive function, high versus low adherence to the Mediterranean diet significantly maintained total brain volume over the 3-year period, demonstrating for the first time that diet may impact brain volume in longitudinal fashion.

Nutrient and Flavanol Studies in Cognitive Function and Cognitive Disorders

Omega-3

It had been previously established that breastfeeding infants improves cognitive development and performance of children, in part because breast milk is a natural source of DHA. Indeed, when gestating and breastfeeding mothers increase DHA consumption through DHA-rich foods or supplements, children have improved performance in cognitive tasks and IQ.

Drover et al. (2009) completed three double-blind randomized controlled trials (*N*=29) that demonstrated improved cognitive performance at 9 months when formula-fed infants were given supplements of DHA and arachidonic acid, provided that the supplementation began at age 6 weeks or earlier.

Later in life, cognitive decline and dementia share qualities with schizophrenia in that maintaining brain volume is a primary concern for reducing pathology. Because DHA, rather than EPA, is the omega-3 fatty acid that localizes as structural brain volume, the majority of omega-3 research in cognition has been focused on DHA. Yurko-Mauro et al. (2015) completed a meta-analysis of 15 double-blind randomized controlled trials that tested DHA and episodic memory. Episodic memory was significantly improved in patients with mild cognitive impairment who received DHA (*P*=0.004), but DHA was ineffective in people with no complaints of cognitive impairment. Subgroup analysis suggested that greater than 1-g daily doses of combined DHA-EPA (*P*=0.04) or greater than 500-mg doses of DHA alone were required for significant improvement (*P*≤0.038). However, the effect size of omega-3 on episodic memory was small (0.114).

Yassine et al. (2017) provided a review of the history of research into DHA supplementation for cognitive decline, dementia, and Alzheimer's disease. Briefly, DHA supplementation for clinical Alzheimer's disease is ineffective. However, there is clinical evidence that high-dose supplementation (≥1 g/day) appears to be effective in preventing the onset of Alzheimer's disease in *APOE4* carriers. There is ample mechanism evidence to support this hypothesis. *APOE4* carriers have aberrant metabolism of DHA, including increased catabolism of DHA by the liver, decreased transport of DHA across the blood-brain barrier, decreased integration of DHA in neurons, and increased oxidation of DHA. DHA supplementation in *APOE4* carriers may help to stabilize these mechanisms and thereby increase DHA availability to maintain brain volume.

Folate

Durga et al. (2007) completed a large 3-year double-blind randomized controlled trial (*N*=819, ages 50–70 years) evaluating the impact of folate supplementation on age-related cognitive decline. Whereas previous randomized controlled trials using folate as an intervention to improve cognition did not produce significant results, this study included patients only if homocysteine levels were elevated and B_{12} levels were within normal limits. Because both low folate and low B_{12} can increase homocysteine levels, this ensured that the elevated homocysteine levels were due to folate insufficiency.

Compared with placebo, folate demonstrated significant improvements in global cognitive function, memory, sensorimotor speed, and information processing speed and nonsignificant improvements in complex speed and word fluency. The effect size of the intervention was equal to 1.5 years of aging for global cognitive function, 4.7 years for memory, 6.9 years for delayed memory, 1.7 years for sensorimotor speed, and 2.1 years for information processing speed. Although these results are promising, the intervention applies to a select group of patients who have folate-mediated elevated homocysteine levels and normal B_{12} levels. Additionally, only seven patients in the trial had a Mini-Mental State Examination score lower than 24, so the study results may not be applicable to patients with established clinical cognitive impairment.

Berries and Berry Extracts

Flavonoids have a wide range of antioxidant and anti-inflammatory neuronal mechanisms. Anthocyanidins, the blue-red compounds found in berries, cross the blood-brain barrier and localize in areas of the brain related to learning and memory. Devore et al. (2012) published a prospective cohort study (N=16,010) analyzing the effects of flavonoid consumption, including blueberries and strawberries, on cognitive decline in women ages 70 years and older. After accounting for sociodemographics, alcohol intake, BMI, and physical activity, high berry consumption (blueberries ≥ 1 serving per week vs. <1 serving per month and/or strawberries ≥ 2 servings per week vs. <1 serving per week) was significantly associated with improved cognitive function, with an effect size equal to up to 2.5 years of cognitive aging.

There have been several human randomized controlled trials in nonclinical and clinical populations with blueberry, cherry, or strawberry freeze-dried extracts or juice (Miller et al. 2018). All of the trials have been small and short term. In each trial, one or a few cognitive domains improved, whereas the remaining cognitive domains did not improve compared with placebo. These results may be an indication that larger and longer trials are needed to produce convincing outcomes.

Cacao, Chocolate, and Chocolate Flavanols

Clinical research into flavonoid berry extracts has been preliminary, but research into chocolate flavonoids has been more robust. Chocolate contains compounds that increase endothelial nitric oxide production in a use-dependent fashion, causing vasodilation. For instance, after consuming high-flavanol chocolate, when cardiac output increases, coronary blood vessels dilate, and when cognitive activity increases, blood vessels to the areas of the brain being used vasodilate more than they would without chocolate. Two nearly identical double-blind randomized controlled trials were conducted by Mastroiacovo et al. (2015) and Desideri et al. (2012) testing the effect of cacao flavanols on cognitive and cardiometabolic measures in elderly individuals. The two trials deviated in that Mastroiacovo and colleagues tested elderly individuals without evidence of cognitive impairment, and Desideri and colleagues tested patients with mild cognitive impairment. In both trials, 90 individuals were randomly assigned to high flavanol (993 mg), intermediate flavanol (520 mg), or low flavanol (48 mg) daily for 8 weeks. The intervention groups produced a dose-dependent response compared with the control groups. Patients with mild cognitive impairment had trend-level improvement on the Mini-Mental State Examination ($P=0.13$) and significant improvements on Trail Making Tests A and B and Verbal Fluency ($P \leq 0.018$) scores in response to flavonoids. Nonclinical elderly individuals had significant improvements on Trail Making Test A and B scores and Verbal Fluency scores ($P \leq 0.0001$). The intervention groups also had significant improvements in blood pressure, insulin resistance, and lipid levels.

Brickman et al. (2014) made use of high-definition functional magnetic resonance imaging demonstrating that the degradation of the dentate gyrus in the hippocampus was the most reliable brain region related to age-related cognitive decline and that cocoa flavanols may improve blood flow to, and activation of, the dentate gyrus, thereby improving cognition. They conducted a 3-month double-blind randomized controlled trial ($N=37$) with a high-flavanol intake group versus a low-flavanol intake group. Compared with the low-flavanol group, the high-flavanol group had significant improvement ($P=0.038$) on dentate gyrus–related cognitive performance, with a large effect size (0.816), and showed significant increases in cerebral blood flow to the dentate gyrus. Chocolate flavanols can be reduced through processing. For example, processing cocoa with alkali effectively eliminates flavanol content, and this processed cocoa is used for low-flavanol chocolate control groups. In commercial products, traditionally processed dark chocolate and raw cacao have the highest flavanol content.

Dietary Randomized Controlled Trials and Cognitive Function

In the PREDIMED-NAVARRA trial ($N=522$), Martínez-Lapiscina et al. (2013) published results from the first long-term (average 6.5 years) randomized controlled trial evaluating the cognitive effects of the Mediterranean diet on individuals with cardiovascular risk factors. The trial population was a subset of the PREDIMED trial ($N=7,447$)—the largest dietary lifestyle trial in the history of research—that randomly assigned patients at high cardiovascular risk to a Mediterranean diet supplemented by extra virgin olive oil (MedDiet+olive oil) or 30 g of walnuts, almonds, and hazelnuts per day (MedDiet+nuts) versus a low-fat control group. At the end of the trial, cognitive testing was performed with the Mini-Mental State Examination and the Clock Drawing Test. The MedDiet+olive oil and MedDiet+nuts groups had significantly higher scores on both tests compared with the low-fat control group after accounting for confounding factors ($P \leq 0.045$). The results remained consistent after further accounting for depression in the subset of individuals who were screened for depression ($n=268$; $P \leq 0.045$).

Valls-Pedret et al. (2015) improved on the PREDIMED-NAVARRA trial with the addition of baseline and follow-up cognitive testing on 334 patients (average age 66.8 years at baseline), with an average follow-up time of 4.1 years. The trial was nearly identical in design to the earlier trial because both studies were subsets of the PREDIMED trial. In the fully adjusted model, the MedDiet+olive oil and the MedDiet+nuts intervention groups versus the low-fat control group produced significant or trend-level improvements in composite scores for memory, executive function, and global cognition, with the exception of executive function in the MedDiet+nuts versus control group, which improved but did not reach statistical association ($P=0.221$).

CONCLUSION

A comprehensive diet based on freshly prepared, minimally processed natural foods provides nutrient-rich and antioxidant-rich sources of nourishment that can aid everyone on their journey toward better health (see Table 13–2 for a list of dietary recommendations). This advice is particularly pertinent for people with bipolar spectrum disorders and schizophrenia spectrum disorders who disproportionately suffer morbidity from cardiometabolic diseases. In some individuals, improvements in diet quality, nutrient status, and microbiome diversity and decreases in diet-related neuro-oxidative damage and neuroinflammatory cascades might help prevent the onset of, and act as adjuvant treatment for, psychiatric disorders. Regarding supplemental-nutrient double-blind randomized controlled trials, there have been both promising and inconsistent results in terms of efficacy in the treatment of core psychiatric symptoms. One might consider that individual nutrients are necessary, but not sufficient, if the remainder of an individual's diet and lifestyle choices produce an obesogenic, pro-oxidative, and proinflammatory milieu in his or her bodily systems. However, even the best diets may require supplementation if there are genetic factors that inhibit efficient use of individual nutrients.

TABLE 13–2. Dietary recommendations for psychiatric health

Global recommendation

Epidemiological evidence suggests that whole-food diets that emphasize whole grains, beans, vegetables, mushrooms, nuts, seeds, fruits, olive oil, and fish and deemphasize processed foods and artificial ingredients may be preventive for depression; bipolar disorder; schizophrenia; and developmental, pediatric, and cognitive disorders.

Depressive disorders recommendations

Adjuvant EPA omega-6 fatty acids may improve depressive symptoms.

Adjuvant zinc may improve depressive symptoms in patients.

L-Methylfolate is FDA approved for suboptimal folate levels in depressed patients; 15 mg L-methylfolate adjuvant to an SSRI may improve depressive symptoms.

The Mediterranean diet may improve depressive symptoms and increase remission when used in addition to standard of care in patients with baseline poor dietary status.

Bipolar spectrum disorders recommendations

Omega-3 supplementation may be beneficial for depressive symptoms.

60 g of BCAA daily for 1 week as adjuvant to standard of care may reduce acute mania symptoms. Concomitant use of BCAA and valproate is contraindicated because of potential liver damage.

There are case reports of a ketogenic diet benefiting bipolar symptoms.

Schizophrenia spectrum disorders recommendations

Adjuvant *N*-acetylcysteine may be effective in treating negative symptoms.

Adjuvant folate and L-methylfolate may improve core symptoms of schizophrenia, particularly in patients with aberrant folate metabolism. L-Methylfolate is FDA approved for hyperhomocysteinemia in patients with schizophrenia.

DHA-EPA omega-3 fatty acids may have benefit in core symptoms in nonacute schizophrenia patients. Patients in acute psychosis should avoid omega-3 supplementation.

Insufficient gestational and perinatal cholecalciferol is associated with risk for schizophrenia.

ADHD recommendations

Artificial colors and preservatives increase hyperactivity in children.

Broad-spectrum micronutrients may improve inattention and mood dysregulation in children and adults.

Restricted elimination diets may improve core ADHD symptoms.

TABLE 13–2.	Dietary recommendations for psychiatric health *(continued)*

ASD recommendations

Prepregnancy overweight and insufficient gestational cholecalciferol levels are associated with risk for ASD.

Cholecalciferol insufficiency may continue in childhood; the effects of cholecalciferol supplementation on core symptoms of ASD are inconclusive but may be dose dependent.

Cognitive function and disorders recommendations

Early-life DHA improves cognitive function in children.

DHA omega-3 may benefit adults with mild cognitive impairment, but the effect size is small.

DHA omega-3 may benefit *APOE4* carriers.

Long-term folate supplementation may improve cognition in patients with folate-deficiency hyperhomocysteinemia.

High-flavanol chocolate increases blood flow to the brain and improves cognitive performance.

The Mediterranean diet may inhibit cognitive decline by improving cardiovascular health.

Abbreviations. ADHD=attention-deficit/hyperactivity disorder; *APOE4*=apolipoprotein E4; ASD=autism spectrum disorder; BCAA=branched-chain amino acids; DHA=docosahexaenoic acid; EPA=eicosapentaenoic acid; FDA=U.S. Food and Drug Administration; SSRI=selective serotonin reuptake inhibitor.

DISCUSSION QUESTIONS

1. When would you consider a nutritional intervention to help a patient with treatment-resistant symptoms?
2. What laboratory testing might help you to use nutritional interventions more precisely?
3. How would you engage a patient in making sustained dietary changes to support his or her psychiatric treatment?

RECOMMENDED READINGS

Jacka FN, O'Neil A, Opie R, et al: A randomised controlled trial of dietary improvement for adults with major depression (the "SMILES" trial). BMC Medicine 15(1):23, 2017

Malhi GS, Bassett D, Boyce P, et al: Royal Australian and New Zealand College of Psychiatrists Clinical Practice Guidelines for Mood Disorders. Aust N Z J Psychiatry 49(12):1087–1206, 2015

Sarris J, Logan AC, Akbaraly TN, et al: Nutritional medicine as mainstream in psychiatry. Lancet Psychiatry 2(3):271–274, 2015

REFERENCES

Akbaraly TN, Brunner EJ, Ferrie JE, et al: Dietary pattern and depressive symptoms in middle age. Br J Psychiatry 195(5):408–413, 2009 19880930

Amminger GP, Schäfer MR, Papageoriou K, et al.: Long-chain omega-3 fatty acids for indicated prevention of psychotic disorders: a randomized, placebo-controlled trial. Arch Gen Psychiatry 67(2):146–154, 2010 20124114

Amminger GP, Schäfer MR, Schlögelhofer M, et al: Longer-term outcome in the prevention of psychotic disorders by the Vienna omega-3 study. Nat Commun 6:7934, 2015 26263244

Anastasiou CA, Yannakoulia M, Kosmidis MH, et al: Mediterranean diet and cognitive health: initial results from the Hellenic Longitudinal Investigation of Ageing and Diet. PLoS One 12(8):e0182048, 2017 28763509

Berk M, Copolov DL, Dean O, et al: N-acetyl cysteine for depressive symptoms in bipolar disorder: a double-blind randomized placebo-controlled trial. Biol Psychiatry 64(6):468–475, 2008a 18534556

Berk M, Copolov D, Dean O, et al: N-acetyl cysteine as a glutathione precursor for schizophrenia: a double-blind, randomized, placebo-controlled trial. Biol Psychiatry 64(5):361–368, 2008b 18436195

Berk M, Dean OM, Cotton SM, et al: Maintenance N-acetyl cysteine treatment for bipolar disorder: a double-blind randomized placebo controlled trial. BMC Med 10:91, 2012 22891797

Bozzatello P, Brignolo E, De Grandi E, et al: Supplementation with omega-3 fatty acids in psychiatric disorders: a review of literature data. J Clin Med 5(8):67, 2016 27472373

Brickman AM, Khan UA, Provenzano FA, et al: Enhancing dentate gyrus function with dietary flavanols improves cognition in older adults. Nat Neurosci 17(12):1798–1803, 2014 25344629

Brinkworth GD, Buckley JD, Noakes M, et al: Long-term effects of a very low-carbohydrate diet and a low-fat diet on mood and cognitive function. Arch Intern Med 169(20):1873–1880, 2009 19901139

Brinkworth GD, Luscombe-Marsh ND, Thompson CH, et al: Long-term effects of very low-carbohydrate and high-carbohydrate weight-loss diets on psychological health in obese adults with type 2 diabetes: randomized controlled trial. J Intern Med 280(4):388–397, 2016 27010424

Delichatsios HK, Leonard MM, Fasano A, et al: Case records of the Massachusetts General Hospital. case 14-2016: a 37-year-old woman with adult-onset psychosis. N Engl J Med 374(19):1875–1883, 2016 27168437

Desideri G, Kwite-Uribe C, Grassi D, et al: Benefits in cognitive function, blood pressure, and insulin resistance through cocoa flavanol consumption in elderly subjects with mild cognitive impairment: the Cocoa, Cognition, and Aging (CoCoA) study. Hypertension 60(3):794–801, 2012 22892813

Devore EE, Kang JH, Breteler MMB, et al: Dietary intakes of berries and flavonoids in relation to cognitive decline. Ann Neurol 72(1):135–143, 2012 22535616

Do KQ, Trabensinger MK, Lauer CJ, et al.: Schizophrenia: glutathione deficit in cerebrospinal fluid and prefrontal cortex in vivo. Eur J Neurosci 12(1):3721–3728, 2000 11029642

Dohan FC, Grasberger JC: Relapsed schizophrenics: earlier discharge from the hospital after cereal-free, milk-free diet. Am J Psychiatry 130(6):685–688, 1973 4739849

Drover J, Hoffman DR, Castañeda YS, et al: Three randomized controlled trials of early long-chain polyunsaturated fatty acid supplementation on means-end problem solving in 9-month-olds. Child Dev 80(5):1376–1384, 2009 19765006

Durga J, van Boxtel MP, Schouten EG, et al: Effect of 3-year folic acid supplementation on cognitive function in older adults in the FACIT trial: a randomised, double blind, controlled trial. Lancet 369(9557):208–216, 2007 17240287

Ellengaard PK, Licht RW, Poulsen HE, et al: Add-on treatment with N-acetylcysteine for bipolar depression: a 24-week randomized double-blind parallel group placebo-controlled multicentre trial (NACOS-study protocol). J Bipolar Disord 6(1):11, 2018 29619634

Farokhnia M, Azarkolah A, Adinehfar F, et al: N-acetylcysteine as an adjunct to risperidone for treatment of negative symptoms in patients with chronic schizophrenia: a randomized, double-blind, placebo-controlled study. Clin Neuropharmacol 36(6):185–192, 2013 24201233

Gu Y, Brickman AM, Stern Y, et al: Mediterranean diet and brain structure in a multiethnic elderly cohort Neurology 85(20):1744–1751, 2015 26491085

Hallahan B, Ryan T, Hibbeln JR, et al: Efficacy of omega-3 highly unsaturated fatty acids in the treatment of depression. Br J Psychiatry 209(3):192–201, 2016 27103682

Howard AL, Robinson M, Smith GJ, et al: ADHD is associated with a "Western" dietary pattern in adolescents. J Atten Disord 15(5):403–411, 2011 20631199

Hyman SL, Stewart PA, Foley J, et al: The gluten-free/casein-free diet: a double-blind challenge trial in children with autism. J Autism Dev Disord 46(1):205–220, 2016 26343026

Jacka FN, Pasco JA, Mykletun A, et al: Diet quality in bipolar disorder in a population-based sample of women. J Affect Disord 129(1–3):332–337, 2011a 20888648

Jacka FN, Kremer PJ, Berk M, et al: A prospective study of diet quality and mental health in adolescents. PLoS One 6(9):e24805, 2011b 21957462

Jacka FN, Ystrom E, Brantsaeter AL, et al: Maternal and early postnatal nutrition and mental health of offspring by age 5 years: a prospective cohort study. J Am Acad Child Adolesc Psychiatry 52(10):1038–1047, 2013 24074470

Jacka FN, O'Neil A, Opie R, et al: A randomised controlled trial of dietary improvement for adults with major depression (the "SMILES" trial). BMC Med 15(1):23, 2017 28137247

Janowitz D, Wittfeld K, Terock J, et al: Association between waist circumference and gray matter volume in 2344 individuals from two adult community-based samples. Neuroimage 122:149–157, 2015 26256530

Kaplan BJ: Clinical trial of a nutritional supplement in adults with bipolar disorder (NCT00109577). Calgary, Alberta, Canada, University of Calgary, 2012. Available at: https://clinicaltrials.gov/ct2/show/NCT00109577. Accessed October 20, 2017.

Kaplan BJ, Simpson JSA, Ferre RC, et al: Effective mood stabilization with a chelated mineral supplement: an open-label trial in bipolar disorder. J Clin Psychiatry 62(12):936–944, 2001 11780873

Kelly D: Randomized controlled trial of a gluten free diet in patients with schizophrenia who are gliadin-positive (NCT01927276). Catonsville, MD, University of Maryland, 2017. Available at: https://clinicaltrials.gov/ct2/show/NCT01927276. Accessed December 14, 2018.

Kelly D: Confirmatory efficacy trial of a gluten-free diet in a subgroup of persons with schizophrenia who have high levels of IgG anti-gliadin antibodies (AGA IG) (NCT03183609). Catonsville, MD, University of Maryland, 2018. Available at: https://clinicaltrials.gov/ct2/show/NCT03183609. Accessed December 14, 2018.

Kien CL, Bunn JY, Tompkins CL, et al: Substituting dietary monounsaturated fat for saturated fat is associated with increased daily physical activity and resting energy expenditure and with changes in mood. Am J Clin Nutr 97(4):689–697, 2013 23446891

Kinney DK, Teixeira P, Hsu D, et al: Relation of schizophrenia prevalence to latitude, climate, fish consumption, infant mortality, and skin color: a role for prenatal vitamin d deficiency and infections? Schizophr Bull 35(3):582–595, 2009 19357239

Knivsberg AM, Reichelt KL, Høien T, Nødland M: A randomised, controlled study of dietary intervention in autistic syndromes. Nutr Neurosci 5(4):251–261, 2002 12168688

Levine J, Stahl Z, Sela BA, et al: Homocysteine-reducing strategies improve symptoms in chronic schizophrenic patients with hyperhomocysteinemia. Biol Psychiatry 60(3):265–269, 2006 16412989

Liu T, Lu Q-B, Yan L, et al: Comparative study on serum levels of 10 trace elements in schizophrenia. PLoS One 10(7):e0133622, 2015 26186003

Ino M, Corley J, Cox SR, et al: Mediterranean-type diet and brain structural change from 73 to 76 years in a Scottish cohort. Neurology 88(5):449–455, 2017 28053008

Malhi GS, Bassett D, Boyce P, et al: Royal Australian and New Zealand College of Psychiatrists Clinical Practice Guidelines for Mood Disorders. Aust N Z J Psychiatry 49(12):1087–1206, 2015

Martínez-González MA, Garcia-Arellano A, Toledo E: A 14-item Mediterranean diet assessment tool and obesity indexes among high-risk subjects: the PREDIMED trial. PLoS One 7(8):e43134 2012 22905215

Martínez-Lapiscina EH, Clavero P, Toledo E, et al: Mediterranean diet improves cognition: the PREDIMED-NAVARRA randomised trial. J Neurol Neurosurg Psychiatry 84(12):1318–1325, 2013 23670794

Mastroiacovo D, Kwik-Uribe C, Grassi D, et al: Cocoa flavanol consumption improves cognitive function, blood pressure control, and metabolic profile in elderly subjects: the Cocoa, Cognition, and Aging (CoCoA) Study—a randomized controlled trial. Am J Clin Nutr 101(3):538–548, 2015 25733639

McCann D, Barrett A, Cooper A, et al: Food additives and hyperactive behaviour in 3-year-old and 8/9-year-old children in the community: a randomised, double-blinded, placebo-controlled trial. Lancet 370(9598):1560–1567, 2007 17825405

McEvoy CT, Guyer H, Langa KM, et al: Neuroprotective diets are associated with better cognitive function: the Health and Retirement Study. J Am Geriatr Soc 65(8):1857–1862, 2017 28440854

McGorry PD, Nelson B, Markulev C, et al: Effect of omega-3 polyunsaturated fatty acids in young people at ultrahigh risk for psychotic disorders: the NEURAPRO randomized clinical trial. JAMA Psychiatry 74(1):19–27, 2017 27893018

McGrath JJ, Eyles DW, Pedersen CB, et al: Neonatal vitamin D status and risk of schizophrenia: a population-based case-control study. Arch Gen Psychiatry 67(9):889–894, 2010 20819982

Miller MG, Hamilton DA, Joseph JA, Shukitt-Hale B: Dietary blueberry improves cognition among older adults in a randomized, double-blind, placebo-controlled trial Eur J Nutr 57(3):1169–1180, 2018 28283823

Nanri A, Mizoue T, Poudel-Tandukar K, et al: Dietary patterns and suicide in Japanese adults: the Japan Public Health Center-based Prospective Study. Br J Psychiatry 203(6):422–427, 2013 24115342

Noaghiul S, Hibbeln JR: Cross-national comparisons of seafood consumption and rates of bipolar disorders. Am J Psychiatry 160(12):2222–2227, 2003 14638594

Palmer CM: Ketogenic diet in the treatment of schizoaffective disorder: two case studies. Schizophr Res 189:208–209, 2017 28162810

Papakostas GI, Shelton RC, Zajecka JM, et al: l-Methylfolate as adjunctive therapy for SSRI-resistant major depression: results of two randomized, double-blind, parallel-sequential trials. Am J Psychiatry 169(12):1267–1274, 2012 23212058

Pawełczyk T, Grancow-Grabka M, Kotlicka-Antczak M, et al: A randomized controlled study of the efficacy of six-month supplementation with concentrated fish oil rich in omega-3 polyunsaturated fatty acids in first episode schizophrenia. J Psychiatr Res 73:34–44, 2016 26679763

Peet M: Diet, diabetes and schizophrenia: review and hypothesis. Br J Psychiatry Suppl 47:S102–S105, 2004a 15056602

Peet M: International variations in the outcome of schizophrenia and the prevalence of depression in relation to national dietary practices: an ecological analysis. Br J Psychiatry 184:404–408, 2004b 15123503

Pelsser LM, Frankena K, Toorman J, et al: Effects of a restricted elimination diet on the behaviour of children with attention-deficit hyperactivity disorder (INCA study): a randomised controlled trial. Lancet 377(9764):494–503, 2011 21296237

Perry BI, McIntosh G, Weich S, et al: The association between first-episode psychosis and abnormal glycaemic control: systematic review and meta-analysis. Lancet Psychiatry 3(11):1049–1058, 2016 27720402

Potkin SG, Weinberger D, Kleinman J, et al: Wheat gluten challenge in schizophrenic patients. Am J Psychiatry 138(9):1208-1211, 1981 7270725

Psaltopoulou T, Sergentanis TN, Panagiotakos DB, et al: Mediterranean diet, stroke, cognitive impairment, and depression: a meta-analysis. Ann Neurol 74(4):580–591, 2013 23720230

Raine A, Mellingen K, Liu J, et al: Effects of environmental enrichment at ages 3–5 years on schizotypal personality and antisocial behavior at ages 17 and 23 years. Am J Psychiatry 160(9):1627–1635, 2003 12944338

Ríos-Hernández A, Alda JA, Farran-Codina A, et al: The Mediterranean diet and ADHD in children and adolescents. Pediatrics 139(2):e20162027, 2017 28138007

Roffman JL, Petruzzi LJ, Tanner AS, et al: Biochemical, physiological and clinical effects of L-methylfolate in schizophrenia: a randomized controlled trial. Mol Psychiatry 23(2):316–322, 2018 28289280

Rucklidge JJ, Frampton CM, Gorman B, et al: Vitamin-mineral treatment of attention-deficit hyperactivity disorder in adults: double-blind randomised placebo-controlled trial. Br J Psychiatry 204:306–315, 2014 24482441

Rucklidge JJ, Eggleston MJF, Johnstone JM, et al: Vitamin-mineral treatment improves aggression and emotional regulation in children with ADHD: a fully blinded, randomized, placebo-controlled trial. J Child Psychol Psychiatry 59(3):232–246, 2018 28967099

Sanchez CE, Barry C, Sabhlok A, et al: Maternal pre-pregnancy obesity and child neurodevelopmental outcomes: a meta-analysis. Obes Rev 19(4):464–484, 2018 29164765

Sánchez-Villegas A, Galbete C, Martinez-González MÁ, et al: The effect of the Mediterranean diet on plasma brain-derived neurotrophic factor (BDNF) levels: the PREDIMED-NAVARRA randomized trial. Nutr Neurosci 14(5):195–201, 2011 22005283

Sarris J, Mischoulon D, Schweitzer I: Omega-3 for bipolar disorder: meta-analyses of use in mania and bipolar depression. J Clin Psychiatry 73(1):81–86, 2012 21903025

Sarris J, Logan AC, Akbaraly TN, et al: Nutritional medicine as mainstream in psychiatry. Lancet Psychiatry 2(3):271–274, 2015 26359904

Sarris J, Murphy J, Mischoulon D, et al: Adjunctive nutraceuticals for depression: a systematic review and meta-analyses. Am J Psychiatry 173(6):575–587, 2016 27113121

Sathe N, Andrews JC, McPheeters ML, et al: Nutritional and dietary interventions for autism spectrum disorder: a systematic review. Pediatrics 139(6):e20170346, 2017 28562286

Scarna A, Gijsman HJ, McTavish SFB, et al: Effects of a branched-chain amino acid drink in mania. Br J Psychiatry 182:210–213, 2003 12611783

Schröder H, Fitó M, Estruch R, et al: A short screener is valid for assessing Mediterranean diet adherence among older Spanish men and women. J Nutr 141(6):1140–1145, 2011 21508208

Singh K, Connors SL, Macklin EA, et al: Sulforaphane treatment of autism spectrum disorder (ASD). Proc Natl Acad Sci USA 111(43):15,550–15,555, 2014 25313065

Singh MM, Kay SR: Wheat gluten as a pathogenic factor in schizophrenia. Science 19(4225):401–402, 1976 1246624

Sonuga-Barke EJ, Brandeis D, Cortese S, et al: Nonpharmacological interventions for ADHD: systematic review and meta-analyses of randomized controlled trials of dietary and psychological treatments. Am J Psychiatry 170(3):275–289, 2013 23360949

Stahl ST, Albert SM, Dew MA, et al: Coaching in healthy dietary practices in at-risk older adults: a case of indicated depression prevention. Am J Psychiatry 171(5):499–505, 2014 24788282

Valls-Pedret C, Sala-Vila A, Serra-Mir M, et al: Mediterranean diet and age-related cognitive decline: a randomized clinical trial. JAMA Intern Med 175(7):1094–1103, 2015 25961184

Vinkhuyzen AAE, Eyles DW, Burne THJ, et al: Gestational vitamin D deficiency and autism-related traits: the Generation R Study. Mol Psychiatry 23(2):240–246, 2018 27895322

Wang T, Shan L, Du L, et al: Serum concentration of 25-hydroxyvitamin D in autism spectrum disorder: a systematic review and meta-analysis. Eur Child Adolesc Psychiatry 25(4):341–350, 2016 26514973

Whiteley P, Haracopos D, Knivsberg AM, et al: The ScanBrit randomised, controlled, single-blind study of a gluten- and casein-free dietary intervention for children with autism spectrum disorders. Nutr Neurosci 13(2):87–100, 2010 20406576

Woo HD, Kim DW, Hong YS, et al: Dietary patterns in children with attention deficit/hyperactivity disorder (ADHD). Nutrients 6(4):1539–1553, 2014 24736898

Wu D-M, Wen X, Han X-R, et al: Relationship between neonatal vitamin D at birth and risk of autism spectrum disorders: the NBSIB study. J Bone Miner Res 33(3):458–466, 2018 29178513

Yassine HN, Braskie MN, Mack WJ, et al: Association of docosahexaenoic acid supplementation with Alzheimer disease stage in apolipoprotein E e4 carriers: a review. JAMA Neurol 74(3):339–347, 2017 28114437

Yurko-Mauro K, Alexander DD, Van Elswyk ME: Docosahexaenoic acid and adult memory: a systematic review and meta-analysis. PLoS One 10(3):e0120391, 2015 25786262

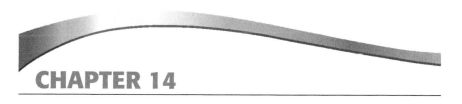

CHAPTER 14

The Gut-Brain Axis and Microbiome in Psychiatric Disorders

Emeran A. Mayer, M.D.

Hyo Jin Ryu, B.S.

E. A. Mayer has been supported by grants from the National Institute of Diabetes and Digestive and Kidney Diseases (DK048351, DK064539, and DK096606).

KEY POINTS

- Bidirectional communication occurs within the brain-gut microbiome axis via multiple mechanisms.
- Preclinical science supports a role of gut microbes in emotion and behavior.
- Recent clinical studies implicate alterations in gut microbiome brain signaling in psychiatric disorders.
- Treatment recommendations are emerging on the basis of altered brain-gut microbiome interactions.

Largely on the basis of studies in experimental animals, significant progress has been made in the past decade in illuminating the role of bidirectional interactions between the nervous system, the gastrointestinal tract, and the gut microbiome. Studies performed in experimental animal models have confirmed the role of the gut microbiome in modulating affective, social, nociceptive, and ingestive behaviors, yet causality and translation of these findings into healthy humans and patients with psychiatric disorders have been limited, and the effectiveness of specific gut microbiome–targeted treatments remains to be established. Despite these limitations, the new brain-gut microbiome (BGM) science has spawned a considerable effort in academia and industry to determine if prebiotic, probiotic, and postbiotic interventions may be beneficial either as primary or as adjuvant therapy in disorders such as autism spectrum disorders, anxiety, depression, Alzheimer's disease, Parkinson's disease, schizophrenia, and epilepsy. Such therapies could be in the form of special diets, dietary supplements (prebiotics and probiotics), novel probiotics, novel molecules targeting gut microbial signaling molecules (postbiotics), or biotics that confer mental health benefits (psychobiotics).

In this chapter, we first briefly review the key findings that demonstrate the existence of bidirectional signaling between the brain and gut microbiota in both animals and humans and then review the evidence for the role of BGM communication channels in psychiatric disorders. Finally, we discuss possible therapeutic implications of such communication within the BGM axis.

SIGNALING FROM THE BRAIN TO THE GUT MICROBIOTA

There are more than 40 years of literature demonstrating the effect of stress on the community structure of the gut microbiome; this research has been reviewed elsewhere (Cryan and Dinan 2012; Rhee et al. 2009). A consistent effect observed in different models involves a transient stress-induced reduction in the abundance of the genus *Lactobacillus* in stool microbiota. As summarized in Table 14–1 and shown in Figure 14–1, multiple mechanisms, primarily mediated through the autonomic nervous system, result in the modulation of the microbial environment and microbial gene expression and behavior. These stress-induced changes in gut physiology change the gut microbial habitat, which can lead to a modulation of microbiota composition and/or activity. A recent study using a chronic variable stress mouse model showed a reduction in *Lactobacillus* in the feces and a shift in tryptophan metabolism from serotonin toward the kynurenine pathway (Marin et al. 2017). These preclinical findings suggest that chronic stress-induced gut dysbiosis in humans may result in the modulation of brain function by microbial metabolites (see next section, "Signaling From the Gut Microbiota to the Brain").

TABLE 14–1. Mechanisms mediating the effect of stress on gut microbiome

Area	Mechanisms
Microbial environment	Gastrointestinal motility (regional alterations in intestinal transit)
	Intestinal permeability
	Paneth cell secretion (antimicrobials)
	Intestinal fluid and mucus secretion
	Gastric/bile acid secretion
	Intraintestinal pH
	Epithelial and blood-brain barrier permeability
Microbiome	Direct modulation of microbial gene expression and virulence by luminally released norepinephrine
	Stress-induced signaling molecules released into gut lumen, such as serotonin and opioids

Note. These mechanisms are reviewed extensively by Mayer 2011 and Rhee et al. 2009.

In addition to such indirect effects of brain influences on the gut microbiome, direct modulation of microbial virulence gene expression by norepinephrine in the gut lumen has been demonstrated in animal models of stress (Hughes and Sperandio 2008). Although autonomic nervous sys-

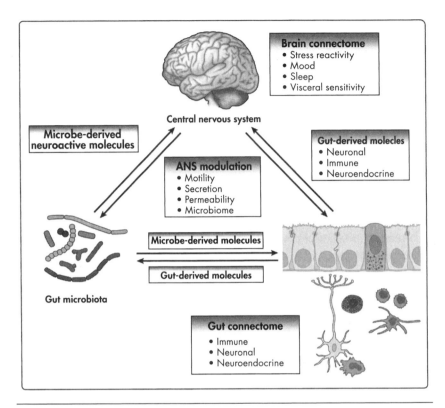

FIGURE 14–1.   Systems biological model of brain-gut microbiome interactions.

Gut microbes communicate with the gut via microbial metabolites, and changes in gut function can modulate gut microbial behavior. Through the autonomic nervous system (ANS), the brain can alter gut microbial composition and function indirectly by modulating the gut microbial environment in the gut. The brain can also alter the function of gut microbes directly by modulating gene expression profiles via the sympathetic nervous system. The gut microbes can communicate to the brain indirectly via gut-derived molecules or directly via microbe-generated signals. Alterations in the gain of these bidirectional interactions in response to perturbations such as psychosocial or gut-directed (e.g., diet, medications, infection) stress can change the behavior of this system, manifesting as brain-gut disorders.

Source.   Fung TC, Olson CA, Hsiao EY: "Interactions Between the Microbiota, Immune and Nervous Systems in Health and Disease." *Nature Neuroscience* 20(2):145–155, 2017. Adapted with permission from Springer Nature. Copyright ©2017.

tem effects on various gut functions have been studied primarily for stress, older observational studies in humans have shown similar effects in relationship to certain emotional states, such as fear, anger, and sadness. For example, whereas fear and anxiety are associated with accelerated intestinal transit, reduced intestinal motility has been observed with sadness (Mayer 2011).

SIGNALING FROM THE GUT MICROBIOTA TO THE BRAIN

Preclinical Studies

Current evidence indicates that bottom-up modulation of the central nervous system (CNS) by the gut microbiome occurs primarily through neuroimmune and neuroendocrine mechanisms, often involving the vagus and possibly spinal nerves. Experimental models and interventions used to demonstrate gut microbial influences on brain and behavior are shown in Table 14–2. This communication is mediated by several microbe-derived molecules, including short-chain fatty acids (SCFAs), secondary bile acids, and tryptophan metabolites, which act on enteroendocrine cells in the gut or can enter the systemic circulation, in particular in the context of increased gut permeability.

TABLE 14–2. Experimental strategies in preclinical models to study gut microbial influences on brain and behavior

Strategy	Significance
Germ-free	Germ-free phenotype can be reversed by recolonization with specific pathogen-free, human-derived, and synthetic microbiota.
Antibiotics	Antibiotics induced transient changes to the composition and diversity of fecal microbiota and increased exploratory behavior and brain-derived neurotrophic factor expression in the hippocampus.
	Long-term treatment in adult mice reduced hippocampal neurogenesis and resulted in deficits in novel object recognition tasks through a mechanism dependent on circulating monocytes. Adoptive transfer of Ly6C^{hi} monocytes or voluntary exercise and probiotic treatment rescued these phenotypes.
Probiotics	Probiotics reduced basal or induced anxiety-like behavior in animal models with normal gut microbiota.
	Probiotic supplementation improved memory and learning in diabetic mice.

Note. These findings are summarized by Bercik et al. (2012) and Mayer et al. (2015).
Abbreviation. Ly6C^{hi}=lymphocyte antigen 6 complex locus C, in high levels.

In addition to these metabolites, the microbiota can generate a number of neuroactive molecules, including but not limited to γ-aminobutyric acid (GABA), serotonin, norepinephrine, and dopamine (Cryan and Dinan 2012; Mayer et al. 2015). Interactions between gut microbial metabolites and enteroendocrine cells have been described in the regulation of satiety and hunger and likely play a role in other functions. Both preclinical and clinical data have demonstrated that microbiota-derived SCFAs, generated from host dietary resistant starch and nonstarch polysaccharides, stimulate L-cells located at the distal ileum to secrete peptide YY and glucagon-like peptide-1 and peptide-2, which induce satiety and behavioral changes (Holzer and Farzi 2014). The widespread distribution of G-protein-coupled SCFA receptors on enteroendocrine cells involved in the regulation of food intake and digestion is consistent with the important role of the gut microbes in the regulation of food intake and in obesity.

One of the best-characterized examples of microbial host interaction is between microbes, enterochromaffin cells, and the brain. Tryptophan is a key molecule in the BGM axis because it is the precursor to the neurotransmitter serotonin (5-hydroxytryptophan) and a number of other metabolites that contribute to the neuroendocrine signaling within the BGM axis (Ruddick et al. 2006). Serotonin is produced by the enterochromaffin cells of the gastrointestinal tract, with 95% of the body's serotonin stored in enterochromaffin cells and enteric neurons and only 5% in the brain (Kim and Camilleri 2000). The gut microbiota is essential in the peripheral availability of tryptophan, which is imperative to the brain's synthesis of serotonin.

Although the exact mechanisms of peripheral tryptophan regulation are unknown, some evidence suggests that the microbiota can modulate the degradation of dietary tryptophan down the kynurenine pathway (Schwarcz et al. 2012). In a mouse model of chronic variable stress, the administration of the probiotic *L. reuteri* normalized stress-induced behavioral changes and was associated with a reduction of circulating kynurenine levels resulting from microbially derived H_2O_2 inhibition of indoleamine 2,3-dioxygenase 1 (*IDO1*) mRNA expression. These findings suggest a possible role of kynurenine in modulating brain and behavior (Marin et al. 2017).

Commensal bacteria are known to shape the host immune system and affect signaling of peripheral immune cells to the CNS (Fung et al. 2017). Recently, it has been demonstrated that gut microbiota can also influence the development and function of CNS-resident immune cells, especially microglia (Erny et al. 2015). Germ-free mice have compromised microglia maturation and morphology, leading to weakened early responses to pathogen exposure (Erny et al. 2015). This phenotype can be normalized by postnatal SCFA supplementation or colonization with a complex microbial community. In addition to the crucial role of microbial signaling in programming the BGM axis during early life, gut microbe–to–brain signaling is required throughout adulthood to preserve microglial maturation (Erny et al. 2015).

There are two natural barriers to signaling within the BGM axis: the intestinal barrier and the blood-brain barrier. Permeability of these two barriers is not static because stress, inflammation, and the gut microbes themselves are able to modulate the permeability of both structures. Thus, the amount of information reaching the brain from the gut is highly variable depending on the state of the host.

Clinical Studies

A small number of clinical studies has successfully demonstrated the association of gut microbial community structure with brain parameters and subjective outcomes of interventions with probiotics and prebiotics. Probiotic supplementation in humans does not appear to change gut microbial composition but induces its effect on the brain via modification of the collective microbiome transcriptional state. Examination of microbial community functional dynamics and metabolomics will help refine the underlying mechanisms responsible for these effects and can help identify putative targets for therapeutic intervention. No high-quality controlled studies in humans have reported the effects of other microbiome-targeted interventions, such as antibiotics or fecal microbial transplants, on the brain or behavior.

DEVELOPMENTAL ASPECTS OF BRAIN-GUT MICROBIOME INTERACTIONS

As shown in Figure 14–2, there are multiple factors that shape the programming of the BGM during the first 3 years of life, including gestation. During this time period, the community structure of the gut microbiota is being established, and the interactions of the evolving microbiome with the developing CNS are being programmed. After this programming period, the gut microbiota and the BGM are fairly stable and much less susceptible to perturbations throughout adult life. On the basis of this time course, it is plausible that several neurodevelopmental disorders may be positively affected by interference with the normal programming by maternal infections, dietary influences, and medications, in particular, antibiotics.

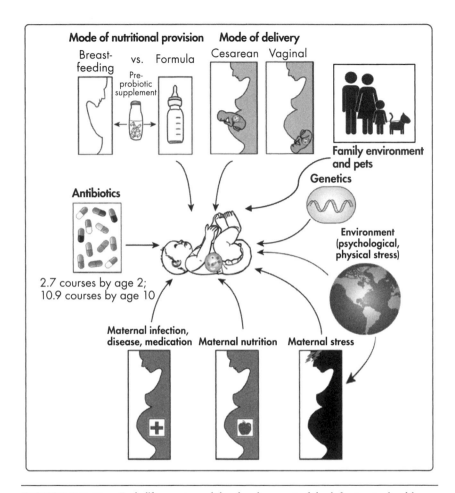

FIGURE 14–2. Early life events and the development of the infant gut microbiome.

Early life represents a particularly vulnerable period for the infant gut microbiome because the microbiome is highly responsive to numerous factors. In addition to genetics, prenatal influences (e.g., maternal nutrition, stress, overall health), mode of delivery, early life nutrition (breastfeeding, formula feeding), physical and psychological environments, and antibiotic use all influence the infant gut microbiome.

Source. Reprinted from Borre YE, O'Keeffe GW, Clarke G, et al: "Microbiota and Neurodevelopmental Windows: Implications for Brain Disorders." *Trends in Molecular Medicine* 20(9):509–518, 2014, with permission from Elsevier.

ALTERED BRAIN-GUT MICROBIOME INTERACTIONS IN PSYCHIATRIC AND NEUROLOGICAL DISEASES

A systematic review of clinical studies of the microbiome in people with schizophrenia and bipolar disorder suggests that these disorders are associated with reduced microbial diversity and show global community differences compared with nonpsychiatric comparison samples (Dickerson et al. 2017). In some reports, specific microbial taxa were associated with clinical disease characteristics, including physical health, depressive and psychotic symptoms, and sleep, but little information was available on the functional potential of those community changes. A plausible mechanism by which microbial dysbiosis may impact systemic physiological as well as brain functioning may include altered intestinal permeability resulting in low-grade systemic immune activation, which may also affect the brain.

Depression and Anxiety

Preclinical studies have demonstrated the microbiota's ability to modulate emotional behaviors (Table 14–3) and influence parameters significant to depression pathogenesis and severity, including levels of neurotransmitters and neuromodulators serotonin, brain-derived neurotrophic factor, synaptogenesis, and synapse maturation (Diaz Heijtz et al. 2011). Furthermore, major depressive disorder–associated gut dysbiosis is corroborated by the abnormal serum immunological parameters of subsets of depressed patients (Maes et al. 2008). For example, an increased toll-like receptor 4 expression and enhanced immunoglobulin-mediated immune response to lipopolysaccharides of specific commensal bacteria implicate a "leaky gut," or increased intestinal permeability, and problematic management of bacterial translocation (Kelly et al. 2016a). Although studies characterizing the gut microbiome of individuals with major depressive disorder versus healthy control subjects have yielded marginally distinct assemblage correlations, three different studies have reported results suggesting causality: depressed human-to-rodent fecal microbial transplants have induced depression-like behaviors in the animal models (Kelly et al. 2016b; Zheng et al. 2016); prebiotic and probiotic administration to healthy control subjects has improved anxiety and mood (Steenbergen et al. 2015); and incidences of *Escherichia coli* subtype outbreaks in Canada and Germany led to rises in depression and anxiety-related symptoms among the affected population (Kelly et al. 2016a). A recently published nested control study using a large, population-based database in the United Kingdom showed a significantly increased risk for depression and anxiety after antibiotic therapy (Lurie et al. 2015).

TABLE 14–3.   Role of gut microbiome in brain and behavior

Brain and behavioral changes	Findings
Stress responsiveness	Stress-induced corticosterone was reduced by *Lactobacillus rhamnosus*.
	Bifidobacterium infantis treatment reversed maternal separation–induced decrease in swim behavior and mobility, decrease in brain noradrenaline, and increase in peripheral IL-6 and amygdala corticotropin-releasing factor mRNA levels.
Depression- and anxiety-like behavior	Behaviors were reduced via treatment with *L. rhamnosus*.
	B. breve and *B. longum* reduced anxiety; *B. longum* induced antidepressant-like behavior.
	Behaviors were reduced via germ-free or antibiotic-induced depletion of microbiota, which can be reversed with the restoration of the intestinal microbiota.
	Behaviors were induced in germ-free maternal separation mice when non–maternal separation microbiota was transferred and modified by the colonic environment of the maternal separation mice.
	Fecal microbiota transplantation from patients with depression to microbiota-depleted rats induced anxiety- and depression-like behavior.
Nociceptive response	Antibiotic-induced disruption of gut microbiota during the postnatal period was associated with increased visceral sensitivity in adulthood.
	Reduced hypernociception was associated with increased IL-10 on stimulation and was reversible by anti-IL-10 antibody treatment.
	Lactobacillus increased expression of μ opioid and cannabinoid receptors in intestinal epithelial cells and modulated gastrointestinal analgesic functions.

TABLE 14–3. Role of gut microbiome in brain and behavior *(continued)*

Brain and behavioral changes	Findings
Nociceptive response *(continued)*	*L. farciminis* produced antinociceptive effects, including prevention of stress-induced hypersensitivity, increase in colonic paracellular permeability, and colonocyte myosin light chain phosphorylation.
	L. reuteri prevented hyperexcitability of colonic dorsal root ganglion neurons on harmful stimuli and increased the excitability of colonic after-hyperpolarization neurons.
Feeding behavior, taste preference, and metabolic consequences	Increased caloric intake and fat preference and decreased satiation signaling were observed in gut microbiota–depleted mice.
	Deficiency in toll-like receptor 5 was associated with hyperphagia and typical symptoms of metabolic syndrome.
	L. johnsonii La1 was associated with decrease in blood pressure by altering autonomic neurotransmission via the central histaminergic nerves and suprachiasmatic nucleus.
Brain neurochemistry	Altered cortical and hippocampal brain-derived neurotrophic factor levels were observed.
	Reduced hippocampal 5-HT_{1A} receptor expression was observed.
	Increased striatal monoamine turnover and reduced synaptic plasticity gene expression were observed.

Note. These findings are summarized by Bercik et al. (2012), Cryan and Dinan (2012), Mayer et al. (2014, 2015), and Vuong and Hsiao (2017).
Abbreviations. 5-HT_{1A} =serotonin type 1A; IL=interleukin.

Autism Spectrum Disorder

The wide-ranging and variable core symptoms of autism spectrum disorder include difficulty with social and communicative behavior, repetitive behavior, and restricted interests (see Chapter 10, "Physical Exercise in the Management of Autism Spectrum Disorders"). Often, associated comorbidities include intellectual disability, sleep disruption, feeding difficulty, anxiety, and gastrointestinal symptoms. The prevalence of gastrointestinal symptoms is 9%–90% (Vuong and Hsiao 2017), and children affected by autism spectrum disorder are nearly eight times more likely to have at least one gastrointestinal symptom (Chaidez et al. 2014). Moreover, gastrointestinal symptom severity is strongly correlated with severity of autism spectrum disorder symptoms. These symptoms are also highly correlated with anxiety and sensory hyperresponsiveness conditions modulated by gut microbiota in preclinical models (Vuong and Hsiao 2017). Gut dysbiosis is an increasingly documented finding in patients with autism spectrum disorder, but results from different studies are highly variable, and, similar to other clinical conditions, causality remains limited to intriguing, albeit untested, hypotheses. The promising recent results of Kang et al. (2017) showed that in a noncontrolled study, transfer of a standardized human gut microbiota led to reductions in gastrointestinal and behavioral symptoms, with a concordant maintenance of gut eubiosis, which persisted 8 weeks after the fecal microbial transplant. Randomized double-blind clinical trials are essential in order to verify a causative role of the gut microbiota as an effective therapeutic target for maintenance of symptoms related to autism spectrum disorder.

Obesity and Food Addiction

A dysregulation of feeding behavior plays an important role in the current obesity epidemic (Pedram et al. 2013). The gut microbiota plays an important role in the modulation of satiety signals (see earlier discussion in section "Signaling From the Gut Microbiota to the Brain") and eating behaviors (Arora et al. 2012). In preclinical studies, fecal transplantation from hyperphagic, obese mice to germ-free mice induced hyperphagic behavior and weight gain in the recipients (Turnbaugh et al. 2006; Vijay-Kumar et al. 2010). In addition, the gut microbiome has been associated with changes in brain microstructure in obesity, and distinct microbial-brain signatures were able to differentiate obese from lean subjects (Fernandez-Real et al. 2015). The gut microbiota is able to produce several neuroactive compounds, including several indole-containing metabolites and serotonin. The administration of probiotics modifies brain function (Tillisch et al. 2013) and even brain metabolites, including GABA and glutamate (Janik et al. 2016). A handful of studies point to a dramatic change in gut microbial composition after bariatric surgery (Damms-Machado et al. 2015; Furet et al. 2010; Graessler et al. 2013; Li et al. 2011; Zhang et al. 2009). Remarkably, fecal transplantation from subjects after bariatric surgery was able to transmit the weight loss effects of bariatric surgery to a germ-free, nonoperated recipient, inducing weight loss and reduced food intake (Tremaroli et al. 2015).

Parkinson's Disease

Although the clinical hallmarks of Parkinson's disease are motor deficits, there are numerous nonmotor symptoms that greatly compromise patients' quality of life. These nonmotor symptoms include problems related to dysfunctional autonomic and enteric nervous systems (e.g., slow transit constipation), sensory alterations, and psychiatric symptoms. The risk of developing Parkinson's disease increases with infrequency of bowel movement and greater constipation severity, and there is a significant comorbidity of Parkinson's and irritable bowel syndrome–like symptoms (Mertsalmi et al. 2017). Moreover, constipation is among the earliest features of Parkinson's disease, appearing up to 20 years before motor dysfunction (Fasano et al. 2015). Thus, early and new-onset gastrointestinal symptoms may be prodromal, making the gut microbiota a promising source of information for diagnosis, prognosis, and, potentially, pathogenesis. To date, clinical studies of gut microbiota in people with Parkinson's remain limited to characterizing an assemblage of differences against healthy control subjects, although some of the reported differences may actually be a consequence of impaired colonic transit. The first study to suggest a causality was that of Sampson et al. (2016), who demonstrated that the physical impairments in a rodent model were enhanced by microbiota from Parkinson's patients but not from healthy control subjects.

Epilepsy

There is currently limited scientific evidence supporting a causative role of the gut microbiome in epilepsy. One study reported significant differences in gut microbial architecture in epileptic infants (Xie et al. 2017). The reported therapeutic benefits of a ketogenic diet on patients with therapy-resistant epilepsy suggests a possible role of diet-induced changes in gut microbial function. After a week of the ketogenic diet treatment, 64% of epileptic infants showed obvious improvement, with a 50% decrease in seizure frequency (Xie et al. 2017).

Schizophrenia

Only one study has investigated the gut microbiome in people with schizophrenia and related psychotic disorders (Schwarz et al. 2018). The authors observed that compared with nonpsychiatric control subjects, patients with first-episode psychosis exhibited an altered gut microbial signature, and gut microbial composition was associated with severity of psychotic symptoms and global functioning in patients at the time of hospitalization for first-episode psychosis. First-episode patients who showed the greatest alterations in gut microbial composition at the time of hospitalization showed lower rates of disease remission at 1-year follow-up.

THERAPEUTIC INTERVENTIONS

Microbiome-targeted therapies include prebiotic, probiotic, and postbiotic interventions and dietary changes, which can directly modulate the gut microbiome, metabolic, immune, and hormonal systems that may be disturbed in psychiatric disorders (Figure 14–3). The best evidence to date supports a positive role of Mediterranean-type diets in terms of both prevention and treatment responses in depression (Jacka et al. 2017). To date, there is limited evidence for benefits of probiotic interventions (Wallace and Milev 2017) and no evidence from high-quality, controlled clinical trials to show significant benefits of postbiotic interventions in the form of dietary supplements mimicking gut microbial products.

Depression

Associations between healthy dietary patterns and a reduced prevalence of and risk for depression and anxiety have been reported in several randomized controlled trials (Opie et al. 2015). Results from the large European Prevención con Dieta Mediterránea (PREDIMED) study (Sánchez-Villegas et al. 2013) showed a strong trend toward a reduced risk for incident depression for individuals randomly assigned to a Mediterranean diet rich in plant-based foods and high in polyphenols and omega-3 fatty acids. Similarly, adhering to a Mediterranean-type diet with fish oil for 3 months decreased depression scores and increased mental health quality of life in people with self-reported depression (Parletta et al. 2017), and higher adherence to a vegetable-based dietary pattern or Mediterranean-type diets was positively associated with high measures of psychological resilience among 10,812 people in southern Italy (Bonaccio et al. 2018). In addition, dietary counseling greatly improved diet score while decreasing depression symptoms in people experiencing a major depressive episode (Jacka et al. 2017).

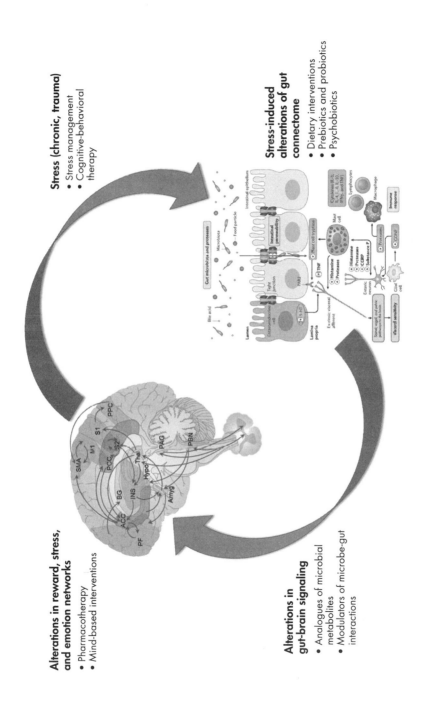

FIGURE 14–3. Therapeutic targets within the brain-gut microbiome (BGM) axis (*previous page*).

Stress-induced changes in the gut connectome result in the production of microbial metabolites and other signaling molecules that can signal back to the brain, modulating specific brain networks. Such stress-induced brain modulation via the BGM axis is likely involved in several psychiatric disorders. Possible targets for therapeutic interventions at different levels of the BGM axis are shown in the bullet points.

Abbreviations. ACC=nucleus accumbens; Amyg=amygdala; BG=basal ganglia; CDNF=cerebral dopamine neurotrophic factor; Hypo=hypothalamus; IfNγ=interferon gamma; interleukin; INS=insula; PAG=periaqueductal gray; PBN=parabrachial nuclei; PF=prefrontal cortex; PPC=posterior parietal cortex; M1=primary motor cortex; S1=primary somatosensory cortex; S2=secondary somatosensory cortex; SMA=supplementary motor area; Thal=thalamus; TNF=tumor necrosis factor.

Source. Enck P, Aziz Q, Barbara G, et al: "Irritable Bowel Syndrome." *Nature Reviews Disease Primers* 2:16,014, 2016 and Mayer EA, Labus JS, Tillisch K, et al: "Towards a Systems View of IBS." *Nature Reviews Gastroenterology and Hepatology* 12(10):592–605, 2015. Adapted with permission from Springer Nature. Copyright ©2016, 2015.

Schizophrenia, Epilepsy, and Alzheimer's Disease

Some researchers have speculated that the unhealthy dietary intake (especially high fat and low fiber) that is characteristic of many people with schizophrenia may result in gut microbial imbalance or dysbiosis, increased intestinal permeability, and systemic low-grade immune activation (Henderson et al. 2006). However, a direct beneficial effect of dietary changes in schizophrenia has not been established. In therapy-refractory epilepsy, some evidence suggests benefit from a ketogenic diet (Nei et al. 2014), and on the basis of mouse experiments (Olson et al. 2018), this beneficial effect may be mediated by the gut microbiome. High adherence to a Mediterranean DASH Intervention for Neurodegenerative Delay (MIND) diet, which is similar in composition to the Mediterranean diet, has been shown to reduce the risk of cognitive decline (Morris et al. 2015).

Maternal and early life nutrition is also emerging as a determinant of later mental health outcomes in children, and severe macronutrient deficiencies during crucial developmental periods have long been implicated in the pathogenesis of both depressive and psychotic disorders. However, a mediating role of the gut microbiome in these dietary benefits has not been established.

Case Example

Letitia is a 40-year-old woman with a history of mild constipation and recurring episodes of lower abdominal pain. According to her mother, she was delivered by cesarean section and was formula fed. Because of recurrent respiratory tract infections, she had received at least four courses of antibiotics by age 3 years.

During the past 2 years, Letitia has had chronically recurring sinus infections that were repeatedly treated with broad-spectrum antibiotics. During the course of antibiotics, she developed more frequent, loose bowel movements. She also had been given a diagnosis of panic attacks and more recently had noticed an increase in her general anxiety level. The intake of a probiotic for 10 days resulted in the complete resolution of her gastrointestinal symptoms as well as an improvement of her anxiety symptoms.

Letitia's psychiatrist encouraged her to switch to a traditional Mediterranean diet, high in plant-based foods; to regularly consume a variety of naturally fermented foods, such as sauerkraut, kimchi, and yogurt; and to continue to take her probiotic for at least 1 year. The goal of these dietary measures was to increase the diversity of Letitia's gut microbiota, which may have been compromised during her early life experiences, including the repeated administration of antibiotics. Letitia also received instruction in the practice of abdominal breathing and mindfulness-based stress reduction. The combined therapeutic approach resulted in a more than 60% reduction in both gastrointestinal and anxiety symptoms, and Letitia rarely required an as-needed clonazepam dose.

CONCLUSION

On the basis of available data, the emerging BGM science has the potential to improve conventional therapies for several psychiatric disorders. Although animal experimental studies suggest a possible therapeutic role for certain probiotics (psychobiotics), well-controlled clinical trials in humans are needed to confirm the therapeutic value of currently available microbiome-targeted therapies. Several ongoing clinical trials are evaluating the role of diet in the treatment of depression and degenerative brain disorders, and such interventions may be useful as prophylactic or adjuvant therapies to existing pharmacological treatments.

DISCUSSION QUESTIONS

1. What are the main channels of communication between the gut microbiota and the brain?
2. What role does the interaction between the brain, the gut, and the gut microbiome play in psychiatric conditions?
3. As a practicing clinician, how do you aim to introduce and integrate your knowledge of the significance of a disrupted gut-brain axis in psychiatric disorders?

RECOMMENDED READINGS

Cryan JF, Dinan TG: Mind-altering microorganisms: the impact of the gut microbiota on brain and behaviour. Nat Rev Neurosci 13(10):701–712, 2012

Fung TC, Olson CA, Hsiao EY: Interactions between the microbiota, immune and nervous systems in health and disease. Nat Neurosci 20(2):145–155, 2017

Martin CR, Osadchiy V, Kalani A, et al: The brain-gut-microbiome axis. Cell Mol Gastroenterol Hepatol 6(2):133–146, 2018

Mayer EA: Gut feelings: the emerging biology of gut-brain communication. Nat Rev Neurosci 12(8):453–466, 2011

Mayer EA, Knight R, Mazmanian SK, et al: Gut microbes and the brain: paradigm shift in neuroscience. J Neurosci 34(46):15490–15496, 2014

REFERENCES

Arora T, Loo RL, Anastasovska J, et al: Differential effects of two fermentable carbohydrates on central appetite regulation and body composition. PLoS One 7(8):e43263, 2012 22952656

Bercik P, Collins SM, Verdu EF: Microbes and the gut-brain axis. Neurogastroenterol Motil 24(5):405–413, 2012 22404222

Bonaccio M, Di Castelnuovo A, Costanzo S, et al: Mediterranean-type diet is associated with higher psychological resilience in a general adult population: findings from the Moli-sani study. Eur J Clin Nutr 72(1):154–160, 2018 28952609

Chaidez V, Hansen RL, Hertz-Picciotto I: Gastrointestinal problems in children with autism, developmental delays or typical development. J Autism Dev Disord 44(5):1117-1127, 2014 24193577

Cryan JF, Dinan TG: Mind-altering microorganisms: the impact of the gut microbiota on brain and behaviour. Nat Rev Neurosci 13(10):701–712, 2012 22968153

Damms-Machado A, Mitra S, Schollenberger AE, et al: Effects of surgical and dietary weight loss therapy for obesity on gut microbiota composition and nutrient absorption. BioMed Res Int 2015:806248, 2015 25710027

Diaz Heijtz R, Wang S, Anuar F, et al: Normal gut microbiota modulates brain development and behavior. Proc Natl Acad Sci USA 108(7):3047–3052, 2011 21282636

Dickerson F, Severance E, Yolken R: The microbiome, immunity, and schizophrenia and bipolar disorder. Brain Behav Immun 62:46–52, 2017 28003152

Erny D, Hrabe de Angelis AL, Jaitin D, et al: Host microbiota constantly control maturation and function of microglia in the CNS. Nat Neurosci 18(7):965–977, 2015 26030851

Fasano A, Visanji NP, Liu LWC, et al: Gastrointestinal dysfunction in Parkinson's disease. Lancet Neurol 14(6):625–639, 2015 25987282

Fernandez-Real JM, Serino M, Blasco G, et al: Gut microbiota interacts with brain microstructure and function. J Clin Endocrinol Metab 100(12):4505–4513, 2015 26445114

Fung TC, Olson CA, Hsiao EY: Interactions between the microbiota, immune and nervous systems in health and disease. Nat Neurosci 20(2):145–155, 2017 28092661

Furet JP, Kong LC, Tap J, et al: Differential adaptation of human gut microbiota to bariatric surgery-induced weight loss: links with metabolic and low-grade inflammation markers. Diabetes 59(12):3049–3057, 2010 20876719

Graessler J, Qin Y, Zhong H, et al: Metagenomic sequencing of the human gut microbiome before and after bariatric surgery in obese patients with type 2 diabetes: correlation with inflammatory and metabolic parameters. Pharmacogenomics J 13(6):514–522, 2013 23032991

Henderson DC, Borba CP, Daley TB, et al: Dietary intake profile of patients with schizophrenia. Ann Clin Psychiatry 18(2):99–105, 2006 16754415

Holzer P, Farzi A: Neuropeptides and the microbiota-gut-brain axis. Adv Exp Med Biol 817:195–219, 2014 24997035

Hughes DT, Sperandio V: Inter-kingdom signalling: communication between bacteria and their hosts. Nat Rev Microbiol 6(2):111–120, 2008 18197168

Jacka FN, O'Neil A, Opie R, et al: A randomised controlled trial of dietary improvement for adults with major depression (the "SMILES" trial). BMC Med 15(1):23, 2017 28137247

Janik R, Thomason LAM, Stanisz AM, et al: Magnetic resonance spectroscopy reveals oral Lactobacillus promotion of increases in brain GABA, N-acetyl aspartate and glutamate. Neuroimage 125:988–995, 2016 26577887

Kang DW, Adams JB, Gregory AC, et al: Microbiota transfer therapy alters gut ecosystem and improves gastrointestinal and autism symptoms: an open-label study. Microbiome 5(1):10, 2017 28122648

Kelly JR, Clarke G, Cryan JF, Dinan TG: Brain-gut-microbiota axis: challenges for translation in psychiatry. Ann Epidemiol 26(5):366–372, 2016a 27005587

Kelly JR, Borre Y, O' Brien C, et al: Transferring the blues: depression-associated gut microbiota induces neurobehavioural changes in the rat. J Psychiatr Res 82:109–118, 2016b 27491067

Kim DY, Camilleri M: Serotonin: a mediator of the brain-gut connection. Am J Gastroenterol 95(10):2698–2709, 2000 11051338

Li JV, Ashrafian H, Bueter M, et al: Metabolic surgery profoundly influences gut microbial-host metabolic cross-talk. Gut 60(9):1214–1223, 2011 21572120

Lurie I, Yang YX, Haynes K, et al: Antibiotic exposure and the risk for depression, anxiety, or psychosis: a nested case-control study. J Clin Psychiatry 76(11):1522–1528, 2015 26580313

Maes M, Kubera M, Leunis JC: The gut-brain barrier in major depression: intestinal mucosal dysfunction with an increased translocation of LPS from gram negative enterobacteria (leaky gut) plays a role in the inflammatory pathophysiology of depression. Neuroendocrinol Lett 29(1):117–124, 2008 18283240

Marin IA, Goertz JE, Ren T, et al: Microbiota alteration is associated with the development of stress-induced despair behavior. Sci Rep 7:43859, 2017 28266612

Mayer EA: Gut feelings: the emerging biology of gut-brain communication. Nat Rev Neurosci 12(8):453–466, 2011 21750565

Mayer EA, Knight R, Mazmanian SK, et al: Gut microbes and the brain: paradigm shift in neuroscience. J Neurosci 34(46):15490–15496, 2014 25392516

Mayer EA, Tillisch K, Gupta A: Gut/brain axis and the microbiota. J Clin Invest 125(3):926–938, 2015 25689247

Mertsalmi TH, Aho VTE, Pereira PAB, et al: More than constipation—bowel symptoms in Parkinson's disease and their connection to gut microbiota. Eur J Neurol 24(11):1375–1383, 2017 28891262

Morris MC, Tangney CC, Wang Y, et al: MIND diet associated with reduced incidence of Alzheimer's disease. Alzheimers Dement 11(9):1007–1014, 2015 25681666

Nei M, Ngo L, Sirven JI, Sperling MR: Ketogenic diet in adolescents and adults with epilepsy. Seizure 23(6):439–442, 2014 24675110

Olson CA, Vuong HE, Yano JM, et al: The gut microbiota mediates the anti-seizure effects of the ketogenic diet. Cell 174(2):497, 2018 30007420

Opie RS, O'Neil A, Itsiopoulos C, et al: The impact of whole-of-diet interventions on depression and anxiety: a systematic review of randomised controlled trials. Public Health Nutr 18(11):2074–2093, 2015 25465596

Parletta N, Zarnowiecki D, Cho J, et al: A Mediterranean-style dietary intervention supplemented with fish oil improves diet quality and mental health in people with depression: a randomized controlled trial (HELFIMED). Nutr Neurosci (Dec 7):1–14, 2017 29215971

Pedram P, Wadden D, Amini P, et al: Food addiction: its prevalence and significant association with obesity in the general population. PLoS One 8(9):e74832, 2013 24023964

Rhee SH, Pothoulakis C, Mayer EA: Principles and clinical implications of the brain-gut-enteric microbiota axis. Nat Rev Gastroenterol Hepatol 6(5):306–314, 2009 19404271

Ruddick JP, Evans AK, Nutt DJ, et al: Tryptophan metabolism in the central nervous system: medical implications. Expert Rev Mol Med 8(20):1–27, 2006 16942634

Sampson TR, Debelius JW, Thron T, et al: Gut microbiota regulate motor deficits and neuroinflammation in a model of Parkinson's disease. Cell 167(6):1469–1480, 2016 27912057

Sánchez-Villegas A, Martínez-González MA, Estruch R, et al: Mediterranean dietary pattern and depression: the PREDIMED randomized trial. BMC Med 11:208, 2013 24229349

Schwarcz R, Bruno JP, Muchowski PJ, et al: Kynurenines in the mammalian brain: when physiology meets pathology. Nat Rev Neurosci 13(7):465–477, 2012 22678511

Schwarz E, Maukonen J, Hyytiäinen T, et al: Analysis of microbiota in first episode psychosis identifies preliminary associations with symptom severity and treatment response. Schizophr Res 192:398–403, 2018 28442250

Steenbergen L, Sellaro R, van Hemert S, et al: A randomized controlled trial to test the effect of multispecies probiotics on cognitive reactivity to sad mood. Brain Behav Immun 48:258–264, 2015 25862297

Tillisch K, Labus J, Kilpatrick L, et al: Consumption of fermented milk product with probiotic modulates brain activity. Gastroenterology 144(7):1394–1401, 2013 23474283

Tremaroli V, Karlsson F, Werling M, et al: Roux-en y gastric bypass and vertical banded gastroplasty induce long-term changes on the human gut microbiome contributing to fat mass regulation. Cell Metab 22(2):228–238, 2015 26244932

Turnbaugh PJ, Ley RE, Mahowald MA, et al: An obesity-associated gut microbiome with increased capacity for energy harvest. Nature 444(7122):1027–1031, 2006 17183312

Vijay-Kumar M, Aitken JD, Carvalho FA, et al: Metabolic syndrome and altered gut microbiota in mice lacking Toll-like receptor 5. Science 328(5975):228–231, 2010 20203013

Vuong HE, Hsiao EY: Emerging roles for the gut microbiome in autism spectrum disorder. Biol Psychiatry 81(5):411–423, 2017 27773355

Wallace CJK, Milev R: The effects of probiotics on depressive symptoms in humans: a systematic review. Ann Gen Psychiatry 16:14, 2017 28239408

Xie G, Zhou Q, Qiu CZ, et al: Ketogenic diet poses a significant effect on imbalanced gut microbiota in infants with refractory epilepsy. World J Gastroenterol 23(33):6164–6171, 2017 28970732

Zhang H, DiBaise JK, Zuccolo A, et al: Human gut microbiota in obesity and after gastric bypass. Proc Natl Acad Sci USA 106(7):2365–2370, 2009 19164560

Zheng P, Zeng B, Zhou C, et al: Gut microbiome remodeling induces depressive-like behaviors through a pathway mediated by the host's metabolism. Mol Psychiatry 21(6):786–796, 2016 27067014

CHAPTER 15

Managing Sleep for Optimal Performance, Brain Function, and Mental Health

Scott Kutscher, M.D.

Fiona Barwick, Ph.D.

KEY POINTS

- Homeostatic sleep drive, or process S, accumulates the longer we are awake and the more active we are during the day. High sleep drive helps us fall asleep more quickly and stay asleep more soundly.

- Circadian rhythms, or process C, fluctuate across 24 hours, helping us stay awake during the day as sleep drive increases and stay asleep during the night as sleep drive decreases. They are influenced by zeitgebers, including food, activity, and especially light.

- Healthy adult sleep is characterized by multiple cycles in and out of lighter and deeper stages of sleep throughout the night, with non–rapid eye movement deep sleep occurring predominantly in the first half of the night and longer periods of rapid eye movement sleep occurring in the second half.

- Insomnia and poor sleep hygiene are the most common sleep problems in psychiatric disorders, but hypersomnia, circadian dysregulation, obstructive sleep apnea, and restless legs syndrome also occur. Insomnia and poor sleep hygiene are best addressed using cognitive-behavioral therapy (CBT) techniques.

- The most effective CBT techniques for improving insomnia teach people to spend only as much time in bed as they typically sleep (time-in-bed restriction) and to sleep only in bed and do wakeful activities elsewhere (bed reassociation training).

- Practicing strategies to calm the mind and relax the body will smooth the path to sleep far better than blunt efforts to try to sleep, which are ineffectual and counterproductive because they activate the mind and body and block the path to sleep.

Sleep is critical for maintaining healthy biological function and optimal performance. Sleep may be disrupted for many reasons—sleep disorders such as insomnia or sleep apnea, medical conditions such as chronic pain or diabetes, and psychiatric problems such as depression or bipolar disorder. In fact, sleep disturbance is associated with almost all psychiatric disorders and their pharmacological treatments. Disrupted sleep can lead to impaired cognition, poorer athletic performance, dysregulated mood, increased cardiovascular disease, altered metabolism, lower immune functioning, and greater incidence of cancer. In order to promote healthy sleep, it is important to understand the processes involved in normal sleep, know how to identify the presence of disordered sleep, and learn the techniques for correcting the physiological and psychological factors that contribute to abnormal sleep. Although medications and devices can resolve some sleep disorders, effective therapies for improving sleep often rely on cognitive-behavioral techniques. These techniques not only reduce the medication burden so common in psychiatric illness but also promote healthy behaviors that work synergistically to increase energy, enhance mood, strengthen coping, and improve sleep.

NORMAL ADULT SLEEP

Normal adult sleep can be described by the overall structure of sleep and the processes that drive sleep. These processes and their interaction determine when we naturally feel sleepy or wakeful. They also affect daily fluctuations in alertness, metabolism, and performance. These processes can become disrupted or degraded in abnormal sleep and so are often the targets of therapy to improve sleep.

Process S

The principle behind *process S*—also called the homeostatic sleep drive is simple: we accumulate a sleep drive, or sleep debt, as we stay awake. The longer we stay awake, the more sleep drive we build, until it reaches the point where it overwhelms our waking systems, driving us to sleep. Process S is like a roller coaster, accumulating potential energy on its upward climb and then expending it during the thrilling downward plunge. Process S is associated with an increase in various metabolites, most notably adenosine. After reaching a critical level, adenosine activates the primary sleep center in the hypothalamus, the ventrolateral preoptic nucleus, and initiates the process of sleep. Caffeine, the world's most popular exogenous substance, suppresses process S by blocking adenosine receptors.

Process C

Despite the buildup of sleep drive, most people do not feel linearly sleepier during the day. Instead, feelings of sleepiness vary because of the actions of *process C,* the circadian process of sleep and wakefulness. Process C is regulated by the suprachiasmatic nucleus, a pair of nuclei situated directly above the optic chiasm in the hypothalamus. It is marked by variations in melatonin, which is released in the pineal gland and regulated by light and core body temperature. These markers are inversely correlated, so low melatonin and high core body temperature indicate increased alertness, whereas high melatonin and low core body temperature denote greater sleepiness. Melatonin reaches its nadir and core body temperature peaks in the late afternoon and early evening, inhibiting process S and allowing us to stay awake for prime-time television. Melatonin levels start to rise, and core body temperature starts to fall, when darkness descends because light no longer suppresses melatonin release. This release disinhibits process S and enables sleep onset. Melatonin levels continue to rise during the night, peaking 2–3 hours before final waking and helping to promote continued sleep in the early morning hours, when process S is not as strong. Process C continues to fluctuate during the day and can be influenced or augmented by multiple factors called *zeitgebers*, including food, exercise, and, most profoundly, light.

Sleep Architecture

Just as normal sleepiness is the product of multiple processes, healthy adult sleep is a dynamic system involving multiple neurotransmitters and brain regions. It is divided into rapid eye movement (REM) sleep and non–rapid eye movement (NREM) sleep. NREM sleep is further divided into stages N1, N2, and N3.

NREM sleep, despite being named for what it is not, makes up the majority of sleep, with N2 alone composing 50% of a normal night of sleep. The predominant neurotransmitter during NREM sleep is γ-aminobutyric acid (GABA), and its increase is associated with progressively slower brain activity, from theta range during N1 into delta range during N3. There is a correlated increase in parasympathetic activity, with metabolism, blood pressure, and heart rate all dropping significantly, a phenomenon known as *dipping*.

REM sleep, or dream sleep, is mediated by acetylcholine in the reticular activating system and comprises brain activity in the theta or alpha range. Sympathetic tone is elevated relative to NREM sleep, including increased metabolism and greater variability in heart rate and blood pressure. To prevent enactment of dreams, there is general muscle paralysis, apart from phasic bursts of muscle activity such as the fast, lateral eye movements that give REM sleep its name.

A healthy adult will cycle through different sleep stages multiple times, starting in light N1, going through moderate N2 and deeper N3, and lightening again before entering REM for the first time, about 90 minutes after sleep onset. The process continues throughout the night, with four or five cycles on average during a single night. Deeper N3 sleep, or slow-wave sleep, occurs predominantly in the first half of the night, with progressively longer periods of REM sleep toward early morning. The architecture of sleep is relatively preserved across the adult lifespan, except for a marked reduction in N3 sleep.

ABNORMAL ADULT SLEEP

Addressing Common Sleep Problems

A comprehensive sleep history should be part of every mental health evaluation because sleep behaviors and symptoms often inform diagnosis. For example, a person who complains of excessive fatigue or sleepiness while allowing himself or herself only 4 hours of sleep a night would be treated differently from someone with the same complaint who is sleeping 10 hours. Sleep disorders are common, and their symptoms often overlap with psychiatric disorders. Someone who reports difficulty with memory and concentration may meet criteria for attention-deficit/hyperactivity disorder (ADHD), but further report by bed partners of loud snoring and witnessed gasping may suggest sleep apnea instead.

A full sleep history includes delineation of the sleep period or periods, estimation of sleep and wake times during these periods, description of behaviors or activities during sleep, and perceived impact on daytime performance or function. Because the historian is usually, well, asleep, supporting information from bed partners or housemates can be helpful. Validated surveys such as the Epworth Sleepiness Scale (Johns 1991), STOP-BANG survey (Chung et al. 2008), or Morningness-Eveningness Questionnaire (Horne and Östberg 1976) are readily available to assist in screening for sleep disorders. When more detailed measurement is required for diagnosis of specific sleep disorders, polysomnography is the gold standard, but additional tools available include ambulatory sleep monitoring, actigraphy, and sleep diaries.

Any co-occurring medical disorders that might be impacting sleep should also be identified and treated appropriately. Conditions that can lead to disrupted sleep include chronic pain, especially fibromyalgia and chronic fatigue; obesity, allergies, and chronic obstructive pulmonary disease, all of which can cause breathing difficulties at night; gastrointestinal distress, such as gastroesophageal reflux or irritable bowel syndrome; and other conditions such as late-stage diabetes and chronic kidney disease.

Insufficient Sleep

Much of what we know about the consequences of abnormal adult sleep is focused on sleep loss—either partial or complete. The American Academy of Sleep Medicine recommends at least 7 hours of sleep per night for optimal health and safety in otherwise healthy adults, but as many as 40% of U.S. adults are not meeting this goal (Watson et al. 2015). As sleep loss climbs, so does sleep burden from process S. Increased sleep burden leads to greater reported and measured sleepiness, slower reaction time, lapses in attention, poorer executive function, increased negative mood states, and even hallucinations after 3–4 days of total sleep deprivation (Durmer and Dinges 2005). Chronic partial sleep deprivation results in similar levels of impairment, often without conscious awareness. Besides impaired neurocognitive performance, total or partial sleep loss affects other organ systems, with cardiovascular and metabolic functioning exhibiting marked deterioration (Knutson et al. 2007). This adverse impact on mental and physical health highlights the need to prioritize sleep where possible so that essential sleep needs are met.

Insomnia

In contrast to the hypersomnolence caused by insufficient sleep, hyperarousal characterizes insomnia. Insomnia is one of the most common sleep disorders, with annual incidences in the United States estimated at 30% acute and 10% chronic insomnia (Ohayon 2002). Symptoms include difficulty with initiation and maintenance of sleep. Although perceived fatigue and associated impairment in daytime function are present, hypersomnolence is typically absent, and people with insomnia are unable to sleep despite opportunity. Insomnia can be a primary symptom, but it often co-occurs with a psychiatric or medical disorder. The Spielman model of insomnia (also known as the 3P behavioral model) theorizes predisposing factors that create risk for insomnia, a precipitating stressor or stressors that provoke acute insomnia, and perpetuating factors that lead to chronic insomnia (Spielman et al. 1987a). Cognitive-behavioral therapy (CBT) is the recommended treatment for insomnia (Qaseem et al. 2016) because it targets perpetuating factors and leads to significant and sustained improvement in 70%–80% of individuals who complete therapy. This therapy is effective even when insomnia co-occurs with psychiatric disorders such as depression, anxiety, and posttraumatic stress disorder (PTSD; Edinger et al. 2009), with some evidence suggesting that it can enhance psychiatric outcomes as well as improve sleep (Manber et al. 2008; Talbot et al. 2014).

Sleep-Disordered Breathing

Obstructive sleep apnea (OSA) is a breathing disorder in which repeated episodes of either partial (hypopneas) or complete (apneas) airway collapse occur during sleep. OSA is diagnosed by polysomnography or ambulatory monitoring when the combination of apneas and hypopneas, as measured by the apnea hypopnea index, is five or more per hour. OSA is highly prevalent in the general population, with up to 25% of men and 10% of women diagnosed with the disorder (Young et al. 1993). Although

OSA often is associated with obesity, upper airway anatomy can create genetic predisposition for sleep apnea in the absence of obesity in 50% of cases. Repetitive airway collapse can disrupt sleep, leading to chronic partial sleep deprivation, and decrease blood oxygen. It can also disrupt nearly every organ system through multiple pathways, especially cardiovascular, metabolic, neurocognitive, and hormonal systems. Mood symptoms are also common because of chronic sleep deprivation. Recommended treatment for OSA is positive airway pressure, which is effective in 95% of the individuals who use it as prescribed.

Circadian Rhythm Disorders

The constellation of circadian rhythm disorders can be explained by irregularities in process C. Natural circadian rhythms are slightly longer than 1 full day, so they must be entrained, or yoked, to the 24-hour clock by external cues, called zeitgebers. The most powerful zeitgeber is light, and its signal is sent to the suprachiasmatic nucleus via specialized melanopsin receptors in the retina, which are most sensitive to short wavelengths of blue-green light. When internal circadian rhythms are out of alignment with the external environment, a mismatch occurs between endogenous sleep-wake rhythms and desired or required sleep-wake schedules. This mismatch causes conflict with school and work schedules as well as social activities. For example, shift work disorder occurs when work schedules intrude on or overlap with natural sleep periods. Jet lag syndrome is a temporary dissociation between internal rhythms and external cues caused by crossing three or more time zones.

Delayed and advanced sleep phase disorders, in which process C is shifted later or earlier, are two sides of the same coin. In delayed sleep phase disorder, commonly seen in adolescence, process C is shifted later, so sleep phase may not start until early morning and may extend until afternoon. In advanced sleep phase disorder, which can occur in the elderly, process C is shifted earlier, so sleep phase begins in the late afternoon or early evening and ends in the early morning. If process C runs free because circadian rhythms are not entrained by zeitgebers, non-24-hour circadian disorder results, in which bedtime shifts later and later each night until the sleep period moves fully around the clock. This disorder usually occurs in individuals who are blind or whose melanopsin pathways have been injured or destroyed. If process C deteriorates or is destroyed, as in neurodegenerative conditions such as dementia, irregular sleep-wake disorder results, wherein sleep occurs erratically in short bouts throughout the day and night. Although rare, irregular sleep-wake disorder can also occur in psychotic disorders such as schizophrenia.

Restless Legs Syndrome

Restless legs syndrome (RLS) is the most common movement disorder and is diagnosed clinically with the presence of four distinct features: 1) an uncomfortable urge to move the legs that is 2) worse at rest and 3) worse in the evening and 4) relieved by movement. Patients with RLS often complain of insomnia, but further questions will show that sleep difficulties are tied directly to leg discomfort. RLS is often associated with low serum ferritin levels, which should be checked in every patient. It is also associated with periodic limb movements in sleep (PLMS), semirhythmic limb activity that can be identified on polysomnography. Despite the overlap, PLMS is clinically distinct and not a part of the diagnostic criteria for RLS in adults.

RLS has a higher prevalence in people with neuropathy and kidney failure as well as in pregnant women. It is also associated with certain psychiatric disorders, such as ADHD, possibly because low ferritin levels dysregulate dopaminergic pathways, where iron is a required cofactor for tyrosine hydroxylase in dopamine production (Cortese et al. 2005). RLS complicates management of psychiatric disorders, particularly depression, because medication classes used to treat depression (selective serotonin reuptake inhibitors [SSRIs], serotonin-norepinephrine reuptake inhibitors [SNRIs], tricyclic antidepressants [TCAs], and monoamine oxidase inhibitors) often exacerbate RLS symptoms and because medication classes used to treat RLS (dopamine agonists, low-dose opioids) can exacerbate psychiatric symptoms.

Case Example

Brandon, a 22-year-old college graduate, reports difficulty falling asleep and unrefreshing sleep on waking. In college he stayed up late studying and scheduled all his classes in the afternoon. Now he needs to be awake at 6 A.M. to commute to his job. Despite getting into bed as early as 9 P.M. to ensure sufficient sleep time, Brandon does not fall asleep until 2 or 3 A.M. He finds himself increasingly anxious about how lack of sleep is affecting his performance at work and has started using alcohol to fall asleep. On a recent family vacation, however, he reverted to his college pattern of going to bed at 4 A.M. and waking at noon, and he felt completely rested and refreshed.

Delayed sleep phase disorders are common among young adults and are characterized by sleep schedules that are significantly later than normal. These individuals appear to have sleep onset insomnia, but the issue self-resolves when they can sleep in their natural sleep window. Although anxiety and substance use are often present, they may be secondary to the sleep complaint.

ABNORMAL ADULT SLEEP IN PSYCHIATRIC DISORDERS

Overview of Common Sleep Problems

Changes in sleep—including changes in sleep need, sleep consolidation, total sleep time, and sleep architecture—are associated with almost all psychiatric disorders as well as their pharmacological treatments. This strong association highlights the need to screen for sleep problems in people with psychiatric disorders, especially because psychiatric conditions commonly coexist. The causal relationship between sleep and psychiatric disorders is likely bidirectional and complex, with psychiatric disorders causing or contributing to disturbed sleep, and insufficient or disrupted sleep increasing risk for and exacerbation of psychiatric problems. Interestingly, studies of normal and abnormal sleep show that neural and stress response systems involved in mood and anxiety regulation are also involved in sleep-wake regulation, pointing to possible shared etiological pathways. Effective management of psychiatric disorders should include empirically supported treatments for reported sleep complaints. Education about normal sleep, behavioral techniques that teach healthy sleep habits, and cognitive techniques that correct unhelpful behaviors or beliefs around sleep can support better sleep and management of psychiatric symptoms.

Major Depressive Disorder

Disrupted sleep—including insomnia, hypersomnia, and OSA—is so widespread in depression that it is one of the diagnostic criteria. Subjective and objective sleep disturbances precede and predict future depressive episodes, including postpartum depression. Sleep problems are further exacerbated because depressed individuals tend to spend more time in bed, which decreases sleep drive and lowers sleep quality. Objective changes in sleep architecture have been identified, such as decreased N3 or slow-wave sleep, reduced REM sleep latency, and increased REM sleep time. Not surprisingly, most antidepressant medications suppress REM sleep and delay its onset. Although not specific enough to function as biomarkers, these sleep abnormalities can persist after remission, raising the possibility that sleep disturbance might represent a biological susceptibility to depression (Minkel et al. 2017).

The effects of antidepressant medications can compound sleep disturbance in depression. For example, TCAs and the atypical antidepressants trazodone and mirtazapine are sedating, whereas SSRIs, SNRIs, and the atypical antidepressant bupropion are usually activating. TCAs and SSRIs may also precipitate or exacerbate RLS. To counter these effects, sedating medications should be taken at bedtime, whereas activating medications should be taken in the morning.

Sleep complaints often remain after other depressive symptoms resolve, and their persistence predicts increased severity and recurrence of depression. CBT is an empirically supported treatment for mild to moderate depression and can be delivered in combination with CBT for insomnia to achieve synergistic benefit for patients (Asarnow et al. 2014). Similarly, bright-light therapy has proven effective for seasonal depression and hypersomnia, and proper treatment of OSA can ameliorate depression symptoms. For example, an individual diagnosed with depression who is spending 10 hours in bed but reports sleeping only 6 hours a night can be encouraged to gradually reduce time in bed to 7 hours to boost sleep drive and increase level of daytime activities, especially social and physical activities that improve mood (see section "Match Sleep Opportunity to Sleep Ability"). Phototherapy for 45 minutes in the morning after awakening might also be recommended to improve mood and enhance alertness. Interestingly, half of individuals with major depression show rapid symptom improvement after total or partial sleep deprivation, but this technique has adverse effects, and improvements dissipate quickly after recovery sleep.

Bipolar Disorder

Sleep problems are as common in people with bipolar depression as in people with unipolar depression and extend beyond insomnia and hypersomnia to include irregular sleep patterns, delayed sleep phase, and reduced sleep need (Harvey et al. 2017). Delayed sleep phase and circadian dysregulation often result from irregular, inappropriate, or inadequate timing of zeitgebers that regulate circadian rhythms, such as exposure to light, engagement in activities, and scheduling of meals and social events. Sleep disturbances in bipolar disorder worsen current symptoms, increase risk for onset and relapse, and continue between episodes. They likely contribute to the disinhibition of mood, reward, and attention neural circuitry that characterizes bipolar disorder. For example, sleep deprivation can trigger manic or hypomanic episodes, in contrast to the symptom improvement that occurs with unipolar depression. Changes in sleep architecture with bipolar disorder are similar to those seen in major depression, but findings are less consistent.

The timing of medications used to treat bipolar disorder is important. Antidepressants for unipolar depression are also used in bipolar depression and can have similar activating effects (see subsection "Major Depressive Disorder"), with TCAs and SSRIs more likely to precipitate manic episodes. Atypical antipsychotics prescribed specifically for bipolar disorder that have sedating effects, such as quetiapine and olanzapine, should be taken at bedtime. Mood stabilizers such as lamotrigine that affect circadian function by delaying sleep onset should be taken in the morning. As with depression, CBT techniques can work synergistically to improve bipolar symptoms and sleep complaints. In fact, a modified CBT protocol designed to address symptoms of bipolar disorder, insomnia, and circadian dysregulation simultaneously was recently piloted with reported success (Kaplan and Harvey 2013).

Anxiety Disorder

As with other psychiatric disorders, subjective sleep disturbance is included as a diagnostic criterion for generalized anxiety because it occurs so frequently (Krystal et al. 2017). Up to 80% of individuals with anxiety have symptoms consistent with insomnia (Taylor et al. 2005). Sleep problems typically start with the onset of anxiety, but anxiety can also disrupt sleep directly, as in nocturnal panic attacks. These disorders may share causal pathways because individuals with anxiety or insomnia show increased activation in wake-promoting neurotransmitter systems. To date, however, no abnormalities in sleep architecture have been discovered with anxiety.

CBT is the recommended first-line treatment for all anxiety disorders—including panic disorder and generalized anxiety—as well as insomnia. In fact, integrating CBT techniques to address both disorders has been explored (Stanley et al. 2004). Education about normal sleep and healthy sleep habits, along with correction of any maladaptive behaviors or beliefs around sleep, can help to reduce anxiety symptoms and improve sleep. Hence, individuals diagnosed with anxiety often benefit from sleep education; relaxation strategies; and cognitive techniques that limit checking the time at night, encourage the challenging and reframing of inaccurate and unhelpful beliefs about sleep, and cultivate a mindful approach to the experience of being awake at night (see subsections "Relax the Body" and "Calm the Mind" later in the chapter). Although benzodiazepines are often used to treat anxiety disorders because they reduce sleep onset latency, they also suppress REM and N3 sleep.

Posttraumatic Stress Disorder

Subjective sleep disturbance is pervasive in people with PTSD and is one of the diagnostic criteria (Krystal et al. 2017). Sleep problems include difficulty falling and staying asleep (90%) and nightmares (70%), symptoms that reflect the trauma-related domains of reexperiencing and hypervigilance. Nightmares can be exacerbated by OSA, which occurs more often in this population. PTSD should also be differentiated from REM behavior disorder (RBD), a parasomnia in which the normal muscle atonia typical of REM sleep is lost and dreams, often with violent content, are "acted out." Despite these subjective reports of sleep disturbance in PTSD, the only consistent abnormalities in sleep architecture relate to REM sleep, including greater REM density and more frequent transitions from REM sleep.

Individuals with PTSD should be carefully screened for sleep disorders, especially insomnia, nightmares, sleep apnea, and RBD. Identified sleep problems should be treated appropriately because sleep complaints can persist even after successful treatment of PTSD. As noted earlier in the subsection "Insomnia," the most effective treatment for insomnia is CBT. PTSD-related nightmares are better addressed with a validated protocol such as imagery rehearsal therapy (Nadorff et al. 2014). Imagery rehearsal therapy, in which an individual "rescripts" an unpleasant dream to make it more positive and empowering, is an empirically supported treatment that requires practicing the rescripted dream daily but allows individuals to reduce nightmare frequency and/or severity without medication (Morganthaler et al. 2018). Prazosin or clonidine can also help reduce the frequency and severity of nightmares, but other commonly prescribed medications, such as SSRIs, should be used more cautiously because they can be activating and also initiate or exacerbate RBD symptoms.

Schizophrenia Spectrum Disorders

Schizophrenia is associated with various sleep disturbances, including sleeplessness, insomnia, hypersomnia, nightmares, irregular sleep-wake patterns, and circadian dysregulation of all types (Benson and Feinberg 2017; Wulff et al. 2012). Circadian dysregulation may reflect maladaptive sleep-wake behaviors, diminished exposure to effective zeitgebers, and/or changes in melatonin secretion. Worsening sleep predicts aggravation or recurrence of psychotic symptoms as well as impaired coping. Objectively, individuals with schizophrenia show difficulty with sleep onset and maintenance, decreased total sleep time, and reduced REM sleep. Because of circadian dysregulation, individuals with schizophrenia often benefit from efforts to establish a more regular sleep-wake schedule and to support this schedule with additional circadian cues, such as more regular meals and activities both physical and social (see later subsection "Establish and Maintain Good Sleep Hygiene").

Appropriate medication is the cornerstone of treatment for schizophrenia. Antipsychotics, both first and second generation, can improve sleep by reducing time to fall asleep or time awake at night and by increasing total sleep time. However, clozapine and olanzapine can increase nighttime sleep duration to problematic levels (12–14 hours), possibly due to their effects on serotonin, dopamine, norepinephrine, and GABA. Antipsychotic medications can also induce RLS and PLMS as well as parasomnias such as sleepwalking because they work by lowering dopamine levels. CBT techniques are an important adjunctive therapy in this population because they address inaccurate beliefs about sleep and maladaptive sleep-wake behaviors. In fact, a modified CBT-insomnia protocol has been developed to target the varied sleep problems that occur in people with schizophrenia (Freeman et al. 2015).

Attention-Deficit/Hyperactivity Disorder

ADHD is commonly diagnosed in childhood and persists into adulthood in two-thirds of individuals (Cortese and Lecendreux 2017). Sleep disturbance was originally a criterion for the disorder and has reappeared in recent guidelines as a differential diagnostic for sleep apnea or delayed sleep phase. Up to 70% of children with ADHD experience sleep problems—including poor sleep habits, insomnia, delayed sleep phase, sleep apnea, PLMS, and RLS—but prevalence in adults is unclear. The activating effects of stimulant medications used to treat ADHD further complicate the clinical picture. Sleep disorders should be carefully screened, and empirically supported treatments for OSA, RLS, and insomnia should be used where indicated. Evidence for treatment of delayed sleep phase is limited, but phototherapy (Rybak et al. 2006) and melatonin may be helpful (Auger et al. 2015).

Autism Spectrum Disorders

Sleep disturbance is common in children with autism spectrum disorders, with up to 80% experiencing sleep problems, especially sleep onset insomnia (Veatch et al. 2015). Its continuation and course in adulthood are less clear, although insomnia remains common (Goldman et al. 2017). Sleep problems exacerbate symptoms of autism spectrum disorder, worsen daily functioning, and negatively impact family dynamics. Etiology is multifactorial, with neurological (abnormalities in melatonin synthesis), medical and psychiatric (vulnerability to seizures and ADHD), and behavioral (hypersensitivity to stimuli, poor sleep habits) contributors. Behavioral symptoms, such as insensitivity to social cues and preference for electronics, may increase risk for circadian dysregulation. Parasomnia may also be more common in people with autism spectrum disorders, but susceptibility to other sleep disorders such as OSA or RLS is unclear. Sleep education and sleep hygiene are recommended first-line approaches for sleep problems among people with autism spectrum disorders, along with proper treatment of medical and psychiatric conditions that impact sleep. Providers and caretakers should also be aware of how prescribed medications may affect sleep.

Substance Use and Addiction

Most substances that are prone to abuse change sleep patterns and sleep architecture. Specific effects depend on whether substances are sedating or activating. Careful questioning can elicit whether use is for social reasons or for management of sleep-wake difficulties. If the latter, appropriate evaluation and treatment of related sleep, medical, or psychiatric disorders should be recommended, including referral to a substance abuse specialist when necessary (Roehrs and Roth 2017).

Sedatives such as alcohol, benzodiazepines, and opiates can shorten sleep onset in the first half of the night but disrupt sleep because of rebound effects in the second half. They also suppress respiratory drive, which increases risk for OSA and PLMS. Stimulants promote wakefulness by altering neurochemicals: caffeine blocks adenosine, preventing the accumulation of sleep drive, and amphetamines increase the release of dopamine. The activating effects of stimulants cause insomnia at night, followed by sleepiness during the day, which perpetuates the cycle of use. Any substance or medication with a short half-life, such as nicotine, is especially disruptive of sleep because cravings due to withdrawal are more frequent and intense. All substances mentioned here, including cannabis, suppress REM sleep and cause REM sleep rebound if discontinued. Apart from REM suppression, the effects of cannabis on sleep, especially the more potent strains currently cultivated, are still unclear.

Dementia and Neurodegenerative Disorders

The common pathophysiology of neurodegenerative disorders, the destruction of neurons, typically results from neurotoxic accumulation of excessive central nervous system proteins such as β-amyloid (Alzheimer's disease), tau (frontotemporal dementia and chronic traumatic encephalopathy), and α-synuclein (Parkinson's disease and Lewy body dementia). Emerging research suggests that sleep, particularly slow-wave sleep, plays a critical role in proper clearance of these proteins and that impaired sleep may be one mechanism by which these disorders develop (Xie et al. 2013).

Sleep systems and patterns are commonly impaired in neurodegenerative disorders, and various sleep disorders may develop. RLS, PLMS, and RBD are strongly linked to the α-synucleinopathies and may precede frank disease onset by several years (Kutscher et al. 2014). Circadian rhythms can be impaired, and patients often present with advanced phase disturbances in earlier stages of the disorder and irregular sleep-wake patterns in later stages, when individuals sleep and wake intermittently throughout the 24-hour day. Social and physical isolation, limited mobility and activity, and reduced light exposure all aggravate irregular sleep-wake patterns because environmental cues that regulate circadian rhythms are lost. Given dementia-related cognitive impairment, nonmedication treatment should focus on behavioral rather than cognitive strategies to target insomnia and circadian dysregulation, and medications or devices to manage other sleep disorders should be implemented in collaboration with caretakers.

COGNITIVE-BEHAVIORAL STRATEGIES TO IMPROVE SLEEP

Overview of Cognitive-Behavioral Therapy Principles

CBT principles are the foundation for nonmedication approaches to reducing anxiety, enhancing mood, losing weight, and improving management of chronic conditions. Treating sleep problems is no exception. As noted earlier, CBT techniques have proven even more effective than sedative-hypnotic medications at resolving insomnia and sustaining improvements over the long term (Morin et al. 2006).

The fundamental principle underlying any CBT treatment is the connection between thoughts, feelings, behaviors, and the body. Because of this interconnection, changing one component can change others. For example, changing behaviors at bedtime can alter bodily stress and help with relaxation, and changing thoughts about wakefulness at night can transform feelings about this experience. CBT techniques are powerful tools because they change unhelpful sleep habits while taking advantage of sleep drive and circadian biology. In the following subsections, we describe several of the most effective CBT techniques for improving sleep.

Match Sleep Opportunity to Sleep Ability

Individuals who report trouble falling asleep, staying asleep, or both are often spending long periods of time awake at night (>30 minutes). The fastest and most effective way to reduce time awake at night is to match *sleep opportunity* (amount of time spent in bed each night) to *sleep ability* (average amount of sleep each night, which can be estimated by completing a 2-week sleep diary, an example of which can be found at http://yoursleep.aasmnet.org/pdf/sleepdiary.pdf). This behavioral technique essentially eliminates wakefulness from time spent in bed, thus consolidating sleep and improving sleep quality. As wakefulness at night diminishes and sleep quality improves, time in bed is gradually increased each week until optimal sleep duration is reached.

This intervention, known as *sleep restriction* or *time-in-bed restriction* (Spielman et al. 1987b), runs counter to the widely held perception that spending more time in bed will lead to more and better sleep. In fact, for individuals with insomnia, spending more time in bed worsens sleep by decreasing sleep drive, increasing wakefulness at night, exacerbating worry about sleep ability, and promoting sleep effort, all of which interfere with natural sleep. The paradoxical reality, supported by substantial research, shows that *decreasing* time in bed is the most effective way to improve sleep because it increases sleep drive and thereby reduces wakefulness, sleep worry, and sleep effort.

This technique must be applied with caution, however, because restricting time in bed creates a state of mild sleep deprivation because individuals with insomnia almost always overestimate the amount of time they are awake at night and underestimate the amount of time they are asleep. Time in bed should be no less than 5 hours to prevent excessive daytime sleepiness and perhaps more for individuals who are losing sleep because of OSA, RLS, or delayed sleep phase or for individuals at risk for mania, migraines, or seizures. A more gradual restriction might also appeal to individuals who struggle to get out of bed because of depression, psychosis, or low motivation. Finally, providers should keep in mind that psychiatric conditions and psychotropic medications can also affect levels of daytime energy and fatigue, so nonsleep factors will almost certainly need to be addressed to optimize daytime functioning (see other chapters in this volume).

Reassociate Bed and Bedroom With Sleep and Sleepiness

Lying awake at night with nothing to distract or occupy our minds can increase worry about sleep as well as other stressors. This state of worried wakefulness can be associated unconsciously with the bed, bedroom, and bedtime. Rather than operating as cues for sleep and sleepiness, bed, bedroom, and bedtime become conditioned cues for anxious and frustrated wakefulness. When this happens, people may find themselves dozing on the couch near bedtime but waking up when they try to sleep in bed.

The best way to extinguish this nonconscious association is through a behavioral technique known as *stimulus control* or *bed reassociation training* (Bootzin et al. 1991). This approach instructs people to 1) go to bed only when sleepy; 2) get out of bed if awake at night (>20 minutes) and return to bed only when sleepy; 3) sleep only in bed; 4) do wakeful activities (reading, watching television, using phones or laptops) away from the bed or bedroom; and 5) get out of bed at the same time every morning, no matter the duration of sleep the previous night. Rigorous adherence to these instructions helps reinforce the bed, bedroom, and bedtime as cues for sleep and sleepiness.

This technique is most effective when implemented strictly, but it can be modified in individuals with low motivation, chronic pain, or cognitive impairment or those at risk for falls. An alternative approach would create distinct cues for sleep versus wake by allowing people to sit up in bed on top of the covers with lights on when awake while encouraging them to lie down in bed under the covers with lights off when asleep. Individuals may also need help distinguishing between sleepiness (predisposition to fall asleep, as evidenced by heavy eyes, slowed breathing, and nodding head) and tiredness (feeling of physical and mental exhaustion unaccompanied by signs of sleepiness), especially in the context of psychiatric conditions and psychotropic medications. Ensuring that individuals get into bed only when sleepy and not just tired is critical for the successful of this technique.

Establish and Maintain Good Sleep Hygiene

Sleep hygiene refers to environmental factors and health or lifestyle practices that either help or hinder sleep (Hauri 1991). Environmental factors include the establishment of a protected sleep environment. Health practices include appropriate use of alcohol, caffeine, diet, and exercise. Good sleep hygiene can support better sleep but by itself does not usually correct poor sleep. Sleep hygiene includes the following techniques:

- Make sure that the bedroom is dark, cool, quiet, and comfortable, although individual preferences can vary. Mattress and pillows can be firm or soft. A bedroom temperature between 62°F and 68°F is best for sleep. An eye mask, heavy blinds, ear plugs, white noise, an air conditioner, or an electric blanket can all be used to optimize the sleep environment. Electronics and screens should be kept out of the bedroom.
- Ensure that use of substances does not interfere with sleep. Limit caffeine consumption to three or fewer beverages finished at least 12 hours before bedtime. Drink alcohol moderately, finish drinks at least 3–4 hours before bedtime, and do not use alcohol as a sleep aid. Quit smoking for both sleep and health benefits.
- Schedule meals and activities appropriately. Get regular physical activity during the day to build sleep drive but finish at least 3–4 hours before bedtime to allow time to cool down because increased core body temperature is an alerting cue. Eat regular meals throughout the day that align with circadian sleep-wake patterns and that allow sufficient time for digestion before getting into bed. A good rule is to eat within 1 hour of waking up and to not eat within 3–4 hours of bedtime.

Eliminate or Limit Napping

Eliminating daytime naps can boost sleep drive, reinforce appropriate circadian sleep-wake patterns, and strengthen the association between bed and sleep. Some individuals benefit from daytime naps, however, especially given the sedating effects of psychotropic medications. If refraining from daytime naps or adhering to time-in-bed restriction rules is too difficult, a short nap of less than 45 minutes taken 7–9 hours before bedtime will not interfere with sleep the coming night. Additional sleep is not the only strategy that counters daytime sleepiness or sedation. Bright light and physical or social activity reduce daytime sleepiness, with added benefits of boosting sleep drive and improving sleep and mood.

Increase Activity Level

Sleep drive accumulates the longer we are awake, but it also increases with activity level. The more active we are during the day—physically, socially, and mentally—the higher our sleep drive at bedtime. The higher our sleep drive, the faster we are likely to fall asleep and the less likely we are to wake up at night. Finding ways to be more active during the day, even in brief "bursts," can improve sleep at night. As Part II, "Exercise in the Prevention and Management of Specific Psychiatric Disorders," makes abundantly clear, increasing activity not only improves sleep but also reduces anxiety, enhances mood, and improves management of psychiatric disorders.

Relax the Body

Whereas a stressed mind and a tense body put obstacles in the way of sleep, a calm mind and a relaxed body smooth the pathway to sleep. Tense muscles, increased heart rate, rapid shallow breathing, worried thoughts, and negative emotions occur when our sympathetic nervous system is activated. This *fight or flight* response is antithetical to sleep. Activation of the parasympathetic system, conversely, leads to relaxed muscles, slower heart rate, deeper breathing, and a calmer mind. This *rest and digest* response facilitates sleep. When sympathetic activity is low and parasympathetic activity is high, we fall asleep and stay asleep more easily.

The best time to relax and disengage from the stress of the day is during the hour before bedtime. This *wind-down* period should include only relaxing and enjoyable activities rather than productive and goal-oriented activities—no working, paying bills, or engaging in stressful conversations. As noted in previous chapters in Part III, "Healthy Body, Healthy Mind," intentional relaxation is one of the best ways to disengage and destress from the day—in other words, to shift the sympathetic-parasympathetic balance toward sleep. Web-based, app-based, and in-person resources can teach diaphragmatic breathing, body scan, progressive muscle relaxation, visual imagery, meditation, mindfulness, restorative yoga, and biofeedback, which can be incorporated into the prebedtime wind-down period. These approaches take time, however, so patience, persistence, and practice are key. Individuals should practice one technique daily for at least 2–4 weeks before trying others.

Calm the Mind

Stress can be reduced 2–3 hours before bedtime by engaging in *constructive worry* for 20–30 minutes. This strategy requires making a list of worries or concerns that typically come up at night and then 1) *resolving* the worries by writing next to each one a simple but specific step to take the following day or 2) *letting go* of the worries by shredding the paper and throwing it away. This time could also be used to challenge and reframe inaccurate and unhelpful beliefs about sleep, which can help to circumvent the vicious cycle of insomnia that ensues when unhelpful thoughts, negative emotions, and maladaptive behaviors exacerbate and perpetuate sleep disturbance. Common *sleep myths* include believing that sleep should happen quickly and that waking up at night is abnormal, blaming poor sleep for all daytime fatigue and impairment, attributing any mental or physical health problem to poor sleep, and thinking that sleep should be the focal point of daily and nightly efforts.

Changing negative, distressing emotions about sleep or the experience of being awake at night into more positive, accepting ones can also benefit sleep. One way to do this is to not look at the time if awake at night. Although a habit for many people, looking at a clock interferes with sleep because the mental tallying of how much sleep has occurred versus how much sleep remains provokes anxiety and is impossible to prevent. It is far better to set an alarm for the desired wake time before getting into bed and then turn the clock away, set it across the room, or, if necessary, remove it from the room entirely.

Another way to transform the "suffering" that often occurs when awake at night is to adopt a more mindful approach to sleep. This approach encourages letting go of any judgments about the experience ("This is terrible!") or any efforts to make the experience other than what it is ("I need to get back to sleep!"). It requires accepting the experience rather than trying to change it and trusting that your mind and body will give you what you need and self-correct for any sleep loss. A mindful approach reduces anxiety, frustration, and desperation at night. Although this more relaxed emotional state can make it easier to return to sleep, a mindful approach focuses on no goal beyond the experience itself. Cultivating a mindful approach, like learning to relax, requires patience, persistence, and, most of all, practice. As highlighted in other chapters, however, the rewards can be synergistic because mindfulness can improve not only sleep but also mood, energy, coping, and stress tolerance.

CONCLUSION

Sleep problems—including insufficient sleep, insomnia, OSA, circadian rhythm disorders, and RLS—are associated with almost all psychiatric disorders. Because sleep is a fundamental biological process that helps to maintain physical, mental, and emotional resilience and well-being, learning how to support and sustain healthy sleep is crucial for managing psychiatric symptoms and optimizing function. Psychiatric medications are important for symptom management, but they can affect sleep adversely. Effective sleep management not only reduces the medication burden so common in mental illness but, as recent research suggests, works synergistically with other lifestyle interventions to increase energy, improve performance, enhance mood and cognition, and strengthen coping.

DISCUSSION QUESTIONS

1. What are the two biological processes that drive sleep? How does their interaction determine sleepiness and wakefulness, as well as performance fluctuations, across a 24-hour period?
2. What sleep disorders are commonly associated with psychiatric conditions of the individuals you see for clinical care? What are the sleep disturbance symptoms that characterize these disorders?
3. What three behavioral or cognitive techniques could you use to improve sleep in the patients you see? Would you apply these techniques strictly or modify them for certain populations?

RECOMMENDED READINGS

Asarnow LD, Soehner AM, Harvey AG: Basic sleep and circadian science as building blocks for behavioral interventions: a translational approach for mood disorders. Behav Neurosci 128(3):360–370, 2014
Manber R, Carney C: Quiet Your Mind and Get to Sleep: Solutions to Insomnia for Those With Depression, Anxiety, or Chronic Pain. Oakland, CA, New Harbinger, 2009
Walker MP: The role of sleep in cognition and emotion. Ann NY Acad Sci 1156(1):168–197, 2009

REFERENCES

Asarnow LD, Soehner AM, Harvey AG: Basic sleep and circadian science as building blocks for behavioral interventions: a translational approach for mood disorders. Behav Neurosci 128(3):360–370, 2014 24773429

Auger RR, Burgess HJ, Emens JS, et al: Clinical practice guideline for the treatment of intrinsic circadian rhythm sleep-wake disorders: advanced sleep-wake phase disorder (ASWPD), delayed sleep-wake phase disorder (DSWPD), non-24-hour sleep-wake rhythm disorder (N24SWD), and irregular sleep-wake rhythm disorder (ISWRD): an update for 2015—an American Academy of Sleep Medicine clinical practice guideline. J Clin Sleep Med 11(10):1199–1236, 2015 26414986

Benson KL, Feinberg I: Schizophrenia, in Principles and Practice of Sleep Medicine, 6th Edition. Philadelphia, PA, Elsevier, 2017, pp 1370–1379

Bootzin RR, Epstein DR, Wood JM: Stimulus control instructions, in Case Studies in Insomnia. New York, Springer, 1991, pp 19–28

Chung F, Yegneswaran B, Liao P, et al: STOP Questionnaire: A tool to screen patients for obstructive sleep apnea. Anesthesiology 108(5):812–821, 2008 18431116

Cortese S, Lecendreux M: Sleep disturbances in attention-deficit/hyperactivity disorder, in Principles and Practice of Sleep Medicine, 6th Edition. Philadelphia, PA, Elsevier, 2017, pp 1390–1397

Cortese S, Konofal E, Lecendreux M, et al: Restless legs syndrome and attention-deficit/hyperactivity disorder: a review of the literature. Sleep 28(8):1007–1013, 2005 16218085

Durmer JS, Dinges DF: Neurocognitive consequences of sleep deprivation. Semin Neurol 25(1):117–129, 2005 15798944

Edinger JD, Olsen MK, Stechuchak KM, et al: Cognitive behavioral therapy for patients with primary insomnia or insomnia associated predominantly with mixed psychiatric disorders: a randomized clinical trial. Sleep 32(4):499–510, 2009 19413144

Freeman D, Waite F, Startup H, et al: Efficacy of cognitive behavioural therapy for sleep improvement in patients with persistent delusions and hallucinations (BEST): a prospective, assessor-blind, randomised controlled pilot trial. Lancet Psychiatry 2(11):975–983, 2015 26363701

Goldman SE, Alder ML, Burgess HJ, et al: Characterizing sleep in adolescents and adults with autism spectrum disorders. J Autism Dev Disord 47(6):1682–1695, 2017 28286917

Harvey AG, Soehner AM, Buysse DJ: Bipolar disorder, in Principles and Practice of Sleep Medicine, 6th Edition. Philadelphia, PA, Elsevier, 2017, pp 1363–1369

Hauri PJ: Sleep hygiene, relaxation therapy, and cognitive interventions, in Case Studies in Insomnia. New York, Springer, 1991, pp 65–84

Horne JA, Östberg O: A self-assessment questionnaire to determine morningness-eveningness in human circadian rhythms. Int J Chronobiol 4(2):97–110, 1976 1027738

Johns MW: A new method for measuring daytime sleepiness: the Epworth Sleepiness Scale. Sleep 14(6):540–545, 1991 1798888

Kaplan KA, Harvey AG: Behavioral treatment of insomnia in bipolar disorder. Am J Psychiatry 170(7):716–720, 2013 23820830

Knutson KL, Spiegel K, Penev P, et al: The metabolic consequences of sleep deprivation. Sleep Med Rev 11(3):163–178, 2007 17442599

Krystal AD, Stein MB, Szabo ST: Anxiety disorders and posttraumatic stress disorder, in Principles and Practice of Sleep Medicine, 6th Edition. Philadelphia, PA, Elsevier, 2017, pp 1341–1351

Kutscher SJ, Farshidpanah S, Claassen DO: Sleep dysfunction and its management in Parkinson's disease. Curr Treat Options Neurol 16(8):304, 2014 24930678

Manber R, Edinger JD, Gress JL, et al: Cognitive behavioral therapy for insomnia enhances depression outcome in patients with comorbid major depressive disorder and insomnia. Sleep 31(4):489–495, 2008 18457236

Minkel JD, Krystal AD, Benca RM: Unipolar major depression, in Principles and Practice of Sleep Medicine, 6th Edition. Philadelphia, PA, Elsevier, 2017, pp 1352–1362

Morganthaler TI, Auerbach S, Casey KR, et al: Position paper for the treatment of nightmare disorder in adults: an American Academy of Sleep Medicine Position Paper. J Clin Sleep Med 14(6):1041–1055, 2018 29852917

Morin CM, Bootzin RR, Buysse DJ, et al: Psychological and behavioral treatment of insomnia: update of the recent evidence (1998–2004). Sleep 29(11):1398–1414, 2006 17162986

Nadorff MR, Lambdin KK, Germain A: Pharmacological and non-pharmacological treatments for nightmare disorder. Int Rev Psychiatry 26(2):225–236, 2014 24892897

Ohayon M: Epidemiology of insomnia: what we know and what we still need to learn. Sleep Med Rev 6(2):97–111, 2002 12531146

Qaseem A, Kansagara D, Forciea MA, et al: Management of chronic insomnia disorder in adults: a clinical practice guideline from the American College of Physicians. Ann Intern Med 165(2):125–133, 2016 27136449

Roehrs T, Roth T: Medication and substance abuse, in Principles and Practice of Sleep Medicine, 6th Edition. Philadelphia, PA, Elsevier, 2017, pp 1380–1389

Rybak YE, McNeely HE, Mackenzie BE, et al: An open trial of light therapy in adult attention-deficit/hyperactivity disorder. J Clin Psychiatry 67(10):1527–1535, 2006 17107243

Spielman AJ, Caruso LS, Glovinsky PB: A behavioral perspective on insomnia treatment. Psychiatr Clin North Am 10(4):541–553, 1987a 3332317

Spielman AJ, Saskin P, Thorpy MJ: Treatment of chronic insomnia by restriction of time in bed. Sleep 10(1):45–56, 1987b 3563247

Stanley MA, Diefenbach GJ, Hopko DR: Cognitive behavioral treatment for older adults with generalized anxiety disorder: a therapist manual for primary care settings. Behav Modif 28(1):73–117, 2004 14710708

Talbot LS, Maguen S, Metzler TJ, et al: Cognitive behavioral therapy for insomnia in posttraumatic stress disorder: a randomized controlled trial. Sleep 37(2):327–341, 2014 24497661

Taylor DJ, Lichstein KL, Durrence HH, et al: Epidemiology of insomnia, depression, and anxiety. Sleep 28(11):1457–1464, 2005 16335332

Veatch OJ, Maxwell-Horn AC, Malow BA: Sleep in autism spectrum disorders. Curr Sleep Med Rep 1(2):131–140, 2015 26046012

Watson NF, Badr MS, Belenky G, et al: Recommended amount of sleep for a healthy adult: a joint consensus statement of the American Academy of Sleep Medicine and Sleep Research Society. J Clin Sleep Med 11(6):591–592, 2015 25979105

Wulff K, Dijk DJ, Middleton B, et al: Sleep and circadian rhythm disruption in schizophrenia. Br J Psychiatry 200(4):308–316, 2012 22194182

Xie L, Kang H, Xu Q, et al: Sleep drives metabolite clearance from the adult brain. Science 342(6156):373–377, 2013 24136970

Young T, Palta M, Dempsey J, et al: The occurrence of sleep-disordered breathing among middle-aged adults. N Engl J Med 328(17):1230–1235, 1993 8464434

Lifestyle Interventions for Cardiometabolic Health in People With Psychiatric Disorders

Martha C. Ward, M.D.

Robert O. Cotes, M.D.

Stephen J. Bartels, M.D., M.S.

KEY POINTS

- Individuals with psychiatric disorders have a reduced life expectancy, in part due to unhealthy behaviors and comorbid medical conditions.

- Lifestyle interventions show moderate efficacy for improving cardiometabolic health parameters, although several individual, well-designed randomized controlled trials show clinically significant reduction in weight.

- Specific factors increase efficacy of lifestyle interventions: manualized interventions of at least 3 months and employing both education and physical activity.

- Individuals with serious mental illness face unique challenges in engaging in lifestyle interventions, including poverty, access, and psychiatric symptoms.

- It is the prescriber's responsibility to monitor cardiometabolic side effects of psychotropic medication and to make appropriate treatment recommendations or referrals, including lifestyle interventions, when indicated.

Individuals with serious mental illness—including those with schizophrenia, bipolar disorder, severe depression, or posttraumatic stress disorder—have a considerably shorter life expectancy than the general population. Life expectancy for people with serious mental illness is, on average, 10–25 years less than that of the general population, representing one of the nation's greatest single health disparities (Bartels and DiMilia 2017). The causes for this mortality gap are multifactorial and, in part, are related to an increased risk of suicide, violence, accidents, and poverty. However, the greatest cause of early mortality for this high-risk group is due to cardiovascular disease and related chronic medical illnesses (Osborn et al. 2007). Individuals in this group have modifiable behaviors associated with dramatically higher rates of obesity and tobacco use compared with the general population, and in addition, many of the psychotropic medications prescribed to those with serious mental illness are associated with adverse cardiometabolic effects, including weight gain, diabetes, hypertension, and hyperlipidemia (Bak et al. 2014). A recent meta-analysis of more than 3 million individuals with serious mental illness and 113 million control subjects demonstrated that people with serious mental illness have an 85% higher risk of death from cardiovascular disease than regionally matched control subjects (Correll et al. 2017). Further increasing the risk of early mortality, individuals with serious mental illness have difficulties accessing health care and typically receive poorer quality services (Ward et al. 2015).

Promotion of health and wellness is an important component of the recovery process for individuals living with mental illness (Silverstein and Bellack 2008). For obese individuals, a 5% or greater loss in body weight results in improved metabolic function in multiple organ systems (Magkos et al. 2016), and improved fitness can decrease cardiovascular disease risk (Klein et al. 2004). There is an emerging body of evidence to suggest that lifestyle interventions can be effective in reducing cardiovascular disease risk. These interventions include diet, exercise, and behavioral modification. Lifestyle interventions should be considered as a first-line approach to decreasing cardiovascular disease risk for individuals with mental illness.

EFFICACY OF LIFESTYLE INTERVENTIONS FOR PEOPLE WITH MENTAL ILLNESS

Although there have been a number of trials focusing on lifestyle interventions to improve cardiovascular risk in individuals with serious mental illness, study design and results are quite heterogeneous. Interventions that employ both education and physical activity are associated with greater success in achieving clinically significant weight loss (Bartels and Desilets 2012). These two factors have also been shown to be associated with greater success in lifestyle interventions in the general population (Ward et al. 2015). Additional factors that have been associated with greater efficacy of lifestyle interventions in the general population include personalization of the program, more frequent contact with participants, and the use of trained treatment providers (Ward et al. 2015).

In aggregate, the reviews suggest that the magnitude of effect of lifestyle interventions applied to groups of individuals with serious mental illness is modest. For example, limited evidence suggests that trials of lifestyle interventions in individuals with serious mental illness may produce smaller effects than do interventions in the general population. A review by Cabassa et al. (2010) of nine randomized controlled trials in persons with serious mental illness found a mean weight loss of 1.6 kg (95% confidence interval [CI] 0.3–2.9 kg) compared with 3.6–5 kg in the general population.

Several reviews focusing on the population with serious mental illness noted that the modest weight loss attributed to lifestyle interventions may not be clinically relevant because it falls short of the 5%–10% weight loss deemed sufficient to reduce cardiometabolic risk. For instance, Alvarez-Jiménez et al. (2008) examined lifestyle interventions for individuals prescribed atypical antipsychotics and reported a weighted mean difference of –2.56 kg (95% CI –3.20 to –1.92 kg) in reduction in body weight for program participants compared with treatment as usual. However, weight loss in individual studies ranged from 2.5% to 4% of total body weight. Of note, the studies included were limited by inconsistently reported methods and by short follow-up, with a mean of 18.2 weeks (Alvarez-Jiménez et al. 2008).

Additionally, Verhaeghe et al. (2011) demonstrated a weighted average weight change with lifestyle intervention of –1.96 kg (95% CI –0.12 to –3.80 kg) in individuals with serious mental illness. Although weight loss was statistically significant in 11 of 14 reviewed studies, none achieved 5% weight loss (Verhaeghe et al. 2011). Moreover, Bartels and Desilets (2012) reported statistically significant weight loss in 20 of 22 studies included in their review of lifestyle interventions for individuals with serious mental illness, but median percentage of weight loss was 2.6%. Finally, Bonfioli et al. (2012) reported a weight loss of 3.1% of initial body weight in individuals with psychosis after lifestyle intervention. However, the authors noted a relatively short follow-up (mean 18 weeks) and commented on the possibility that weight loss alone does not equate to decreased cardiovascular risk when studying lifestyle interventions for individuals prescribed antipsychotics (Bonfioli et al. 2012).

Despite these general findings, there is increasing evidence that lifestyle interventions for people with serious mental illness that are of sufficient intensity and duration can have a substantive impact on key cardiovascular risk factors. A review by Gabriele et al. (2009) suggested a correlation between weight loss and intervention duration; the mean weight loss was 2.63 kg for 12- to 16-week interventions, 4.24 kg for 6-month interventions, and 3.05 kg for 12- to 18-month interventions. Of note, the 12- to 18-month intervention category included just two studies. The authors also noted evidence of improved hemoglobin A1c and insulin regulation in the studies examined, emphasizing the importance of effects other than weight loss in decreasing metabolic and cardiovascular risk (Gabriele et al. 2009).

A recent meta-analysis by Naslund et al. (2017) evaluated outcomes in 17 randomized trials of lifestyle interventions focused on weight loss for persons with serious mental illness. This systematic review found that lifestyle interventions are effective for treating overweight and obesity among this group. Interventions of 12 months' duration or longer compared with 6 months' duration or shorter achieved more consistent outcomes, although effect sizes were similar for both shorter- and longer-duration interventions.

In summary, available systematic reviews are limited by the small number of studies, small sample sizes, short study duration, variability of the interventions, and heterogeneous research designs. For this reason, an overview of major randomized controlled trials of lifestyle interventions for persons with serious mental illness is particularly informative. In general, these studies suggest that clinically significant changes in weight and other key indicators are feasible.

An early study by Jean-Baptiste et al. (2007) evaluated a 16-week intervention that included exercise planning, behavioral modification, and reimbursement for food in 18 patients with schizophrenia or schizoaffective disorder. The behavioral modification program consisted of 16 weekly hour-long meetings focusing on healthy eating (i.e., food choices, including snacks and dining out; portion control; cooking skills; and reading labels). Problem-solving skills were emphasized throughout, including goal setting, record keeping, motivation for change, and eliminating cues and non-hunger-related eating. The mean difference in weight change for active participants, compared with control subjects, was –5.6 kg.

Wu et al. (2007) conducted a randomized controlled trial of a lifestyle intervention in Taiwan targeting 53 obese patients with schizophrenia who were taking clozapine. The intervention included consumption of lower-calorie foods and increased physical activity. Mean weight change was –5.2 kg in the active treatment arm compared with control subjects, and participants who engaged in the intervention had a 5.4% reduction in their body mass index (Wu et al. 2007).

In 2006, McKibbin and colleagues randomly assigned 57 individuals with schizophrenia and diabetes to a lifestyle intervention or usual care plus information. The intervention was a 24-week diabetes awareness and rehabilitation training (DART), focusing on education concerning exercise and nutrition. Subjects in the active treatment arm showed a mean weight change of –5.4 kg compared with control subjects (McKibbin et al. 2006).

In addition, several key trials have demonstrated clinically significant weight loss (greater than 5% of baseline weight) in subgroups of enrolled subjects. The Randomized Trial of Achieving Healthy Lifestyles in Psychiatric Rehabilitation (ACHIEVE) randomly assigned 291 overweight or obese adults with serious mental illness to a lifestyle intervention or a control group that received information on nutrition and physical activity. The intervention consisted of 18 months of cognitive-behavioral weight management sessions as well as scheduled exercise. At 18 months, 37.8% of participants had lost 5% or more of their initial weight, compared with 22.7% of control subjects (Daumit et al. 2013).

The STRIDE trial, based on the PREMIER lifestyle intervention and Dietary Approaches to Stop Hypertension (DASH), randomly assigned 200 obese individuals prescribed antipsychotic medication to a lifestyle intervention or usual care. The intervention promoted dietary changes (including calorie restriction) and physical activity. At 6 months, 40% of the intervention participants, compared with 17% of control subjects, had lost 5% of their body weight; at 12 months, nearly half (47%) of intervention participants had lost at least 5% of their body weight versus 36% of control subjects (Green et al. 2015).

Finally, the In SHAPE intervention has been shown to be associated with clinically significant reduction in cardiovascular risk in an initial randomized trial (Bartels et al. 2013) and in a subsequent replication trial (Bartels et al. 2015), clearly demonstrating evidence of effectiveness in different populations and settings. The In SHAPE program consists of 1 year (12 months) of weekly sessions with a coach, who assists with fitness training and dietary education. In the first randomized trial of In SHAPE conducted in a largely ethnically homogenous sample in Concord, New Hampshire, 133 overweight or obese adults with serious mental illness were randomly assigned to either lifestyle modification (In SHAPE program) or 1 year of fitness club membership and education (Bartels et al. 2013). Of the intervention participants, 49% achieved clinically significant weight loss (5% or greater). Moreover, twice the proportion of In SHAPE participants (40% vs. 20%) achieved clinically significant increase in fitness.

In a subsequent randomized trial of In SHAPE involving 210 overweight or obese adults with serious mental illness conducted in an ethnically diverse urban setting (46% nonwhite), 51% of In SHAPE participants experienced clinically significant reduction in cardiovascular risk (Bartels et al. 2015). In addition to demonstrating replication of clinically significant reduction in cardiovascular risk, this study also demonstrated sustained benefit at 18-month follow-up. Having established In SHAPE as an evidence-based practice with a replication trial, Bartels and colleagues conducted a subsequent implementation research study involving four community mental health centers. This study confirmed that similar clinically significant outcomes can be achieved when lifestyle interventions are implemented by usual-care providers in public mental health centers (Bartels et al. 2018).

KEY FACTORS TO ADDRESS FOR LIFESTYLE INTERVENTIONS IN MENTAL ILLNESS

Individuals with mental illness often face considerable barriers to accomplishing their wellness goals, and we recommend tailoring interventions in this population (Ward et al. 2015). Personalizing nutritional interventions for individuals in the general population has been shown to be a promising strategy to improve the diets of adults (Eyles and Mhurchu 2009). Additionally, interventions should be culturally and linguistically appropriate for their participants (Kreuter et al. 2003). In this section, we discuss several specific barriers relevant to individuals with mental illness and some strategies to address them.

Patient Factors

Persistent psychiatric symptoms can prevent patients from accomplishing their fitness and nutritional goals. For example, amotivation (lack of motivation or capacity to initiate behaviors), a common symptom in psychotic and depressive disorders, can limit the ability of individuals to effectively participate in lifestyle programs. To address this barrier, group formats may help individuals develop a sense of cohesion and accountability. Using rewards such as gift cards can help to incentivize participants (Erickson et al. 2016). Programs that teach participants to self-monitor their diet and exercise can be helpful (Baker and Kirschenbaum 1993), as can including members of the individual's support network (Wing and Jeffery 1999). Although there are limited interventions for negative symptoms of schizophrenia, depression is common in the illness, and effective treatment of depression may help to improve patients' ability to engage in health behavior changes (Conley et al. 2007).

Individuals with serious mental illness also have cognitive symptoms, with impairments in memory, executive functioning, attention, and processing speed (Reichenberg et al. 2009). For individuals with schizophrenia, the degree of cognitive deficits is often the best predictor of functional outcome (Bowie and Harvey 2006). To overcome these challenges, programs have sought to enhance retention of material by simplifying information, using larger font sizes, using mnemonics, creating educational games, and reading material aloud (Cabassa et al. 2010). Prescribers should also review their patients' pharmacological regimen and consider removing unnecessary medications that can worsen cognitive function (Eum et al. 2017). Physical exercise has also been shown to improve negative, cognitive, and mood symptoms in people with serious mental illness (see Chapter 3, "Physical Exercise in the Management of Major Depressive Disorders," and Chapter 6, "Physical Exercise in the Management of Schizophrenia Spectrum Disorders"), which may support adherence to goals over time.

Psychotropic medications, including mood stabilizers and antipsychotic medication, can cause side effects that may interfere with a lifestyle intervention program. Sedation may reduce motivation to participate and can lead to difficulties paying attention during educational sessions. As a solution, group meetings can be scheduled at times when individuals are feeling less fatigued. Additionally, many psychotropic medications have anticholinergic side effects that can lead to dry mouth. Providers can suggest sugar-free hard candies or water instead of the sugary beverages that patients often use to manage this issue. Finally, antipsychotic medications can be associated with dramatic weight gain, diabetes, and hyperlipidemia. In addition to switching from high- to low-weight-gain-propensity agents and treating hyperlipidemia with appropriate lipid-lowering agents, augmenting lifestyle interventions with metformin has been associated with significant reductions in weight and improved metabolic outcomes for persons with serious mental illness (Wu et al. 2008).

Finally, key social determinants of health have major impact on the adverse outcomes often experienced by people with serious mental illness. For example, these individuals are often disproportionally affected by poverty (Saraceno et al. 2005) and might not have access to clothing or shoes that are appropriate for fitness activities. Additionally, access to fitness facilities can be problematic. Poverty is also associated with poor diet (Leung et al. 2012), and individuals with mental illness typically eat fewer fruits and vegetables and whole grains and more saturated fat than the general population (Brown et al. 1999; Strassnig et al. 2003). One possible solution is to take participants to grocery stores or restaurants to assist with their food choices (Bradshaw et al. 2005).

Setting Factors

As previously discussed in the section "Efficacy of Lifestyle Interventions for People With Mental Illness," studies of longer duration (at least 3 months) have been associated with greater success in lifestyle interventions in both individuals with mental illness and the general population. Additionally, higher frequency of patient contact, independent of the length of treatment, has been shown to be associated with greater effects in lifestyle interventions in the general population (Ali et al. 2012). Ultimately, the greatest success in reducing cardiometabolic risk will likely come from patients incorporating lasting behavioral changes that can be sustained in their home environment, and everyday life, past the duration of any active intervention.

Moreover, data from studies in the general population have consistently shown that face-to-face interactions are associated with greater efficacy than are virtual meetings (Venditti and Kramer 2012). However, access to lifestyle interventions for those with mental illness may be limited by transportation difficulties associated with poverty (McCabe and Leas 2008), and patient-centered problem-solving concerning transportation needs may be essential to ensure program feasibility (Galletly and Murray 2009). When possible, lifestyle modification programs should offer public transit vouchers, rideshares, or other reduced-cost transportation options. Program leaders may also assist participants with applications for reduced-fare public transportation. Alternatively, sessions may be brought to the consumers, with meetings held in locations that are more convenient than the medical setting. Lifestyle modification programs involving other underserved populations have successfully staged sessions in community centers, local schools, and churches (Johnson et al. 2011).

Efforts aimed at improving uptake and sustainability of lifestyle interventions have explored the role of peer specialists in providing lifestyle interventions. Peer specialists are individuals successfully living with mental illness who complete formal training and provide behavioral health counseling to patients. Peer specialists often use their own life experiences to relate to and motivate patients (Bartels and Desilets 2012). In the Health and Recovery Program (HARP) study, Druss et al. (2010) randomly assigned 80 participants with serious mental illness to usual care or to a six-session intervention based on the Chronic Disease Self-Management Program, delivered by peer specialists. At 6 months, study participants showed greater patient activation than did those in usual care (7.7% relative improvement vs. 5.7% decline) and additionally showed a trend toward greater physical activity, medication adherence, and physical health–related quality of life. Additionally, O'Hara et al. (2017) engaged 14 individuals with serious mental illness living in supported housing in a 12-week peer-based group lifestyle balance curriculum. In surveying the participants, the study authors found the intervention both feasible and acceptable to the study participants (O'Hara et al. 2017). Finally, a series of recent pilot studies suggested that a combination of peer support and technology has substantial promise in advancing the practical delivery, impact, and sustainability of lifestyle interventions for persons with mental illness (Aschbrenner et al. 2016; Naslund et al. 2016). In addition to wearable devices and mobile technology, social media interventions—including the use of Facebook and text messaging—may have a significant role in supporting sustained lifestyle changes (Naslund et al. 2018).

Provider Factors

For individuals taking medications from high-risk classes, prescribers should choose medications judiciously and avoid polypharmacy when possible. Prescribers often rely on a complex set of rules in order to select an antipsychotic (Hamann et al. 2005), and in survey data, prescribers have reported that they are generally concerned about cardiometabolic side effects of antipsychotics and would make changes if metabolic side effects emerged (Newcomer et al. 2004). However, in real-world settings, prescribers and their patients often weigh the perceived balance of efficacy and metabolic side effects of a medication (Hermes et al. 2013). We strongly encourage providers to systematically follow the American Diabetes Association et al. (2004) guidelines for cardiometabolic monitoring for people taking antipsychotic medications. Cardiometabolic screening often occurs at a less-than-desirable rate (Morrato et al. 2008).

Educating and empowering the next generation of prescribers is essential to improving the overall health of individuals with serious mental illness. The mental health setting may often be the only setting in which an individual is receiving medical services. Psychiatric residents should 1) take ownership of the overall health of their patients, 2) learn how to initially assess and treat uncomplicated medical conditions such as diabetes and hypertension, 3) make referrals to primary care physicians and specialists when indicated, and 4) gain experience working in integrated mental health and primary care settings when feasible. Management of medical problems does not require completion of a combined internal medicine and psychiatry residency; general psychiatry residency programs are increasingly educating trainees on the management of common medical problems (Druss and Walker 2011).

CONCLUSION

An extensive literature cites the wide mortality gap for individuals with psychiatric disorders, with the majority of deaths from natural causes, including cardiovascular disease. In order to address this, we recommend a combination of strategies to reduce cardiovascular risk in this population.

Much of the increased cardiovascular risk is due to adverse health behaviors, and thus, lifestyle interventions are a first-line approach. When considering intervention design, we recommend employing the factors that have been shown to be associated with greater efficacy in individuals with serious mental illness: longer duration (3 or more months), a manualized approach, and multifactorial design, focusing on both nutrition and physical activity (Bartels and Desilets 2012). Increasing evidence also points to the feasibility and acceptability of employing peer specialists in such interventions (Druss et al. 2010). We also recommend including personalization, more frequent contact, and trained treatment providers. Unique challenges faced by patients with mental illness must also be addressed when creating such interventions. We recommend considering socioeconomic status, access to services (including availability of transportation and convenience of location), psychiatric symptoms, cognitive impairment, and medication side effects when tailoring lifestyle interventions for persons with mental illness (Ward et al. 2015).

In addition to addressing adverse health behaviors, we recommend thoughtful pharmacology for people with psychiatric disorders. Appropriate monitoring for and recognition of metabolic abnormalities is essential. In addition to appropriate monitoring, we recommend prescribing of psychotropic medications that are associated with less significant adverse metabolic effects when possible. Informed consent should include information about weight gain and a plan to mitigate metabolic effects. Use of minimum effective dosage of certain antipsychotics and appropriate dosage-reduction strategies is recommended. Polypharmacy should be avoided when feasible and monitored when necessary. In patients who have gained more than 7% of pretreatment weight or have developed hyperglycemia, hyperlipidemia, or hypertension, physical benefits of switching drugs must be considered with the patient while weighing risk of psychiatric decompensation with adverse medical outcomes (De Hert et al. 2012). In such instances, we also recommend considering lifestyle interventions that can counteract antipsychotic-induced metabolic abnormalities.

Mental health clinics are often the principal connection that patients with serious mental illness have to the health care system, and thus, psychiatrists may be the only physicians these persons encounter. The American Psychiatric Association (2015) released a position statement advocating for the expansion of the psychiatrist's scope of practice to include general health conditions. In line with these recommendations, psychiatrists may employ various integrated care models, within a continuum of level of involvement, in order to meet the medical needs of individuals with serious mental illness. On one end of this continuum, psychiatrists may manage medical conditions themselves, and on the other, they may arrange for integration of primary care providers in their clinical setting.

When direct care of the medical needs of patients with serious mental illness is not feasible, we recommend prompt referral to primary care or appropriate subspecialty physicians. Referrals are often more successful when facilitated by a care manager or other allied health professional. Such facilitation may ensure that patients are able to navigate the complexities of the health care system and allows for clear communication and collaboration between the medical specialist and the mental health provider.

Case Example

Rick is a 28-year-old man with a diagnosis of schizophrenia who started taking olanzapine to target symptoms of auditory hallucinations, disorganization, and aggressive behavior in the context of severe paranoia. On previous hospitalizations, Rick's schizophrenia proved refractory to aripiprazole and risperidone. He comes to the outpatient clinic with his psychiatric symptoms well controlled on olanzapine 20 mg, but he has gained approximately 40 pounds over the previous year since starting the medication. His body mass index is now 40.8, and he has developed diabetes mellitus, with a hemoglobin A1c of 6.9%.

Rick agrees to enroll in the healthy living group at a community mental health center, which is co-led by a psychologist and a certified peer specialist who has undergone whole health action management training with the Substance Abuse and Mental Health Services Administration. The intervention lasts 8 weeks, and Rick is scheduled to return to the clinic in 10 weeks to check in.

At his next clinic appointment, Rick reports having engaged in the program and having picked up some healthy eating tips, including portion control, label reading, and mindfulness surrounding eating (not watching television while eating). He states that he initially lost 4 pounds but has gained it back since the last clinic appointment. He has stopped exercising (he was previously walking for about 30 minutes every other day). The clinician engages Rick in a conversation about employing the skills he learned previously, and Rick reports that 30 minutes of walking every other day was too much. He states that he is confident that he can walk 45 minutes twice weekly. He also agrees to fill out a food log and to record his exercise for the next week.

Rick returns 1 week later and brings in his food log and exercise log. He has successfully walked for 45 minutes twice that week and thinks he could also go to the YMCA with a friend once weekly. His food log reveals that he is eating out more than previously. Rick and the clinician review healthy choices at his regular restaurants using online menus, and Rick agrees to take a Tupperware container when he eats out so that he can control portions. Rick and the clinician also review some of the healthy plate information that he learned in his healthy living class. The clinician arranges for Rick to meet one on one with a certified peer specialist to set further goals for eating and exercise for the next 4 weeks and arranges to see him back in the clinic in 6 weeks.

At the next clinic visit, Rick is doing well and has lost 8 pounds. He is incorporating many of the techniques that he learned from his clinician, the group intervention, and the peer specialist. The clinician discusses the possibility of starting metformin to assist with weight loss, but Rick declines and states that he thinks he can lose the weight using lifestyle changes alone.

DISCUSSION QUESTIONS

1. What is the role of psychiatrists in addressing medical comorbidities in their patients?
2. How can lessons learned from large-scale clinical trials about lifestyle interventions for people with mental illness be applied to real-world clinical settings?
3. How can providers best engage patients in genuine shared decision making about the cardiometabolic risks of treatment and health optimization?

RECOMMENDED READINGS

Bartels S, Desilets R: Health promotion programs for people with serious mental illness (prepared by the Dartmouth Health Promotion Research Team). Washington, DC, SAMHSA-HRSA Center for Integrated Health Solutions, 2012

Bartels SJ, Pratt SI, Aschbrenner KA, et al: Clinically significant improved fitness and weight loss among overweight persons with serious mental illness. Psychiatr Serv 64:729–736, 2013

Green CA, Yarborough BJ, Leo MC, et al: The STRIDE weight loss and lifestyle intervention for individuals taking antipsychotic medications: a randomized trial. Am J Psychiatry 172:71–81, 2015

Ward MC, White DT, Druss BG: A meta-review of lifestyle interventions for cardiovascular risk factors in the general medical population: lessons for individuals with serious mental illness. J Clin Psychiatry 76(4):e477–e486, 2015

REFERENCES

Ali MK, Echouffo-Tcheugui J, Williamson DF: How effective were lifestyle interventions in real-world settings that were modeled on the Diabetes Prevention Program? Health Aff (Millwood) 31(1):67–75, 2012 22232096

Alvarez-Jiménez M, Hetrick SE, González-Blanch C, et al: Non-pharmacological management of antipsychotic-induced weight gain: systematic review and meta-analysis of randomised controlled trials. Br J Psychiatry 193(2):101–107, 2008 18669990

American Diabetes Association, American Psychiatric Association, American Association of Clinical Endocrinologists, North American Association for the Study of Obesity: Consensus development conference on antipsychotic drugs and obesity and diabetes. J Clin Psychiatry 65(2):267–272, 2004 15003083

American Psychiatric Association: Position Statement on the Role of Psychiatrists in Reducing Physical Health Disparities in Patients with Mental Illness. Arlington, VA, American Psychiatric Association, 2015. Available at: www.psychiatry.org/File%20Library/About-APA/Organization-Documents-Policies/Policies/Position-2015-Role-of-Psychiatrists-in-Reducing-Physical-Health-Disparities-in-Patients-with-Mental-Illness.pdf. Accessed February 13, 2018.

Aschbrenner KA, Naslund JA, Bartels SJ: Technology-supported peer-to-peer intervention for people with serious mental illness. Psychiatr Serv 67(8):928–929, 2016 27476896

Bak M, Fransen A, Janssen J, et al: Almost all antipsychotics result in weight gain: a meta-analysis. PLoS One 9(4):e94112, 2014 24763306

Baker RC, Kirschenbaum DS: Self-monitoring may be necessary for successful weight control. Behav Ther 24(3):377–394, 1993

Bartels S, Desilets R: Health Promotion Programs for People With Serious Mental Illness (Prepared by the Dartmouth Health Promotion Research Team). Washington, DC, SAMHSA-HRSA Center for Integrated Health Solutions, 2012

Bartels SJ, DiMilia P: Why serious mental illness should be designated a health disparity and the paradox of ethnicity. Lancet Psychiatry 4(5):351–352, 2017 28330588

Bartels SJ, Pratt SI, Aschbrenner KA, et al: Clinically significant improved fitness and weight loss among overweight persons with serious mental illness. Psychiatr Serv 64(8):729–736, 2013 23677386

Bartels SJ, Pratt SI, Aschbrenner KA, et al: Pragmatic replication trial of health promotion coaching for obesity in serious mental illness and maintenance of outcomes. Am J Psychiatry 172(4):344–352, 2015 25827032

Bartels SJ, Aschbrenner KA, Pratt SI, et al: Implementation of a lifestyle intervention for people with serious mental illness in state-funded mental health centers. Psychiatr Serv 69(6):664–670, 2018 29606077

Bonfioli E, Berti L, Goss C, et al: Health promotion lifestyle interventions for weight management in psychosis: a systematic review and meta-analysis of randomised controlled trials. BMC Psychiatry 12:78, 2012 22789023

Bowie CR, Harvey PD: Cognitive deficits and functional outcome in schizophrenia. Neuropsychiatr Dis Treat 2(4):531–536, 2006 19412501

Bradshaw T, Lovell K, Harris N: Healthy living interventions and schizophrenia: a systematic review. J Adv Nurs 49(6):634–654, 2005 15737224

Brown S, Birtwistle J, Roe L, et al: The unhealthy lifestyle of people with schizophrenia. Psychol Med 29(3):697–701, 1999 10405091

Cabassa LJ, Ezell JM, Lewis-Fernández R: Lifestyle interventions for adults with serious mental illness: a systematic literature review. Psychiatr Serv 61(8):774–782, 2010 20675835

Conley RR, Ascher-Svanum H, Zhu B, et al: The burden of depressive symptoms in the long-term treatment of patients with schizophrenia. Schizophr Res 90(1–3):186–197, 2007 17110087

Correll CU, Solmi M, Veronese N, et al: Prevalence, incidence and mortality from cardiovascular disease in patients with pooled and specific severe mental illness: a large-scale meta-analysis of 3,211,768 patients and 113,383,368 controls. World Psychiatry 16(2):163–180, 2017 28498599

Daumit GL, Dickerson FB, Wang N-Y, et al: A behavioral weight-loss intervention in persons with serious mental illness. N Engl J Med 368(17):1594–1602, 2013 23517118

De Hert M, Yu W, Detraux J, et al: Body weight and metabolic adverse effects of asenapine, iloperidone, lurasidone and paliperidone in the treatment of schizophrenia and bipolar disorder: a systematic review and exploratory meta-analysis. CNS Drugs 26(9):733–759, 2012 22900950

Druss BG, Walker ER: The Synthesis Project: Mental Disorders and Medical Comorbidity. Research Synthesis Report No 21, Princeton, NJ, Robert Wood Johnson Foundation, 2011. Available at: www.integration.samhsa.gov/workforce/mental_disorders_and_medical_comorbidity.pdf. Accessed February 13, 2018.

Druss BG, Zhao L, von Esenwein SA, et al: The Health and Recovery Peer (HARP) program: a peer-led intervention to improve medical self-management for persons with serious mental illness. Schizophr Res 118(1–3):264–270, 2010 20185272

Erickson ZD, Mena SJ, Pierre JM, et al: Behavioral interventions for antipsychotic medication-associated obesity: a randomized, controlled clinical trial. J Clin Psychiatry 77(2):e183–e189, 2016 26930534

Eum S, Hill SK, Rubin LH, et al: Cognitive burden of anticholinergic medications in psychotic disorders. Schizophr Res 190:129–135, 2017 28390849

Eyles HC, Mhurchu CN: Does tailoring make a difference? A systematic review of the long-term effectiveness of tailored nutrition education for adults. Nutr Rev 67(8):464–480, 2009 19674343

Gabriele JM, Dubbert PM, Reeves RR: Efficacy of behavioural interventions in managing atypical antipsychotic weight gain. Obes Rev 10(4):442–455, 2009 19389059

Galletly CL, Murray LE: Managing weight in persons living with severe mental illness in community settings: a review of strategies used in community interventions. Issues Ment Health Nurs 30(11):660–668, 2009 19874094

Green CA, Yarborough BJ, Leo MC, et al: The STRIDE weight loss and lifestyle intervention for individuals taking antipsychotic medications: a randomized trial. Am J Psychiatry 172(1):71–81, 2015 25219423

Hamann J, Kolbe G, Cohen R, et al: How do psychiatrists choose among different antipsychotics? Eur J Clin Pharmacol 61(11):851–854, 2005 16235042

Hermes ED, Sernyak MJ, Rosenheck RA: Prescription of second-generation antipsychotics: responding to treatment risk in real-world practice. Psychiatr Serv 64(3):238–244, 2013 23241613

Jean-Baptiste M, Tek C, Liskov E, et al: A pilot study of a weight management program with food provision in schizophrenia. Schizophr Res 96(1–3):198–205, 2007 17628437

Johnson M, Everson-Hock E, Jones R, et al: What are the barriers to primary prevention of type 2 diabetes in black and minority ethnic groups in the UK? A qualitative evidence synthesis. Diabetes Res Clin Pract 93(2):150–158, 2011 21752486

Klein S, Burke LE, Bray GA, et al: Clinical implications of obesity with specific focus on cardiovascular disease: a statement for professionals from the American Heart Association Council on Nutrition, Physical Activity, and Metabolism: endorsed by the American College of Cardiology Foundation. Circulation 110(18):2952–2967, 2004 15509809

Kreuter MW, Lukwago SN, Bucholtz RD, et al: Achieving cultural appropriateness in health promotion programs: targeted and tailored approaches. Health Educ Behav 30(2):133–146, 2003 12693519

Leung CW, Ding EL, Catalano PJ, et al: Dietary intake and dietary quality of low-income adults in the Supplemental Nutrition Assistance Program. Am J Clin Nutr 96(5):977–988, 2012 23034960

Magkos F, Fraterrigo G, Yoshino J, et al: Effects of moderate and subsequent progressive weight loss on metabolic function and adipose tissue biology in humans with obesity. Cell Metab 23(4):591–601, 2016 26916363

McCabe MP, Leas L: A qualitative study of primary health care access, barriers and satisfaction among people with mental illness. Psychol Health Med 13(3):303–312, 2008 18569898

McKibbin CL, Patterson TL, Norman G, et al: A lifestyle intervention for older schizophrenia patients with diabetes mellitus: a randomized controlled trial. Schizophr Res 86(1–3):36–44, 2006 16842977

Morrato EH, Newcomer JW, Allen RR, et al: Prevalence of baseline serum glucose and lipid testing in users of second-generation antipsychotic drugs: a retrospective, population-based study of Medicaid claims data. J Clin Psychiatry 69(2):316–322, 2008 18251625

Naslund JA, Aschbrenner KA, Scherer EA, et al: Wearable devices and mobile technologies for supporting behavioral weight loss among people with serious mental illness. Psychiatry Res 244:139–144, 2016 27479104

Naslund JA, Whiteman KL, McHugo GJ, et al: Lifestyle interventions for weight loss among overweight and obese adults with serious mental illness: A systematic review and meta-analysis. Gen Hosp Psychiatry 47:83–102, 2017 28807143

Naslund JA, Aschbrenner KA, Marsch LA, et al: Facebook for supporting a lifestyle intervention for people with major depressive disorder, bipolar disorder, and schizophrenia: an exploratory study. Psychiatr Q 89(1):81–94, 2018 28470468

Newcomer JW, Nasrallah HA, Loebel AD: The Atypical Antipsychotic Therapy and Metabolic Issues National Survey: practice patterns and knowledge of psychiatrists. J Clin Psychopharmacol 24(5 suppl 1):S1–S6, 2004 15356414

O'Hara K, Stefancic A, Cabassa LJ: Developing a peer-based healthy lifestyle program for people with serious mental illness in supportive housing. Transl Behav Med 7(4):793–803, 2017 28155109

Osborn DPJ, Nazareth I, King MB: Physical activity, dietary habits and coronary heart disease risk factor knowledge amongst people with severe mental illness: a cross sectional comparative study in primary care. Soc Psychiatry Psychiatr Epidemiol 42(10):787–793, 2007 17721669

Reichenberg A, Harvey PD, Bowie CR, et al: Neuropsychological function and dysfunction in schizophrenia and psychotic affective disorders. Schizophr Bull 35(5):1022–1029, 2009 18495643

Saraceno B, Levav I, Kohn R: The public mental health significance of research on socio-economic factors in schizophrenia and major depression. World Psychiatry 4(3):181–185, 2005 16633546

Silverstein SM, Bellack AS: A scientific agenda for the concept of recovery as it applies to schizophrenia. Clin Psychol Rev 28(7):1108–1124, 2008 18420322

Strassnig M, Brar JS, Ganguli R: Nutritional assessment of patients with schizophrenia: a preliminary study. Schizophr Bull 29(2):393–397, 2003 14552512

Venditti EM, Kramer MK: Necessary components for lifestyle modification interventions to reduce diabetes risk. Curr Diab Rep 12(2):138–146, 2012 22350807

Verhaeghe N, De Maeseneer J, Maes L, et al: Effectiveness and cost-effectiveness of lifestyle interventions on physical activity and eating habits in persons with severe mental disorders: a systematic review. Int J Behav Nutr Phys Act 8:28, 2011 21481247

Ward MC, White DT, Druss BG: A meta-review of lifestyle interventions for cardiovascular risk factors in the general medical population: lessons for individuals with serious mental illness. J Clin Psychiatry 76(4):e477–e486, 2015 25919840

Wing RR, Jeffery RW: Benefits of recruiting participants with friends and increasing social support for weight loss and maintenance. J Consult Clin Psychol 67(1):132–138, 1999 10028217

Wu MK, Wang CK, Bai YM, et al: Outcomes of obese, clozapine-treated inpatients with schizophrenia placed on a six-month diet and physical activity program. Psychiatr Serv 58(4):544–550, 2007 17412858

Wu RR, Zhao JP, Jin H, et al: Lifestyle intervention and metformin for treatment of antipsychotic-induced weight gain: a randomized controlled trial. JAMA 299(2):185–193, 2008 18182600

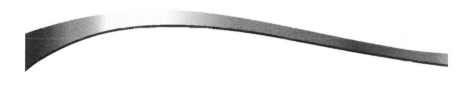

PART IV

Inspiring Healthy Living

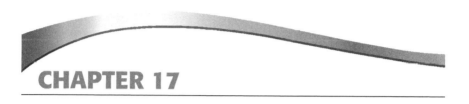

CHAPTER 17

Assessment and Behavioral Change Strategies in Clinical Practice

Alexander Sones, M.D.

Masha Krasnoff, B.A.

Marcus Vicari, B.S.

Donna Ames, M.D.

KEY POINTS

- Implementing behavioral changes in a psychiatric population accustomed to well-ingrained habits can be a challenging but incredibly rewarding experience.

- The comprehensive lifestyle assessment of a psychiatric patient begins with an acknowledgment of the barriers he or she faces in implementing lifestyle changes and is shaped by the mutual understanding between the patient and provider of the patient's recovery.

- A personal recovery plan, composed of individualized strategies to achieve behavioral changes, can increase the likelihood of successful implementation and subsequently can direct the patient on a course toward recovery.

The treatment of mental illness, particularly serious mental illness, is generally focused on prescription of medications that will minimize symptoms. The medical model emphasizes finding a "problem" on the basis of a constellation of symptoms and prescribing treatments to address problems. In contrast to the medical model, we present another approach that uses lifestyle changes and is more holistic and focused on the overall well-being of a person as part of his or her recovery from mental illness. We have found this approach to be inspiring for both the patient and the provider (Tessier et al. 2017).

The time limitations of current psychiatric practice (30-minute medication checks and perhaps 1 hour for an initial assessment) and insurance reimbursement patterns generally inhibit practitioners from approaching the treatment of mental illness in a holistic manner. Furthermore, behavioral changes can be frustratingly difficult to implement in clinical practice. Patients and clinicians alike are aware of the advantages and disadvantages of pharmacotherapy and psychotherapy, and adjunctive therapies such as the ones discussed in this book can be incredibly effective in the treatment of psychiatric illness, enhancing quality of life and well-being, as well as assisting with weight management efforts (Erickson et al. 2016, 2017; Tessier et al. 2017).

However, people are often resistant to modifications to well-ingrained habits and behaviors. In this chapter, we attempt to elucidate the reasons behind the difficulty in modifying behaviors, describe the initial lifestyle assessment of the psychiatric patient, and provide strategies to encourage and support lifestyle changes. This chapter demonstrates how we can empower patients in shared decision making to develop goals and lifestyle changes that will lead to mental health recovery and overall well-being (Joosten et al. 2008). We present lifestyle changes that support a holistic, biopsychosocial-spiritual approach to the treatment of mental illness.

BARRIERS TO OBTAINING LIFESTYLE CHANGES

Individuals with mental illness face many obstacles and barriers to obtaining biopsychosocial-spiritual well-being. Fortunately, many of these obstacles are modifiable in a clinical setting. Clinicians should evaluate all areas of potential barriers to wellness to ensure maximum efficacy of their treatment, and domains outside the medical model of psychiatry should not be avoided. When assessing the barriers to lifestyle changes in the psychiatric patient, it can be helpful to divide these barriers into several identifiable groups: illness-related, clinician-related, and patient-related.

Illness-Related Barriers

The nature of psychiatric illnesses can often act as an obstacle to recovery and implementation of lifestyle changes. Patients with schizophrenia encounter increased difficulty in implementing lifestyle changes relative to individuals without a mental health diagnosis (Smith et al. 1996). Furthermore, the unhealthy lifestyle of some patients with schizophrenia, including poor diet, cigarette and alcohol use, poor physical activity, and high rates of obesity, likely contributes to the life expectancy of an individual with schizophrenia being approximately 20 years shorter than life expectancy in the general population (Laursen et al. 2014). Negative symptoms of schizophrenia can lead to a lack of motivation and drive, inattention to cognitive input, and extreme apathy. Although physical illnesses in individuals with schizophrenia are common, they can be challenging to diagnose and treat partly because of patients' negative symptoms. Furthermore, medications are poor at targeting negative symptoms, preventing other treatment modalities from targeting or accessing the patient's motivational drives.

Similarly, patients with depression frequently have a loss of interest and subsequently a lack of motivation to implement lifestyle changes. Depression leads to lower adherence to medications, decreased likelihood of following clinical recommendations, and diminished self-care (Sumlin et al. 2014; Ziegelstein et al. 2000). Neurocognitive dysfunction may directly result in deficits in motivation and self-awareness, also inhibiting patients' ability to implement lifestyle changes.

Although lifestyle changes can be particularly beneficial in patients with posttraumatic stress disorder (PTSD), cognition overwhelmingly dominated by trauma- and stress-related thoughts may hinder the individuals' ability to implement therapeutic lifestyle changes. Patients with PTSD die 17–18 years earlier, have lower rates of success in weight-loss programs, and report more weight-loss barriers than do individuals without the illness, according to a recent study by Klingaman et al. (2016). Obesity and cardiovascular diseases are overrepresented in patients with PTSD. Similarly, other disorders of cognition such as obsessive-compulsive disorder and anxiety disorders may particularly inhibit individuals' ability to modify well-ingrained lifestyle behaviors.

The implementation of therapeutic lifestyle changes requires a significant amount of work and energy from patients. Individuals must comprehend that their lifestyle choices are causing long-term harm and must have adequate insight regarding their disease as well as their health state. Difficulties with attention and communication may further exacerbate already existing obstacles to achieving lifestyle changes. Motivation is needed to comprehend which foods to eat and which to avoid, and in addition, social skills and comfort being with others are needed for participation in group activities such as tai chi, dance, or yoga (Baker et al. 2015; Meyer et al. 2012; Wilbur et al. 2015).

Medication-Related Barriers

The illness-related barriers to achieving lifestyle changes can be exacerbated by medication nonadherence; however, the medications themselves can also cause barriers to physical, psychological, social, and spiritual health. Notably, antipsychotics can cause significant weight gain, diabetes, hyperlipidemia, obesity, metabolic syndrome, sexual side effects, and osteoporosis (Ames et al. 2016; Erickson et al. 2016, 2017; Tessier et al. 2017). Furthermore, antipsychotics are increasingly prescribed for disorders outside the schizophrenia spectrum, exposing an increasing number of patients to unintended but significant side effects, including weight gain. Although the mechanisms underlying antipsychotic-associated weight gain are not fully understood, it is postulated that antagonism of histamine H_1 and serotonin 2C receptors may adversely influence the experience of satiety and hunger, causing an increase in appetite and food intake. Although mitigation of these effects is possible with diet-modifying interventions and individually tailored nutrition counseling, many patients have limited access to these therapies, and it can be difficult to institute them in a clinical setting (Erickson et al. 2016, 2017).

Patient-Related Barriers

Patient-related factors present another obstacle to obtaining lifestyle changes. Homelessness and financial difficulties, particularly common in people with schizophrenia, are significant obstacles to obtaining adequate exercise and a healthy diet (Klingaman et al. 2016; Lazar et al. 2016). An overwhelmingly high proportion of homeless individuals report food insecurity and physical activity levels below guidelines (Kendzor et al. 2017). Furthermore, many patients live in *food deserts*, urban and often low-income areas devoid of healthful foods such as fresh fruits and vegetables. Individuals living in food deserts often rely on imperishable foods from corner shops rather than fresh foods from supermarkets and subsequently consume a diet rich in processed foods with high levels of fat and sugars. Patients' immediate housing arrangements can also represent an obstacle to obtaining lifestyle changes. For example, they may feel unsafe leaving their belongings to exercise or to try to obtain healthier food options than those provided at their shelter or board and care facility.

Many patients face significant psychosocial constraints in obtaining and maintaining lifestyle changes. Patients may appear to be integrated into their communities yet continue to be unable to access therapeutic interventions. For example, patients may be engaged in work or school yet unable to exercise due to transportation difficulties, child care duties, and other time constraints.

Medical comorbidities can limit patients in obvious and subtle ways, such as the wheelchair-bound patient who is unable to ride a bicycle or the patient whose atrial fibrillation may be triggered by exercise. Patients often are limited by daily routines, unlikely to be described as healthy lifestyles, that are rigid and difficult to alter. Furthermore, those who are socially isolated likely are not be able to rely on friends or family members to offer support in implementing lifestyle changes.

Patients often have a seemingly insurmountable number of obstacles to obtaining biopsychosocial-spiritual well-being through lifestyle changes. Acknowledging the difficulties patients face, the psychiatrist must act as a guide to help patients obtain lifestyle changes. Specific interventions targeting these patient-related factors are discussed in this chapter; however, it is worth noting that the best possible outcomes are achieved by frequent encounters in the medical and mental health systems and with collaboration between psychiatrists, psychologists, primary care physicians, nutritionists, social workers, and exercise professionals.

Case Example 1

Jesse is a 40-year-old man with diagnoses of schizophrenia and substance use disorder. He was living on the streets and had not been in contact with his family for more than 5 years. Eventually, he was connected to a holistic, recovery-oriented mental health program in conjunction with a high-intensity, multidisciplinary, and community-based treatment and case management team. Jesse reconnected with his family, who provided him with housing and a great deal of support. He worked with his treatment team to develop a personal recovery plan that included going back to college to study business, with the ultimate goal of owning a small business. In addition to this vocational goal, Jesse was encouraged to create goals for each of the eight therapeutic lifestyle changes (see section "Holistic Evaluation"). During each meeting with his doctor, Jesse reviewed his progress toward achieving his goals. A therapeutic lifestyle changes worksheet (see Figure 17–2 later in this chapter) was used in conjunction with the personal recovery plan form. Jesse is truly pleased with his progress. He will be graduating next year from the business program, he has stayed sober, and he is exercising regularly. He made friends in his recovery program and has remained connected with his family. He goes to church regularly and studies his Bible daily. Despite being treated with atypical antipsychotic medication, he has not gained weight because he exercises regularly at a gym, walks daily, and is careful about eating well. For neuroprotection, in addition to his antipsychotic medication, his doctor also prescribed vitamin E, magnesium and fish oil, and vitamin D.

COMPREHENSIVE LIFESTYLE ASSESSMENT FOR PEOPLE WITH PSYCHIATRIC DISORDERS

The clinical approach you take with a patient can be open-minded and minimally prejudiced by what others may have diagnosed. It is important to listen to the person when he or she enters your office to hear what matters to him or her. If the patient has already received a diagnosis and is taking medications, the diagnosis may or may not be correct. Position yourself as a fresh pair of eyes willing to work with the patient to consider various options. Explain the holistic, lifestyle-changing, recovery-oriented approach in the first session to introduce the patient to these concepts because past meetings with the psychiatrist may simply have been exchanges of information about symptoms and medications. The dialogue that will begin now in a holistic, recovery-oriented meeting will be noticeably different.

Collaborative information gathering may take a few sessions to be comprehensive. The patient may be given homework to fill out, such as a personal recovery plan (see Figure 17–1 later in the chapter), lifestyle practices diary (see Figure 17–2), or food diary. Evaluation of motivation using a motivation to change interview and/or the University of Rhode Island Change Assessment (URICA; Erickson et al. 2016, 2017) may be helpful for discerning the patient's stage of change. The model for change readiness includes these stages: 1) precontemplation (not thinking about changing), 2) contemplation (ambivalent), 3) preparation (starting to think about changes), 4) action (starting to change), and 5) maintenance (continuing to enact the behavioral change).

A holistic approach encompasses the wellness of a person in biopsychosocial and spiritual realms. When we encounter patients in our offices, they are often in distress. As psychiatrists, we can attempt to discern biological causes of mental distress. Diseases of the body can affect the mind. Similarly, the distress of the mind can manifest itself in bodily dysfunction. In *The Mindbody Prescription*, John Sarno (2001) described the power of the mind to manifest a number of medical conditions. Many patients experience depression, anger, and irritability in the setting of chronic medical illnesses. The psychiatrist must be aware of the symbiotic relationship between mind and body and consider the role of lifestyle behaviors when imbalance emerges.

HOLISTIC EVALUATION

The psychiatrist evaluating a patient in a holistic manner should start with a thorough assessment of the person's medical illnesses, review of systems, vital signs, and current pain level. A timeline of mind-body illnesses and when they started—many illnesses begin in the context of a variety of life stressors—may help the patient gain insight about the link between stress and physical illness in his or her life.

The patient's sleep and eating patterns should be examined. Insomnia may be a symptom of psychiatric illnesses such as anxiety, PTSD, or depression; however, it also can be a manifestation of sleep apnea. Sleep restoration can do a world of good for chronic fatigue and can markedly decrease middle-of-the-night wakening. In a study by Yu et al. (1999), researchers found that standard sleep apnea treatment compared with placebo resulted in improved mood symptoms such as tension, depression, and fatigue.

The comprehensive holistic approach to the treatment of mental illness should include psychoeducation with the patient about the role of nutrition (see Chapter 13, "Diet and Nutrition in the Prevention and Adjuvant Treatment of Psychiatric Disorders") and exercise (Chapters 3–10 in Part II, "Exercise in the Prevention and Management of Specific Psychiatric Disorders") in mental health and well-being. The patient should be given a food and exercise diary to bring back at the next appointment to identify areas that could be improved and to develop goals for change.

To elucidate whether any underlying nutritional deficiencies or metabolic abnormalities are contributing to psychiatric symptoms such as depression or anxiety, the following blood tests can be conducted: hemoglobin A1c, lipid panel, complete blood count, liver function tests, vitamin D, vitamin B_{12}, folate, magnesium, and calcium. To clarify if other conditions such as hypothyroidism may be impacting mental health, thyroid-stimulating hormone should be checked. Nutritional counseling may assist with any abnormalities detected.

It is sometimes difficult to learn everything we want to about a person in the first hour. Our clinical approach in the first hour of meeting a person with mental illness is to introduce the patient to our model of care and to work together with the person to develop a personal recovery plan. In creating a personal recovery plan, the clinician and patient should work together to generate an individualized and outlined document that describes what the patient's goals and preferences are in life, recorded in his or her own words. An example template of a personal recovery plan is provided in Figure 17–1. First, a simple assessment of current life satisfaction is conducted. Validated scales may be valuable in assessing current life satisfaction. The Bio-Psycho-Social-Spiritual Scale (BPSS) is a four-item evaluation created to assess global well-being and has been validated with the World Health Organization Brief Quality of Life Assessment (Erickson et al. 2017; Tessier et al. 2017).

Next, the psychiatrist should use the personal recovery plan to ask the patient about his or her satisfaction with his or her physical health, living circumstances, recreational activities, spiritual life, and sense of meaning or purpose. The patient and psychiatrist should then discuss and envision the patient's journey to recovery and what recovery looks like for that patient. What steps will the patient take to reach recovery? What strengths allow the patient to achieve recovery? What does the patient envision for himself or herself when he or she has achieved recovery?

Deriving meaning from life is a particularly important part of the personal recovery plan. Hungarian neurologist, psychiatrist, and Holocaust survivor Viktor Frankl believed that persons surviving the Holocaust were those who were able to derive meaning in their lives despite their dire circumstances (Frankl 1984). Frankl maintained that having a sense of meaning or purpose is important for humans. Although many people attempt to find "happiness," Frankl maintained that life is not necessarily inherently happy and that if one finds meaning in what one does each day, happiness may be a by-product of finding meaning. Additional studies have examined types of happiness that lead to better health outcomes, especially

My Personal Recovery Plan

Name: _____

Date: _____

Step 1. Satisfaction with areas of my life. Please tell us how satisfied you are with the areas of your life. For each area, rate your level of satisfaction on a scale of 1–5 (1=not satisfied, 3=moderately satisfied, 5=very satisfied) and tell us in a few words why you feel that way.

- **Physical needs** (food, clothing, shelter)
  My level of satisfaction is ___ because of _____
- **Meaningful activities** (work, school, volunteer) in the community
  My level of satisfaction is ___ because of _____
- **Social relationships** (friends, family, intimacy, etc.)
  My level of satisfaction is ___ because of _____
- **Holistic life, spirituality, and wellness** (mind, body, spirit)
  My level of satisfaction is ___ because of _____
- **Recreation, leisure, hobbies, creative expression** (music, art, dance, writing, etc.)
  My level of satisfaction is ___ because of _____
- **Other**
  My level of satisfaction is ___ because of _____

Step 2. What is my overall vision of recovery? If my life could be anything I wanted it to be, what would it look like? What brings meaning to my life? What is meaningful to me?

_____

_____

Step 3. What goals will I set to reach my vision of recovery? I will work on the following goal(s) to improve satisfaction in one or more of the life areas (from step 1):

_____

_____

Step 4. What strengths do I have that will help me achieve my recovery goals? What are the things that I am good at doing? What are some past successes that will help me to achieve my recovery goals? What relationships or associations will help me to achieve my recovery goals?

_____

_____

FIGURE 17–1. Sample template for a personal recovery plan.

Source.   Developed by Tom Fletcher and Richard Martin, Local Recovery Coordinators at the West Los Angeles VA Medical Center, Los Angeles, California.

Step 5. What might prevent me from achieving my recovery goals? Mental health symptoms, substance abuse, addictions, social issues, health issues, family issues, homelessness, unemployment, etc.

_____

_____

Step 6. What steps must I take to reach my recovery goals? What actions, behaviors, and/or responsibilities do I need to take to achieve my goals?

_____

_____

Follow-up visit 1

How much progress have I made to achieve my goal(s) on a scale of 1–5 (1=no progress, 5=goal achieved)?
        ____ Self rating
        ____ Staff rating

Please reevaluate your satisfaction with life areas (see step 1) on a scale of 1–5 (1=not satisfied, 3=moderately satisfied, 5=very satisfied)

        ____ Physical needs
        ____ Meaningful activities
        ____ Social relationships
        ____ Holistic life, spirituality, and wellness
        ____ Recreation, leisure, and hobbies

Follow-up visit 2

How much progress have I made to achieve my goal(s) on a scale of 1–5 (1=no progress, 5=goal achieved)?
        ____ Self rating
        ____ Staff rating

Please reevaluate your satisfaction with life areas (see step 1) on a scale of 1–5 (1=not satisfied, 3=moderately satisfied, 5=very satisfied)

        ____ Physical needs
        ____ Meaningful activities
        ____ Social relationships
        ____ Holistic life, spirituality, and wellness
        ____ Recreation, leisure, and hobbies

FIGURE 17–1. Sample template for a personal recovery plan *(continued)*.

Source. Developed by Tom Fletcher and Richard Martin, Local Recovery Coordinators at the West Los Angeles VA Medical Center, Los Angeles, California.

Follow-up visit 3

How much progress have I made to achieve my goal(s) on a scale of 1–5 (1=no progress, 5=goal achieved)?
___ Self rating
___ Staff rating

Please reevaluate your satisfaction with life areas (see step 1) on a scale of 1–5 (1=not satisfied, 3=moderately satisfied, 5=very satisfied)

___ Physical needs
___ Meaningful activities
___ Social relationships
___ Holistic life, spirituality, and wellness
___ Recreation, leisure, and hobbies

FIGURE 17–1. Sample template for a personal recovery plan *(continued)*.

Source. Developed by Tom Fletcher and Richard Martin, Local Recovery Coordinators at the West Los Angeles VA Medical Center, Los Angeles, California.

within a type of happiness associated with finding a sense of meaning known as *eudaimonic well-being*. Kashdan et al. (2006) and others found that especially among veterans with PTSD, those who adopted a positive affect via gratitude were subject to greater daily eudaimonia and self-esteem.

Once testing is completed and a personal recovery plan is made, the clinician should introduce the concept of therapeutic lifestyle changes. Roger Walsh (2011) outlined eight activities that all psychiatrists should prescribe to patients (Tessier et al. 2017). Specifically, these components are 1) exercise, 2) nutrition and diet, 3) time in nature, 4) relationships, 5) recreation, 6) relaxation and stress management, 7) religious or spiritual involvement, and 8) service and helping others. According to Walsh (2011), these eight activities factor into four categories: biological, psychological, social, and spiritual. Biological prescriptions include changes in nutrition and exercise. Psychological interventions include not only evidence-based psychotherapies but also things the patient can do himself or herself—such as relaxation, stress management, and recreational activities—which can be uplifting. Social therapeutic lifestyle changes that may be prescribed include activities that increase socialization as well as participation in appropriate evidence-based treatments such as social skills training (Smith et al. 1996). Spiritual or religious lifestyle changes include connecting with something greater than oneself and finding meaning. For some people, this connection occurs through religious means: attending church or other religious groups, reading scriptures, meditating, and praying daily; for others, spirituality can be derived by simply spending time in nature. Notably, women attending religious services once a week or more have been found to have an 84% lower risk than those who never attend religious services (Koenig 2016), and frequent religious service attendance has been found to be a long-term protective factor against suicide (Kleiman and Liu 2014).

We have established the utility of a simple sheet of paper—a therapeutic lifestyle changes (TLCs) log—to track these eight lifestyle domains to assist people with a variety of psychiatric disorders (Figure 17–2). We use this behavioral log sheet in individual sessions with patients and have demonstrated a relationship between the number of therapeutic lifestyle changes patients engage in and improvements in quality of life as measured by the BPSS (Ames et al. 2016; Sumlin et al. 2014).

Before prescribing specific therapeutic lifestyle changes, the clinician must examine the patient's personal recovery plan and ensure that suggested changes align with what the patient is interested in accomplishing. For each lifestyle change that is selected by the patient, clear and achievable goals should be established. Typically, we develop a SMART goal for each of the changes that the patient selects. SMART goals are specific, measurable, attainable, realistic, and time-bound (Doran 1981). Commonly used SMART goals include decreasing caloric intake from soft drinks, decreasing food portion size, substituting high-calorie foods with foods that have lower calories, and increasing intake of fruits and vegetables. At each session, the clinician should review the patient's log of how often he or she met the SMART goal for the particular therapeutic lifestyle change, identify the results of that achievement, and then work together with the patient to add additional SMART goals for more changes. Our research suggests that the more lifestyle changes patients participated in, the greater the weight loss as well as the greater the improvement in quality of life (Erickson et al. 2017; Tessier et al. 2017).

Case Example 2

Joe is a 50-year-old man with PTSD and drug-induced psychosis. He is now abstinent from recreational drugs and has come to a clinic for a holistic approach to his mental illness. On his regimen of antipsychotic medications, he gained a tremendous amount of weight. His doctor worked with him to minimize and optimize his medications. He did not want to completely stop the medication but is on the lowest dosage, with good control of most of his symptoms. Joe reports a great deal of stress in his life as a single father, and he has neglected self-care. He met with his psychiatrist, who began to formulate a recovery plan. Joe developed a primary SMART goal of losing 20 pounds in 6 months. During the first month, Joe and his doctor agreed on stopping sugar-laden soft drinks and juices, and Joe was given a pedometer. He lost 7 pounds with these two lifestyle changes. Very pleased with his progress, at the second meeting with his

MY THERAPEUTIC LIFESTYLE PRACTICES DIARY
THE 8 WAYS TO PRACTICE TLCs

First name: _____

Date: _____

My goal is to make little changes for each lifestyle element to improve the quality of my life.

	Specific goals	Sunday	Monday	Tuesday	Wednesday	Thursday	Friday	Saturday
Exercise								
Nutrition and diet								
Time in nature								
Relationships								
Recreation								
Relaxation/stress management								
Relaxation/spiritual involvement								
Service and helping others								

FIGURE 17–2. Eight ways to practice therapeutic lifestyle changes (TLCs).

Source. Greater Los Angeles VA Healthcare System PRRC. Inspired by Tessier et al. 2017; Walsh 2011.

doctor, he added additional SMART goals to work on for the other six life-style changes. At this next session, Joe's doctor encouraged him to seek healthier food options, and the doctor gave Joe a glycemic index list to help with grocery shopping. In addition, Joe has set a goal to treat his stress by listening to music because this relaxes him. He also joined a recovery-oriented group program, where he is able to interact and socialize with others in recovery whom he now considers friends. He has begun to enjoy spending time in nature with his new grandchild. He is planning to return to church because he finds reading the Bible helpful and he wants to positively influence his child and grandchild.

ESTABLISHING, MONITORING, AND SUPPORTING LIFESTYLE CHANGES

The clinician's support of lifestyle changes is an essential component of the patient's recovery and, along with community support, is bound to increase the likelihood of successfully implementing behavioral changes (Erickson et al. 2017). Many patients find it difficult to make changes to long-standing habits such as stopping at the fast food drive-through on the way home from work or watching television on days off. In our experience, it may be overwhelming to make suggestions for all eight therapeutic lifestyle changes at the first session, although some patients enthusiastically jump into this. Alternatively, with the very negative, depressed, withdrawn patient, the clinician can focus on one element at a time, setting a small goal at first and then adding additional goals at future appointments.

Monitoring of lifestyle changes in patients begins at the first visit. Before initiating a recovery-oriented behavioral treatment plan, providers must understand the patient's level of motivation and insight into the need for change. Motivational interviewing can be employed to assess what drives the patient. By consistently discussing what the patient enjoys and finds motivating, the clinician keeps the discussion patient centered and more likely to succeed. Several scales can also be beneficial to assess motivation and insight, such as the URICA and the Self-Appraisal of Illness Questionnaire (SAIQ; Dozois et al. 2004; Marks et al. 2000).

As part of each patient's recovery plan, goals should be set and monitored at each visit, with generous reinforcement for even partial progress toward achieving a goal; examination of the impact of that achievement on symptoms, health, and self-efficacy; and iterative revision of goals to build success (Noordsy et al. 2018). Clinicians should prompt patients to observe improvements in sleep, energy, cognitive clarity, mood, and motivation and the relationship of these improvements to lifestyle changes achieved (Ho et al. 2018). Specific goals should be created for each domain of the recovery plan—physical needs, meaningful activities, social relationships, spirituality, recreation, and any other areas identified in the initial sessions.

Patients begin their process of implementing lifestyle changes at vastly different levels of motivation and ability. Ideally, as part of their recovery journey, people with mental illness will achieve community integration goals such as going back to school, work, work therapy, or volunteerism. More motivated and athletically inclined patients may quickly be able to implement exercise regimens and healthy alterations in their diet. The clinician should discuss with the patient how the goals will be met—whether the patient prefers routine or variety, adventurous or contained settings, group or independent environments, and stimulating or mindful activities.

The emphasis of nutrition counseling should not be on dieting. Although many patients with serious mental illness are overweight as a result of their medications and other risk factors cited earlier (see section "Barriers to Obtaining Lifestyle Changes"), clinicians should emphasize changing the way patients eat, focusing on good-quality food and a healthy plate. In our work with patients, we explain the concept of *healthy plate*, borrowing heavily from the U.S. Department of Agriculture's MyPlate (see www.choosemyplate.gov), and provide a Lifestyle Balance and/or TLC workbook (Erickson et al. 2017; Tessier et al. 2017). Nutrition goals are aimed at improving the intake of vegetables and decreasing intake of non-nutritious foods. High-quality foods are satiating, and patients will lose weight following suggestions for the healthy plate, with the goal of a patient's diet being composed of 50% vegetables and fruit, 20% protein, and 30% healthy grains and carbohydrates. Healthy fats are suggested, as is the reduction of sugary foods and low-quality carbohydrates. For full details of nutritional suggestions, see Chapter 13, Chapter 14, "The Gut-Brain Axis and Microbiome in Psychiatric Disorders," and Erickson et al. (2017)

Food diary tracking is a useful tool that allows for objective analysis of dietary intake and thus may impact weight loss or maintenance, food choices, food allergy identification, and correlation of dietary choices with mood. Although pen and paper journals may be adequate, smartphone applications have made tracking food intake substantially easier because of their convenience as well as added features such as automatic calorie calculations and the ability to directly input food choices by scanning the barcode of the food product. Clinicians can supplement the information in the patient's food journal and provide an objective measure of the patient's progress by tracking in-office weights at each visit in addition to annual hemoglobin A1c levels and cholesterol or lipid levels.

If the patient is unable to achieve lifestyle goals, individualized interventions may be employed to target areas with which the patient is struggling. Patients often encounter difficulty adjusting their behavioral approach toward eating. We encourage providers to inquire about the patient's relationship with food and to determine if there are patterns such as eating during times of emotional distress or *mindless eating*, which is eating without paying attention, often while engaging in other activities such as driving or watching television. Food intake choices can be influenced by seemingly nonrelated factors such as plate size, availability and ease of acquiring types of foods, and time constraints for eating. Patients often benefit from a discussion of being mindful while eating and learning to pay attention to what they eat and at what times of day and night they eat. Patients should set the fork down between bites of food, eat slowly, and chew many times rather than swallowing as much food as possible as quickly as possible.

Family members, close friends, and caregivers may be involved at the patient's discretion because they may provide an additional motivational tool for the patient. If budgeting permits, an additional motivational tool for encouraging patients to meet their exercise goals is to provide small rewards when a goal is attained. For younger patients, a motivational incentive can be found through smartphone applications that encourage individuals to go on scavenger hunts in search of small rewards. These scavenger hunts provide opportunities for exercising, as well as spending time in nature, allowing for one to engage in mindfulness (Tessier et al. 2017). Take-home reminders, such as handouts, pens, or small notes, may be used to provide additional prompting depending on the level of difficulty the patient is facing in implementing lifestyle changes.

Coaching patients to make changes in exercise behaviors often requires SMART goals. In our experience, the easiest exercise to engage patients in is walking. Ideally, we seek to encourage a half-hour to 1 hour of walking per day. We give our patients pedometers, although patients are increasingly using smartphone apps and other digital devices to track steps, running distance, heart rate, and other data regarding their personal health. Before prescribing a vigorous exercise program, we recommend that high-risk patients receive an evaluation from their primary care provider, including an electrocardiogram. An exercise tolerance test can be reassuring for those with most significant cardiovascular risk factors. Exercise may be difficult to do alone, and patients may enjoy classes with others, such as dance or yoga. We have developed yoga and dance classes that were well received by our patients. Ideally, patients pursue such classes not at a mental health program but in the community, in keeping with the emphasis on community reintegration as part of recovery (Meyer et al. 2012; Schulz-Heik et al. 2017; Wilbur et al. 2015). Helpful guidelines for incorporating pedometer use are given in Table 17–1.

In addition to exercise and diet, the therapeutic lifestyle change sheet includes six other areas in which to encourage lifestyle changes. Some pa-

TABLE 17–1. Guidelines for use of pedometers

Help the patient understand how to use a pedometer (where to clip it, how to set it, how to use digital activity tracker).

Make a goal with the patient—anywhere from 10,000 to 25,000 steps depending on how active the person is.

After 1 week, review the data and calculate average steps per day.

After the patient achieves a goal and maintains it, set another goal.

Keep in mind that pedometers may not always be accurate, depending on how the person walks. Compare steps taken by the same person, not those of different people.

tients want to work on all eight lifestyle change areas as soon as possible, whereas others prefer to make one or two lifestyle changes per session. Sometimes, attempts to implement a single lifestyle change can encourage the implementation of others. For example, spending time in nature could also involve exercise and socialization; providers can encourage patients to spend time walking in a park with a friend or family member. As patients achieve success, their confidence and motivation often grow.

Patients who are resistant to dieting or exercising can also make lifestyle changes that can lead to very good outcomes. For example, patients may set the spiritual or religious goal of going to church each week, which may result in more socialization and support. Creative arts can provide relaxation and stress management through enjoyment of music or art activities. We have frequently encouraged patients to attend classes at local community colleges, and they have expressed surprise and delight at their success in joining community college choirs and engaging in writing classes for creative expression.

Establishing, monitoring, and supporting lifestyle changes is a slow, steady, and continual process. Behavioral reinforcement provided by the clinician can be an invaluable resource for patients. The patient and provider should engage in a cycle of lifestyle goal setting, tracking and monitoring progress, reinforcing goals, encouraging and celebrating improvement, and revising goals (see Figure 17–3 for a visual aid of this cycle). Patients and providers should not feel dismayed at the lack of immediate progress; success with the implementation of lifestyle changes results from small, patient-centered changes enacted in a slow and progressive fashion. Ultimately, the limitless success of patients in implementing lifestyle changes is often exciting and rewarding for providers and patients alike.

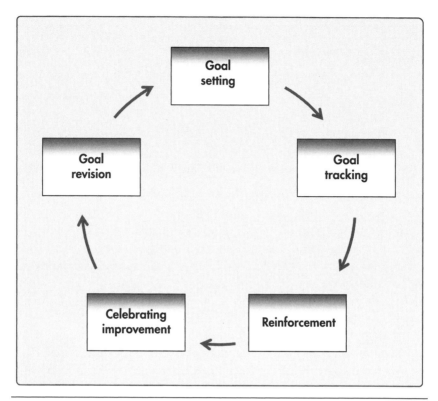

FIGURE 17–3.   Cycle of lifestyle changes.

CONCLUSION

In this chapter we summarized several important concepts in assessment and behavioral change strategy in a clinical setting. Behavioral patterns can be difficult to change, but when achieved, such changes lead to snowballing gains in confidence and self-efficacy. It is our hope that with the methodical, iterative goal setting, appraisal, and reinforcement approach presented here, providers will be better equipped for effectively facilitating lifelong beneficial and therapeutic lifestyle changes for their patients.

DISCUSSION QUESTIONS

1. How does a biopsychosocial approach allow providers to better detect and manage lifestyle changes?
2. What sorts of barriers to implementing lifestyle changes do patients typically face?

3. What factors should be examined in creating and monitoring a patient's personal recovery plan?

RECOMMENDED READINGS

Tessier JM, Erickson ZD, Meyer HB, et al: Therapeutic lifestyle changes: impact on weight, quality of life, and psychiatric symptoms in veterans with mental illness. Mil Med 182(9):e1738–e1744, 2017 28885930

Walsh R: Lifestyle and mental health. Am Psychol 66(7):579–592, 2011 21244124

Jacobson N, Greenley D: What is recovery? A conceptual model and explication. Psychiatr Serv 52(4):482–485, 2001 11274493

REFERENCES

Ames D, Carr-Lopez SM, Gutierrez MA, et al: Detecting and managing adverse effects of antipsychotic medications: current state of play. Psychiatr Clin North Am 39(2):275–311, 2016 27216904

Baker M, Tessier J, Meyer H, et al: Yoga-based classes for veterans with severe mental illness: development, dissemination, and assessment. Fed Pract 32(10):19–25, 2015

Ho PA, Dahle DN, Noordsy DL: Why do people with schizophrenia exercise? A mixed methods analysis among community dwelling regular exercisers. Front Psychiatry 9:596, 2018 30483166

Doran GT: There's a S.M.A.R.T. way to write management's goals and objectives. Management Review 70(11):35–36, 1981

Dozois DJ, Westra HA, Collins KA, et al: Stages of change in anxiety: psychometric properties of the University of Rhode Island Change Assessment (URICA) scale. Behav Res Ther 42(6):711–729, 2004 15081886

Erickson ZD, Mena SJ, Pierre JM, et al: Behavioral interventions for antipsychotic medication-associated obesity: a randomized, controlled clinical trial. J Clin Psychiatry 77(2):e183–e189, 2016 26930534

Erickson ZD, Kwan CL, Gelberg HA, et al: A randomized, controlled multisite study of behavioral interventions for veterans with mental illness and antipsychotic medication-associated obesity. J Gen Intern Med 32(suppl 1):32–39, 2017 28271424

Frankl VE: Man's Search for Meaning: An Introduction to Logotherapy. New York, Simon and Schuster, 1984

Joosten EA, DeFuentes-Merillas L, de Weert GH, et al: Systematic review of the effects of shared decision-making on patient satisfaction, treatment adherence and health status. Psychother Psychosom 77(4):219–226, 2008 18418028

Kashdan TB, Uswatte G, Julian T: Gratitude and hedonic and eudaimonic well-being in Vietnam War veterans. Behav Res Ther 44(2):177–199, 2006 16389060

Kendzor DE, Allicock M, Businelle MS, et al: Evaluation of a shelter-based diet and physical activity intervention for homeless adults. J Phys Act Health 14(2):88–97, 2017 27775471

Kleiman EM, Liu RT: Prospective prediction of suicide in a nationally representative sample: religious service attendance as a protective factor. Br J Psychiatry 204:262–266 2014 24115346

Klingaman EA, Hoerster KD, Aakre JM, et al: Veterans with PTSD report more weight loss barriers than veterans with no mental health disorders. Gen Hosp Psychiatry 39(1):1–7, 2016 26719103

Koenig HG: Association of religious involvement and suicide. JAMA Psychiatry 73(8):775–776, 2016 27367559

Laursen TM, Nordentoft M, Mortensen PB: Excess early mortality in schizophrenia. Annu Rev Clin Psychol 10(1):425–448, 2014 24313570

Lazar CM, Black AC, McMahon TJ, et al: All-data approach to assessing financial capability in people with psychiatric disabilities. Psychol Assess 28(4):362–371, 2016 26146947

Marks KA, Fastenau PS, Lysaker PH, et al: Self-Appraisal of Illness Questionnaire (SAIQ): relationship to researcher-rated insight and neuropsychological function in schizophrenia. Schizophr Res 45(3):203–211, 2000 11042438

Meyer HB, Katsman A, Sones AC, et al: Yoga as an ancillary treatment for neurological and psychiatric disorders: a review. J Neuropsychiatry Clin Neurosci 24(2):152–164, 2012 22772663

Noordsy DL, Burgess JD, Hardy KV, et al: Therapeutic potential of physical exercise in early psychosis. Am J Psychiatry 175(3):209–214, 2018 29490501

Sarno JE: The Mindbody Prescription: Healing the Body, Healing the Pain. New York, Grand Central Publishing, 2001

Schulz-Heik RJ, Meyer H, Mahoney L, et al: Results from a clinical yoga program for veterans: yoga via telehealth provides comparable satisfaction and health improvements to in-person yoga. BMC Complement Altern Med 17(1):198, 2017 28376861

Smith TE, Bellack AS, Liberman RP: Social skills training for schizophrenia: review and future directions. Clin Psychol Rev 16(7):599–617, 1996

Sumlin LL, Garcia TJ, Brown SA, et al: Depression and adherence to lifestyle changes in type 2 diabetes: a systematic review. Diabetes Educ 40(6):731–744, 2014 24939883

Tessier JM, Erickson ZD, Meyer HB, et al: Therapeutic lifestyle changes: impact on weight, quality of life, and psychiatric symptoms in veterans with mental illness. Mil Med 182(9):e1738–e1744, 2017 28885930

Walsh R: Lifestyle and mental health. Am Psychol 66(7):579–592, 2011 21244124

Wilbur S, Meyer HB, Baker MR, et al: Dance for veterans: a complementary health program for veterans with serious mental illness. Arts Health 7(2):96–108, 2015

Yu B-H, Ancoli-Israel S, Dimsdale JE: Effect of CPAP treatment on mood states in patients with sleep apnea. J Psychiatr Res 33(5):427–432, 1999 10504011

Ziegelstein RC, Fauerbach JA, Stevens SS, et al: Patients with depression are less likely to follow recommendations to reduce cardiac risk during recovery from a myocardial infarction. Arch Intern Med 160(12):1818–1823, 2000 10871976

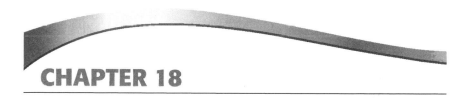

CHAPTER 18

Physician Lifestyle and Health-Promoting Behavior

Debora Holmes, M.E.S.

Erica Frank, M.D., M.P.H.

KEY POINTS

- A majority of people cite their physician as their primary source of information regarding healthy lifestyle decisions; these patients are more likely to adopt a healthy lifestyle when their physician recommends it.

- Physicians and medical students with healthy personal habits more consistently report counseling their patients about these habits, and physicians who personally adopt recommended preventive screenings and interventions have more prevention-adherent patients.

- It is increasingly obvious that medical schools should proactively produce healthy doctors.

- The "Healthy Doc = Healthy Patient" relationship encourages prevention-oriented health care systems to evaluate and support the many positive effects of physicians' health on the health of their patients.

According to a 2000 study, a majority of Americans see their physicians as primary sources of information regarding healthy lifestyle decisions, and patients are more likely to adopt healthy behaviors if their physicians make such recommendations (Abramson et al. 2000). North American physicians and medical students tend to report significantly better health habits when compared with same-age peers. As a group, physicians must continue to encourage exercise and other healthy habits because these behaviors correlate with positive mental and physical health outcomes not only for doctors but also for patients. In this chapter, we discuss this likelihood of habitually healthy physicians promoting these same habits to their patients; this "Healthy Doc = Healthy Patient" relationship (the term was first consistently used by Frank et al. [2005]) is true for many health behaviors. We also highlight the importance of medical school and physician interventions to increase the numbers of physicians (both in training and in practice) adopting and maintaining regular healthy habits, in order to increase the rates of physician-delivered, health-promoting prescriptions in the future.

Many studies in multiple countries have found that physicians and medical students who testify to healthy personal habits more consistently report counseling their own patients about related habits (notably, Duperly et al. 2008a; Frank and Segura 2009; Frank et al. 2000a, 2007a, 2010; Oberg and Frank 2009). Most recently, however, instead of relying solely on physicians' self-reported counseling and preventive practices, the relationship between healthy doctor and healthy patient has been assessed through objectively measured clinical experiences (Frank et al. 2013). In so doing, researchers have further documented consistent, positive relationships between physicians' and patients' preventive health practices.

In this chapter, we also emphasize the importance of cultivating proactive medical doctors in the good soil of responsive medical schools and universities, although, to date, it appears that only one large-scale study (Frank et al. 2005, 2007b) has documented this type of intervention and its efficacy.

PHYSICIAN WELL-BEING AND THE CONNECTION WITH PATIENT HEALTH

Multiple studies have demonstrated that physicians' physical activity, along with other health-promoting activities, can significantly improve the likelihood that these doctors will counsel their own patients about positive changes in diet and exercise (Lobelo et al. 2009). However, barriers—both attitudinal and systemic—exist for many patients (McKenna et al. 1998).

Fortunately, and contrary to many physicians' beliefs that talking to patients about lifestyle change is ineffective (Gould et al. 1995; Pinto et al. 1998), several decades of data show that a physician's advice on either diet or exercise—or both—makes a difference in motivating the patient's own health-related practices. For example, a 1997 Centers for Disease Control and Prevention (CDC) study of 20,847 adult Americans showed that when patients had been given advice from their physicians to exercise, 74.7% of them exercised more; without such advice, only 50.5% were found to be exercising more at follow-up (Centers for Disease Control and Prevention 1999).

Longitudinal monitoring of behavior change with continuous encouragement and goal refinement is helpful to patient success. Between doctor visits, physicians may need to explore more creative options. For instance, with the advent of trackers and smartphone applications to monitor exercise, behavior change techniques—goal setting, feedback, and rewards—are available in small packages. Fitness technology itself has the potential to significantly affect public health, research, and policies, and doctors can be a part of this potential (Sullivan and Lachman 2017).

Physicians may wish to suggest that patients take advantage of their local fitness centers, where trainers and personal exercise records can be a part of goal furtherance. Often, at least in the United States, insurance policies—particularly for seniors—cover or defray the costs of such centers. Of course, if the physician also takes advantage of his or her local fitness center, a great potential exists for conversation regarding such venues.

Encouragement to patients can also come from conveying summaries of current positive research. A recent *Washington Post* article (Burfoot 2018) discussed researchers, including lead researcher Benjamin Levine (Howden et al. 2018), who indicated that cardiovascular health can actually increase in middle age. A "sound bite" (such as the following) from a physician might offer encouragement to a middle-aged patient who could benefit from exercise but feels it is too late for any kind of useful regimen:

> In earlier studies, Levine had shown that older athletes have roughly the same degree of cardiac compliance as young adults. However, he had also discovered that regular exercise couldn't increase the cardiac compliance of subjects over 65. Now he believes he has found the "sweet spot" in time when adults can still enhance their heart function: from ages 45 to 64. "We have demonstrated that if you incorporate regular exercise into your daily life, starting no later than middle age, you can restore the youthfulness of your heart muscle," he says. (Burfoot 2018)

We can see how vital it is to keep the lines of communication open and to provide patients with both new information and feedback about their lifestyles. In their 2014 publication, Drazen and colleagues described the Division of Medical Communications they founded at Brigham and Women's Hospital and the great need for improvement in communication between doctor and patient, stating, "Excellent physician communication skills (physician-to-patient and patient-to-physician) have been found to have a positive impact on patient satisfaction and may positively affect patient health behaviors and health outcomes" (Drazen et al. 2014, p. 1623). Their article offers an expansive discussion of key types of medical communication and best methods of communication.

Data such as those found in the CDC's research (Centers for Disease Control and Prevention 1999) offer compelling reasons to encourage improved exercise (and nutrition and other health) habits among physicians—and this should start with medical students. An intervention study involving senior medical students and 800 standardized patients (Frank et al. 2005, 2007b) found that those students exposed to personal health-promotion curricula (exercise and diet) during medical school were 65% more likely to counsel their patients about exercise and 49% more likely to counsel about diet than medical students who had not been exposed. We expand on student health and intervention in the section "Medical Student Health and the Importance of Cultivating It."

Physicians, Exercise, and Patients

North American physicians tend to live longer than their peers because of healthier habits. Those with the healthiest habits are the most likely to advise their patients about related preventive habits. This is particularly true for exercise (Frank and Holmes 2019). Doctors (and medical students) reporting significantly better exercise habits than their peer groups see a high correlation with positive mental and physical health outcomes—for both physician and patient. As with other healthy habits, findings on exercise highlight the importance of medical school and physician health interventions in order to increase present and future rates of physician-delivered exercise prescriptions (Lobelo et al. 2009).

Good exercise behaviors are strongly normative among North American physicians and medical students. For instance, research has shown that Canadian physicians (Frank and Segura 2009), U.S. women physicians (Frank 1995), and U.S. medical students (Frank et al. 2004a) typically exercise more than their same-age, same-gender peers in the general population. One large national study found that U.S. medical students possess behavioral characteristics that are quite positive overall. Regarding exercise, the students reported a median of 4 hours on average per week, with strenuous exercise preferred (Frank et al. 2006). Similarly, Canadian physicians exercised a mean of 4.7 hours per week (Frank and Segura 2009). A similar relationship between U.S. women doctors and their patients exists: those who comply with American College of Sports Medicine recommendations discuss exercise with their patients significantly more frequently, and these physicians are highly significantly more likely to exhibit confidence in their exercise counseling and training (Lobelo et al. 2009).

Frank and colleagues developed, implemented, and tested a 4-year curricular and extracurricular intervention to promote healthy behaviors among students in the Class of 2003 attending Emory University School of Medicine (EUSM) in Atlanta, Georgia (Frank et al. 2005, 2007b). The objective of this intervention, which focused heavily on physical activity and corresponding classes and sessions (and which we discuss more thoroughly in the section "Medical Student Health and the Importance of Cultivating It"), was to test whether the promotion of medical student health would efficiently improve patient counseling—and, indeed, these students' prevention-related attitudes and counseling practices were positively influenced by the intervention (Frank et al. 2007b).

Other researchers have subsequently assessed physician activity levels and physical activity counseling practices of doctors in training and in practice (e.g., Buffart et al. 2009; van der Ploeg et al. 2007). Physical activity counseling varies by practice setting and specialty; however, some have reported it suboptimal, and numerous barriers may still exist (Burack 1989; Garry et al. 2002).

Collectively, evidence indicates a robust association between personal physical activity behaviors and physical activity counseling practices in both practicing doctors and medical students. We already know how to positively intervene when it comes to exercise and medical students: medical schools are willing to encourage more exercise for their students, and when they do, that correlates with medical students exercising more and telling their patients to do likewise, along with outcomes of more positive personal health. As physicians, we must take care of ourselves as well as our patients: exercising more helps us do a better job with both those responsibilities. The following narrative describes one physician's creative approach to getting a regular dose of workout.

Case Example: For One Physician, Healthy Meets Multitasking

Before laptop computers emerged on the scene, Dr. Erica Frank (chapter coauthor) read journals and books that were not too heavy to hold while she pedaled an exercise bike. However, once she had ridden a few miles with a laptop secured to the front of her stationary bike with a rubber band, she knew she had found her preferred regular exercise modality. Here was a health-promotion activity that satisfied so many criteria simultaneously! She no longer experienced remorse over wasting time getting a special outfit for exercise, getting to and from her place of exercise, or even performing the exercise itself (no longer feeling that her brain and hands and quadriceps should all have higher purposes). Additionally, she no longer stewed in boredom while exercising, a serious impediment to other forms of regular exercise she had attempted previously.

In the thousands of miles ridden since that day, done most days of the year, Dr. Frank learned not only to simultaneously read and write while biking but even to chair conference calls—although the latter usually with the video function turned off. Likewise, she has discovered that it is often an educational and cardiovascular treat to walk around a new urban or biologically rich environment en route to a task. Walking while talking with friends can be fruitful too, whether with a buddy in person or on the phone, with a backward-facing child in a stroller, or as a stroll with a significant other that pays attention to the light, weather, and one's shared ecosystem. This combination allows casual triathleticism at age 55: although Dr. Frank never trains particularly for an event above baseline exercise and usually finishes near last in each category, she always finishes, and without injury or next-day soreness.

Physicians, Diet, and Patients

Because few national studies existed regarding the clinical practices of primary care physicians on overweight and obesity, even in the face of the growing obesity epidemic (National Institute of Diabetes and Digestive and Kidney Diseases 2017), Smith et al. (2011) set out to document patterns among primary care physicians in their practices. The researchers profiled diet, physical activity, and weight control practice patterns via a representative survey of 1,211 primary care physicians sampled from the American Medical Association's Masterfile. Less than 50% of primary care physicians reported that they always provided specific guidance on physical activity, diet, or weight control; those who did most often counseled on physical activity. The researchers concluded that primary care physician assessment and behavioral management of overweight and obesity in adults was inadequate relative to the magnitude of the problem in the United States, given a U.S. overweight/obesity rate of 70% (National Institute of Diabetes and Digestive and Kidney Diseases 2017), and that further research was warranted regarding barriers to care and improved physician engagement in the management of patients' lifestyles.

Realizing that physicians play vital roles in addressing the overweight and obesity epidemic, Pool et al. (2014) analyzed data ($N=5,054$ patients) from the 2005–2008 National Health and Nutritional Examination Survey and reported finding clinically significant patient weight loss associated with physicians discussing their patients' weight status directly. Also in 2014, Dutton and colleagues reported that patients seen by female physicians were more likely to receive obesity counseling or be referred for obesity treatment than were those seen by male physicians (Dutton et al. 2014); their findings add to previous evidence suggesting differences in such counseling practices between male and female physicians (Frank and Harvey 1996).

HEALTHIER PHYSICIAN HABITS: A STUDY OF RESPONSES FROM PATIENTS

As touched on earlier, patients care about physician encouragement surrounding exercise and other preventive practices. Providers who disclose their healthy personal health practices are perceived as more credible and motivating; rates of prevention counseling increase, and patients become more receptive to health promotion counseling from physicians when those physicians demonstrate healthy behaviors themselves. Frank et al. (2000b) conducted a small study ($N=130$) in an Emory University general medical clinic waiting room. They randomly assigned individuals to watch either a standard 2-minute video from Dr. Erica Frank (chapter coauthor) on healthy diet and exercise habits or the standard video plus an extra 30 seconds divulging Dr. Frank's personal health habits regarding diet and exercise. Patients found Dr. Frank in the physician disclosure video to be significantly healthier ($P=0.001$) and also found her more believable and more motivating overall. Specifically, regarding both diet and exercise, patients found that merely 30 extra seconds made Dr. Frank more believable on both diet and exercise ($P=0.006$ and $P=0.002$, respectively) and also more motivating on diet and exercise ($P=0.006$ and $P=0.001$, respectively). These data exhibit that physicians' credibility and ability to motivate patients increases when doctors are clearly viewed as exercising and eating healthy.

MEDICAL STUDENT HEALTH AND THE IMPORTANCE OF CULTIVATING IT

The Healthy Doc = Healthy Patient studies—with more than 100 such studies available from chapter coauthor Erica Frank (see Recommended Readings at the end of the chapter)—exemplify the importance of implementing and testing interventions to promote healthy behaviors during medical school. The objective of the previously mentioned 4-year curricular and extracurricular intervention for promoting healthy behaviors among EUSM students (Frank et al. 2005, 2007b) was to test whether the promotion of medical student health would efficiently improve patient counseling, with the students in the class of 2003 attending EUSM as the intervention group and the class of 2002 as a control.

In general, students receiving the intervention—a personal health promotion curriculum on exercise and diet during their medical school curriculum—perceived the school to be a healthier environment than did the control students, reporting significantly more agreement with school-controlled items such as curricular encouragement of physical activity, emphasis on preventive medicine, provision of extracurricular activities (such as physical activity classes or sessions), and even encouragement of exercising by classmates. Students' prevention-related attitudes and counseling practices were positively influenced by the intervention: students exposed to the curriculum were 65% more likely ($P=0.03$) to counsel their patients about exercise and 49% more likely to counsel ($P=0.04$) regarding diet.

As additional support for encouraging medical student exercise, we note that, those who exercise more are also somewhat more likely to respond that counseling their future patients about exercise would be highly relevant (Frank et al. 2004a) and more likely to actually counsel their current patients about exercise (Frank et al. 2007b). In the latter study, medical students also were shown to be able to appropriately assess their own exercise habits and the need for improvement.

To determine personal and clinical exercise-related attitudes and behaviors of freshmen U.S. medical students, Frank et al. (2004a) looked at 1,906 entering freshman medical students in 17 U.S. medical schools. Students reported high exercise levels—a median of 45 minutes per day of exercise (80 minutes per week each of mild and moderate exercise and

100 minutes per week of strenuous exercise). Nearly all freshman medical students (97.6%) engaged in some moderate or vigorous exercise in a typical week, with 64% complying with U.S. Department of Health and Human Services exercise recommendations. Most freshmen (79%) believed it would be highly relevant to their future practices to counsel patients about exercise; the strongest professional predictor of perceived relevance was the intention to become a primary care provider, and personal predictors included excellent general health, a prevention emphasis by their personal physicians, and performing more strenuous exercise.

A follow-up study by Frank et al. (2007a) reported on predictors of multiple prevention counseling practices among U.S. medical students; overall, those students reporting a healthier medical school environment also reported highly significantly better patient counseling practices. The personal health practices of these students were correlated with the students' perceived relevance of counseling ($P = 0.008$) and also the frequency with which they counseled patients ($P < 0.0001$).

Data from the United States indicate that medical students with healthy personal habits have better attitudes toward preventive counseling, but what about elsewhere? The first major study we know of relating to this association in medical students in low- or middle-income countries examined the association between personal health practices and attitudes toward preventive counseling among first- and fifth-year students from eight medical schools in Bogotá, Colombia (Duperly et al. 2008a, 2009).

In 2006, first- and fifth-year medical students ($N = 661$) completed a culturally adapted Spanish version of the Healthy Doc = Healthy Patient survey (Duperly et al. 2008a, 2009). Logistic regression analyses assessed the association between overall personal practices regarding physical activity, nutrition, weight control, smoking, alcohol use (main exposure variable), and student attitudes toward preventive counseling on these issues (main outcome variable). Data were stratified by year of training and adjusted by gender and medical training–related factors (basic knowledge, perceived adequacy of training, and perception of the school's encouragement of each healthy habit). The median age and percentage of females for the first- and fifth-year students were 21 years and 59.5% and 25 years and 65%, respectively. After controlling for gender and medical training–related factors, consumption of five or more daily servings of fruits and/or vegetables and not being a smoker or binge drinker were associated with positive attitudes toward counseling on nutrition and on alcohol. As with the U.S. physician and medical students, a positive association was found between the personal health habits of Colombian medical students and their corresponding attitudes toward preventive counseling, independent of gender and medical training–related factors.

These findings suggest that within the medical school context, interventions focused on promoting healthy student lifestyles can improve these future physicians' attitudes toward preventive counseling.

HEALTHY DOC = HEALTHY PATIENT CONCEPT AND APPLICATIONS

The Healthy Doc = Healthy Patient initiative (see Frank et al. 2013, Oberg and Frank 2009), a series of studies and programs to improve physicians' prevention counseling via improving their personal health practices, was originally developed in the early 1990s by chapter coauthor Frank. This initiative has ultimately led, among other research, to the research performed at EUSM to improve medical student health, with the hypothesis that this could also improve patient health. The Healthy Doc = Healthy Patient principles, compiled over time, are as follows.

- North American physicians tend to live longer than their peers.
- Physicians live longer because they have healthier habits (including as medical students) than their contemporaries.
- Four behavioral choices (exercise, diet, alcohol use, and tobacco use) account for about 37% of U.S. mortality (Mokdad et al. 2004).
- Physicians and medical students with the healthiest habits are more likely to advise their patients about related preventive habits.
- Appropriate physician revelation about healthy personal habits can make physicians more believable and motivating to patients.
- When medical schools encourage students to be healthy, it positively and significantly influences the students' patient counseling frequency (P=0.002) and the perceived relevance of such counseling (P=0.0007).
- Counseling patients makes a difference in patients' habits and health.
- Physicians do not perform prevention counseling at very high rates.

Analysis and quantitative assessment of the 4-year-long intervention showed that the intervention successfully promoted healthy physical habits among medical students (Frank et al. 2007b). EUSM's class of 2003 was extensively studied after various interventions were performed throughout the students' entire schooling. Specifically, curricular interventions included lectures, problem-based learning discussions, physician case panels, anatomy and exercise manuals, student presentations, an exercise elective and seminar, interventions in all clerkships (dermatology, family medicine, gynecology/obstetrics, internal medicine, pediatrics, psychiatry, and surgery), and shared anonymized data on their class's health practices for use in learning biostatistics. Extracurricular interventions included healthy and quick cooking workshops, personal health prescriptions, provision of healthy breakfasts before exams, group hikes, mountain retreats, monthly walks and runs, weekly yoga classes, a yoga and meditation seminar, a massage talk and demonstration with free lunch, and a wine tasting (added because students initially thought that the researchers were promoting abstemiousness) (Frank et al. 2005).

In this 4-year controlled trial addressing lifestyle behaviors over the course of medical school, intervention-group medical students had some improvement in their personal health practices: male control students reported twice the tobacco use at graduation as reported by males in the intervention group (43% vs. 22%, $P=0.02$), although the two groups had previously reported very similar levels (31% vs. 29%, $P=0.8$) (Frank et al. 2007b; Oberg and Frank 2009). Most importantly, on a population basis, students' diet counseling and exercise counseling practices (as reported by standardized patients) were also strongly positively related to the intervention.

When the Healthy Doc = Healthy Patient principles were postulated to be applicable to medical students and doctors in developing countries, Duperly et al. (2008a, 2008b) decided to test these principles in Colombia—initially collecting data during 2006 from the first- and fifth-year students attending the eight medical schools in Bogotá and more recently expanding that data collection to a nationally representative sample of 24 medical schools. Analysis ($N=661$) confirmed the U.S. findings of a strong association between physical activity and other personal health habits and attitudes toward related preventive counseling. The study found lower rates of compliance regarding physical activity recommendations among Colombian students than among U.S. medical students (50% vs. 61%), but these rates were still better than those of age-matched peers in the Colombian general population. The Colombian Healthy Doc = Healthy Patient study provided further evidence of the strong, consistent, and generalizable association between personal health practices and preventive counseling attitudes among doctors in training.

A Recent Objective View From Israel's Largest Health Maintenance Organization

Beyond merely relying on physicians' self-reported counseling and preventive practices, the relationship between physician health and patient health was recently assessed through objectively measured clinical experiences. Frank et al. (2013) accessed complete vaccination and screening records from Clalit Health Services (CHS), Israel's largest health maintenance organization. This included the electronic medical records of 1) primary care physicians who worked in and were also patients in CHS ($n=1,488$) and 2) those CHS physicians' adult patients ($n=1,886,791$).

Eight prevention-related (screening and immunization practices) quality health indicators used by Clalit as quality metrics were chosen for analysis:

1. Mammography in women ages 50–74 years
2. Colorectal cancer screening in patients ages 50–74 years
3. Low-density lipoprotein measurement every 5 years for patients ages 35–54 years and yearly among patients ages 55–74 years
4. Blood pressure measurement every 5 years for patients ages 40 years and younger
5. Blood pressure measurement every 2 years for patients ages 41–54 years
6. Blood pressure measurement annually for patients 55 years and older
7. Pneumococcal vaccination among patients with a chronic illness and those 65 years and older
8. Annual influenza vaccine among patients with chronic illness and those 65 years and older

For all eight indicators, patients whose physicians were compliant with the preventive practices were more likely ($P<0.05$) to also have undergone these preventive measures than were patients with noncompliant physicians. The investigators also found that more closely related preventive practices showed even more robust relationships.

PREVENTION COUNSELING FOR THE PATIENT

We have already witnessed that physician counseling of patients makes a difference in patients' habits and thus in their overall health and that one of the strongest predictors of health promotion counseling is whether physicians practice healthy behaviors themselves. Conversely, many physicians report difficulties in counseling patients about behaviors they themselves do not practice (Frank 2004; Vickers et al. 2007).

Physicians are key health role models and advisors who often meet with patients during educable moments, and their personal health behaviors affect their credibility and ability to engage their patients in similar healthy behaviors (Frank et al. 2000b). Importantly for busy doctors, it seems that simply talking briefly to patients about their own personal health practices improves the efficiency of health promotion practices for patients (Abramson et al. 2000). Not only is practicing healthy behavior oneself strongly correlated with a physician's counseling of patients on said behavior (Frank 2004), somewhat surprisingly, this may actually hold true regardless of the physician's actual health status: physicians attempting to improve their own poor habits have been found to counsel patients significantly more often than physicians who were not trying to change their own behaviors (Lewis et al. 1986).

Although we are well aware that counseling patients makes a difference in their habits and their health and that North Americans' poor behavioral choices regarding diet, exercise, alcohol, and tobacco account for about 37% of U.S. mortality rates (Mokdad et al. 2004), physicians still do not perform prevention counseling at very high rates (Lobelo et al. 2009). And yet, counter to what we may have learned in medical school, appropriate revelation concerning physicians' own healthy personal exercise and dietary habits can make doctors even more believable and motivating to patients (Frank et al. 2000b). Ultimately, the most important reason for encouraging sufficient medical student and physician exercise, healthy diet, and other health-promoting practices is that this manifestation of the Healthy Doc = Healthy Patient principles makes a difference with patients.

Abramson et al. (2000) surveyed a random sample of 298 primary care physicians and found the following:

- Physicians who perform aerobic exercise regularly are more likely to counsel their patients on the benefits of this type of exercise; the same holds true for physicians who perform strength training.
- Pediatricians and geriatricians counsel a smaller proportion of their patients about aerobic exercise than do family practitioners and internists.
- Counseling regarding strength (versus aerobic) training is less common in all physician groups surveyed and lowest among pediatricians, 50% of whom did not advise strength training for any of their patients.
- Inadequate time was noted by 61% and inadequate knowledge and/or experience by 16% of respondents as the major barriers to counseling regarding aerobic exercise.

Note that these findings, particularly those regarding barriers, suggest strategies that might increase physician exercise counseling behavior.

THE FUTURE OF LIFESTYLE MEDICINE

Medical school deans are quite enthusiastic about the value and appropriateness of encouraging positive health behaviors among their ranks (Frank et al. 2004b). Both deans and students tended to agree with the following statement, taken from the Healthy Doc = Healthy Patient questionnaire survey and scored from 1 (strongly agree) to 5 (strongly disagree): "Medical school faculty members should set a good example for medical students by practicing a healthy lifestyle" (1.4 for deans and 2.1 for medical students). A statement that medical schools should encourage their students and residents to practice healthy lifestyles garnered 1.3 on the scale from deans and 1.9 from students, and a statement that "in order to effectively encourage patient adherence to a healthy lifestyle, a physician must adhere to one him/herself" scored 2.1 and 2.2, respectively.

Case Example: Exercise Vanquishes Stress for One Medical Intern

When she had completed the first half of her medical internship in the oncology department of a large community hospital, Verena had a very hard time leaving behind the suffering and strokes of fate that her patients endured when she stepped through the hospital's exit door each night. In addition, she lived in staff housing in very close proximity to the hospital—her living room faced the windows of the ward in which she worked. She just couldn't seem to get away.

At that point, Verena took up running. Every day after work, she exchanged her scrubs for running tights and a T-shirt and took off into the nearby forest. Sometimes she listened to music, podcasts, or audiobooks; sometimes her brain needed the peace and quiet, and she would simply run and become one with the beautiful natural settings surrounding her. After an hour or so, Verena would return home drenched in sweat but with a peaceful mind. She was able to create the much-needed distance and larger perspective that allowed her to continue working in the medical profession without sacrificing her own well-being.

Seven years later, she still runs, having completed several half-marathons, a marathon, and a half-Ironman-distance triathlon. The sport has given her a healthy body, joy, and her most important outlet for stress. Verena believes that thanks to running, she falls asleep happy and content every night.

More on Well-Being and Interventions for the Physician and Physician in Training

Although physicians' and medical students' personal health practices are better than those of the general population (at least in Canada, Colombia, and the United States), multiple studies still suggest the need to further foster physicians' personal preventive practices, both to promote the personal health of physicians themselves and to improve outcomes for their patients.

Today's physicians often find themselves in a bit of a void when it comes to personal fitness. Even if exercise facilities and healthy foods are present in the immediate vicinity, time itself often presents a big barrier. As doctors and students, we must all consider—and share with coworkers and patients—creative measures and efficient strategies for good health, including multitasking while exercising (recall Dr. Frank's story in this chapter).

We have already touched on technology and various apps to monitor exercise and diet. Fitbits and similar activity trackers, worn on the wrist or otherwise visibly displayed, or a bicycle parked in the office, may open doors to conversations with patients—or, at the very least, convey a physician's personal interest in a healthy lifestyle. These lifestyle changes can feel toughest and most frustrating at their initiation. However, if physicians personally experience this frustration (and especially if they have discovered ways to combat it), the journey's lessons, in turn, can be relayed to patients under their care, along with a dose of motivation, because it comes from a believable source (Frank et al. 2000b). Debora Holmes (chapter coauthor) remembers a point in her life when she lacked the motivation to (among other things) exercise—and then she read the still-accessible *Feeling Good: The New Mood Therapy* (Burns 1980). In a recent blog, author David D. Burns summed up the important points of his book:

> As I wrote in my first book, *Feeling Good: The New Mood Therapy*, highly productive people know that ACTION comes first, followed by motivation. In other words, you have to get started on some task *before* you'll feel motivated. You're not entitled to feel motivated until you've start accomplishing something! Waiting for motivation is the trap that keeps your procrastination alive and prospering. (Burns 2018)

These points made all the difference for Debora at the time, and they continue to do so today. Debora has found that simply stating this principle of action versus motivation to procrastinating individuals changes their worldview and, not surprisingly, reinforces her own. We can all recall words from trusted teachers, doctors, and other professionals—words that really meant something to us and that may even have sent us on new trajectories. Don't underestimate the power of conveying what you, as either a physician or a patient, have personally found motivating and transformative.

The relationship between physician health and patient health most ideally begins at orientation for freshman medical students; medical schools must concentrate on maximizing the growth of these ideals—and individuals— early on. In addition, such programs need to be studied in order to determine how best to actively encourage physician health and, correspondingly, the association between healthy physician and healthy patient. To date, the authors of this chapter know of no such published studies, although a collaboration on such a study is now ongoing between the School of Medicine at Bar-Ilan University (in Safed, Israel) and NextGenU.org that uses NextGen's free, accredited Lifestyle Medicine course. We look forward to encouraging and enabling other such interventions, especially because the findings explored in this chapter suggest that further refinements and broader implementation of interventions are efficient and valuable methods to improve the health of health care professionals, along with the vast populations of patients they serve.

CONCLUSION

At the beginning of every airplane trip, flight attendants or oddly amusing videos lay out guidance for air emergencies. Tucked in the litany is the following familiar sentence: "In case of emergency, oxygen masks will drop from the ceiling. If you are traveling with children, please put on your own mask before helping others." Although perhaps a bit unsettling to parents who value their children's lives above their own, the instruction is based on the logic that we cannot be of use to others unless we are taking care of ourselves. Those of us practicing in medical fields must begin (or continue) to include a focus on optimizing our own lifestyles to best help and inspire our patients and other audiences. If we fail to put on our own mask first, we do a great disservice to those under our care.

We know that the health of North American (and most other studied) physician populations is very good, although there is room for improvement regarding physical and, particularly, mental health among both physicians and medical students. When looking through the lens showing that a healthy doctor is more likely to produce a healthy patient, the physician's health status takes on paramount importance.

The medical and health care communities, along with North American universities, must implement new approaches to achieve these goals. As physicians, we need to 1) discuss ways to simultaneously improve our health and that of our patients and 2) consider the most important new questions to ask regarding physician health. We simply must take care of ourselves as well as our patients; when we do, we will witness more positive personal health outcomes for all concerned.

Although the World Medical Association (2015) passed policy on the importance of encouraging physician well-being, particularly acknowledging the link between healthy doctors and healthy patients, it is unusual to see physician health systematically promoted anywhere on the planet. This suggests that policymakers believe that physicians are already adequately supported and that there are few reasons for them to further support this privileged population. In the few places where support programs for physicians exist, these programs concentrate heavily on suitability and competence to practice, on mental health and illness (especially around burnout and substance abuse), and on practice-related psychological motivation and physical stamina.

Therefore, we urge you—whether provider, patient, or casual reader—to think about your personal habits and then reflect on your advice giving. What kind of correlation do you see? In other words, do you practice what you preach? Physicians and the medical profession at large need to do more in the self-care realm. A failure to create such opportunities is also a failure to efficiently improve the health of everyone in the system. Conversely, the findings and suggestions in this chapter have obvious and pronounced implications for preventing and managing disease on a global scale (see Chapter 20, "Implications of Lifestyle Medicine and Psychiatry for Health Care Systems and Population Health"). We wish you the best in your personal and professional journeys—and in the collective quest for self and global well-being.

DISCUSSION QUESTIONS

1. If you are a physician or other health provider, think about the ways in which your personal health practices (both healthy and less healthy) affect how energetically you pursue health risks with a patient.
2. Whether you are a health provider or not, consider how your own primary care provider's personal health practices may affect your own habits.

RECOMMENDED READINGS

Frank E: STUDENTJAMA. Physician health and patient care. JAMA 291(5):637, 2004

Frank E: Sorted list of physician/medical student health publications. Updated 2019. Available at: https://docs.google.com/spreadsheets/d/1JZeH_L1pK7eMs3R_w6p5mr0h_ZolxkAWJdijXSgbtuY/edit?usp=sharing. Accessed January 23, 2019.

Frank E, Dresner Y, Shani M, et al: The association between physicians' and patients' preventive health practices. CMAJ 185(8):649–653, 2013

Oberg EB, Frank E: Physicians' health practices strongly influence patient health practices. J R Coll Physicians Edinb 39(4):290–291, 2009

Weiss RL (ed): The Handbook of Personal Health and Wellbeing for Physicians and Trainees. New York, Springer, 2018

REFERENCES

Abramson S, Stein J, Schaufele M, et al: Personal exercise habits and counseling practices of primary care physicians: a national survey. Clin J Sport Med 10(1):40–48, 2000 10695849

Buffart LM, van der Ploeg HP, Smith BJ, et al: General practitioners' perceptions and practices of physical activity counselling: changes over the past 10 years. Br J Sports Med 43(14):1149–1153, 2009 18628359

Burack RC: Barriers to clinical preventive medicine. Prim Care 16(1):245–250, 1989 2649905

Burfoot A: Middle age is not too late to increase cardiac fitness, studies show. Washington Post (online), January 29, 2018. Available at: www.washingtonpost.com/lifestyle/wellness/middle-age-is-not-too-late-to-increase-cardiac-fitness-studies-show/2018/01/25/2708d116-faeb-11e7-ad8c-ecbb62019393_story.html?noredirect=on&utm_term=.a3977528b3d9. Accessed May 7, 2018.

Burns DD: Feeling Good: The New Mood Therapy. New York, William Morrow, 1980

Burns DD: Five simple ways to boost your happiness—#2: do something you've been putting off. Feeling Good: The Website of David D. Burns, M.D., February 12, 2018. Available at: https://feelinggood.com/tag/motivation. Accessed May 7, 2018.

Centers for Disease Control and Prevention: Physician advice and individual behaviors about cardiovascular disease risk reduction—seven states and Puerto Rico, 1997. MMWR Morb Mortal Wkly Rep 48(4):74–77, 1999 10023628

Drazen JM, Shields HM, Loscalzo J: A division of medical communications in an academic medical center's department of medicine. Acad Med 89(12):1623–1629, 2014 25186816

Duperly J, Lobelo F, Segura C, et al: Personal habits are independently associated with a positive attitude towards healthy lifestyle counseling among Colombian medical students. Circulation 117:198–291, 2008a

Duperly J, Segura C, Herrera DM, et al: Medical student's knowledge on physical activity counseling is associated with their physical activity levels. Med Sci Sports Exerc 40(5):S251, 2008b

Duperly J, Lobelo F, Segura C, et al: The association between Colombian medical students' healthy personal habits and a positive attitude toward preventive counseling: cross-sectional analyses. BMC Public Health 9:218, 2009 19575806

Dutton GR, Herman KG, Tan F, et al: Patient and physician characteristics associated with the provision of weight loss counseling in primary care. Obes Res Clin Pract 8(2):e123–e130, 2014 24743007

Frank E: The Women Physicians' Health Study: background, objectives, and methods. J Am Med Womens Assoc (1972) 50(2):64–66, 1995 7722210

Frank E: STUDENTJAMA. Physician health and patient care. JAMA 291(5):637, 2004 14762049

Frank E, Harvey LK: Prevention advice rates of women and men physicians. Arch Fam Med 5(4):215–219, 1996 8769910

Frank E, Holmes D: Exercise, in The Art and Science of Physician Wellbeing: A Handbook for Physicians and Trainees. Edited by Trockel M, Roberts LW. New York, Springer International, 2019, in press

Frank E, Segura C: Health practices of Canadian physicians. Can Fam Physician 55(8):810–811.e7, 2009 19675268

Frank E, Rothenberg R, Lewis C, et al: Correlates of physicians' prevention-related practices: findings from the Women Physicians' Health Study. Arch Fam Med 9(4):359–367, 2000a 10776365

Frank E, Breyan J, Elon L: Physician disclosure of healthy personal behaviors improves credibility and ability to motivate. Arch Fam Med 9(3):287–290, 2000b 10728118

Frank E, Galuska DA, Elon LK, et al: Personal and clinical exercise-related attitudes and behaviors of freshmen U.S. medical students. Res Q Exerc Sport 75(2):112–121, 2004a 15209329

Frank E, Hedgecock J, Elon LK: Personal health promotion at US medical schools: a quantitative study and qualitative description of deans' and students' perceptions. BMC Med Educ 4(1):29, 2004b 15581424

Frank E, Smith D, Fitzmaurice D: A description and qualitative assessment of a 4-year intervention to improve patient counseling by improving medical student health. MedGenMed 7(2):4, 2005 16369383

Frank E, Carrera JS, Elon L, et al: Basic demographics, health practices, and health status of U.S. medical students. Am J Prev Med 31(6):499–505, 2006 17169711

Frank E, Carrera JS, Elon L, et al: Predictors of US medical students' prevention counseling practices. Prev Med 44(1):76–81, 2007a 16978687

Frank E, Elon L, Hertzberg V: A quantitative assessment of a 4-year intervention that improved patient counseling through improving medical student health. MedGenMed 9(2):58, 2007b 17955112

Frank E, Segura C, Shen H, et al: Predictors of Canadian physicians' prevention counseling practices. Can J Public Health 101(5):390–395, 2010 21214054

Frank E, Dresner Y, Shani M, et al: The association between physicians' and patients' preventive health practices. CMAJ 185(8):649 653, 2013 23569163

Garry JP, Diamond JJ, Whitley TW: Physical activity curricula in medical schools. Acad Med 77(8):818–820, 2002 12176695

Gould MM, Thorogood M, Iliffe S, et al: Promoting physical activity in primary care: measuring the knowledge gap. Health Educ J 54(3):304–311, 1995

Howden EJ, Sarma S, Lawley JS, et al: Reversing the cardiac effects of sedentary aging in middle age—a randomized controlled trial: implications for heart failure prevention. Circulation 137(15):1549–1560, 2018 29311053

Lewis CE, Wells KB, Ware J: A model for predicting the counseling practices of physicians. J Gen Intern Med 1(1):14–19, 1986 3772565

Lobelo F, Duperly J, Frank E: Physical activity habits of doctors and medical students influence their counselling practices. Br J Sports Med 43(2):89–92, 2009 19019898

McKenna J, Naylor P-J, McDowell N: Barriers to physical activity promotion by general practitioners and practice nurses. Br J Sports Med 32(3):242–247, 1998 9773175

Mokdad AH, Marks JS, Stroup DF, et al: Actual causes of death in the United States, 2000. JAMA 291(10):1238–1245, 2004 15010446

National Institute of Diabetes and Digestive and Kidney Diseases: Overweight and Obesity Statistics. Bethesda, MD, National Institutes of Health, August 2017. Available at: www.niddk.nih.gov/health-information/health-statistics/overweight-obesity. Accessed May 12, 2018.

Oberg EB, Frank E: Physicians' health practices strongly influence patient health practices. J R Coll Physicians Edinb 39(4):290–291, 2009 21152462

Pinto BM, Goldstein MG, Marcus BH: Activity counseling by primary care physicians. Prev Med 27(4):506–513, 1998 9672943

Pool AC, Kraschnewski JL, Cover LA, et al: The impact of physician weight discussion on weight loss in US adults. Obes Res Clin Pract 8(2):e131–e139, 2014 24743008

Smith AW, Borowski LA, Liu B, et al: U.S. primary care physicians' diet-, physical activity-, and weight-related care of adult patients. Am J Prev Med 41(1):33–42, 2011 21665061

Sullivan AN, Lachman ME: Behavior change with fitness technology in sedentary adults: a review of the evidence for increasing physical activity. Front Public Health 4:289, 2017 28123997

van der Ploeg HP, Smith BJ, Stubbs T, et al: Physical activity promotion—are GPs getting the message? Aust Fam Physician 36(10):871–874, 2007 17925913

Vickers KS, Kircher KJ, Smith MD, et al: Health behavior counseling in primary care: provider-reported rate and confidence. Fam Med 39(10):730–735, 2007 17987416

World Medical Association: WMA Statement on Physicians Well-Being. Ferney-Voltaire, France, World Medical Association, October 2015. Available at: www.wma.net/policies-post/wma-statement-on-physicians-well-being. Accessed May 12, 2018.

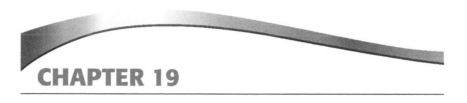

CHAPTER 19

Helping People Find Synergy

The Transformative Potential of Lifestyle Psychiatry

Douglas L. Noordsy, M.D.

Lynn M. Yudofsky, M.D.

KEY POINTS

- Well-being comes from a life that is in balance across multiple lifestyle domains.
- Lifestyle behaviors interact synergistically to reinforce wellness or deteriorate health.
- As people develop dedication to one form of lifestyle behavior (e.g., exercise, meditation), they often develop motivation to improve other lifestyle domains (e.g., nutrition, sleep) to optimize their performance.
- Multimodal lifestyle intervention can help individuals move from targeting an illness to transforming their life and optimizing function.

Throughout this book, you have been learning about evidence regarding the impact of physical exercise, mind-body practices, diet and nutrition, and sleep on the brain and on specific psychiatric disorders. We have also reviewed how to assess lifestyle practices and support people in making behavioral change. The volume of this evidence can be hard for patients and practitioners to keep track of, and new evidence is emerging all the time. Many people have complex disorders with multiple diagnoses and various lifestyle behaviors. In this chapter, we rise above the detail to think about how to help the people you serve achieve more than a simple behavior change—rather, a lifestyle constructed and continually fine-tuned to achieve optimal functioning. In this chapter, we rely on personal and clinical experience more than on data, but it may help to identify useful clinical principles and areas where evidence is needed.

In our experience, many people with psychiatric disorders respond to collaborative lifestyle coaching by making a single lifestyle change or a few changes. Unfortunately, many individuals will periodically lapse into inactivity, staying up too late or overusing substances and then reexperiencing the impact of these behaviors on their well-being. As providers, we help people recognize these relationships and reset goals to maintain their mental well-being and create lasting and sustainable lifestyle changes. As we go through these cycles, we observe whether the individual's underlying belief system and relationship to their behaviors are shifting. We look for openings to raise this question for the patient to consider with us.

The experience of making connections between health-related behaviors and subjective experience may motivate people to expand their behavior change to broad areas of their life in order to achieve an optimal mental state and mind-body balance. This process requires an ability to observe and appreciate relationships between behavior change and subjective experience that unfold slowly over long periods of time; motivation to achieve a sustained, optimal state of mental functioning; an internal locus of control; and a sense of self-efficacy. It may also require a stable, supportive home environment and social network or an ability to create distance from a destructive one.

As we work with people to go beyond specific behavior changes to help resolve identified problems (e.g., exercise and nutrition for an episode of depression), we aim to help them find synergies between interventions and build a vision for self-directed, sustained lifestyle change that can not only resolve the presenting complaint and prevent relapse but also move them to a higher state of well-being. This transformation typically involves patients taking on responsibility for researching and testing ways to expand their health behaviors in multiple domains. We find several consistent themes in this work. Well-being comes from a life that is in balance, and the domains of lifestyle psychiatry help us identify those balance points. However, the journey is personal and unique for each individual.

OBSERVING RELATIONSHIPS

A key step in helping people to move beyond feeling buffeted and overwhelmed by psychiatric symptoms that emerge unexpectedly is to teach individuals how to observe relationships between personal behaviors and subjective state. This process flows naturally from the initial behaviorally focused assessment and can continue throughout care as part of tracking lifestyle interventions and their influence on illness symptoms. The provider takes a curious, nonjudgmental stance, guiding patients in reviewing their health-related behaviors over the prior interval and making connections to symptom severity. For example, consider the temporal relationship between a period of inadequate sleep or inactivity and worsening mood. Consider the potential for two-way or snowballing interactions, such as a night of heavy drinking leading to poor sleep and low motivation, which then leads to inactivity the following day, resulting in lower mood, which may then lead to poor choices about diet and dropping a regular exercise routine, perpetuating the deterioration in sleep and mood. In hindsight, the patient may describe what sounds like a swing into depression with associated impact on sleep and energy. With careful attention to detail, we may disentangle a complex series of interactions that can lead to nuanced awareness of the impact of lifestyle on mood.

This approach can start with simple behavioral observations and experiments. How does the individual feel and function the day after having

6 hours versus 8 hours of sleep? How are concentration and efficiency in school or work after morning exercise? What impacts do nutrition and caffeine have on energy cycles throughout the day? As these relationships build over multiple observations, an appreciation of their interconnections may also emerge. Help the patient to see the synergy that he or she can achieve in combining these effects. Does an efficient day at work allow him or her more time for engagement with family and preparing a nutritious meal without the weight of lingering work tasks?

If approached with a goal of empowerment, the emerging recognition of relationships between health behaviors and experience can be a gift for the patient. It allows people to get ahead of their symptoms rather than being overwhelmed by them. It also allows them to effectively take responsibility for lifestyle management. For example, the individual who has personally observed relationships between his or her health behaviors and mood can more effectively plan a business trip to ensure adequate opportunity for nutrition, exercise, and rest to optimize his or her function, thus reducing anxiety about failure.

WHAT IS A DISORDER AND WHAT IS A TREATMENT?

As people observe connections between their behaviors and their symptoms, a growing recognition of the role of lifestyle in health and well-being often emerges. This creates an opportunity to consider concepts of normality and optimality. Lifestyle is influenced by many social and cultural factors and evolves over time. People may not have considered the lifestyle choices that they make and how these choices influence their health, state of mind, and life satisfaction.

Most psychiatric disorders are defined as a sustained, extreme state of human experience to the degree that they produce distress and functional impairment. Because of a lack of etiological understanding, we define *syndromes* as a cluster of symptoms. Although defining diseases in this way may help with communication, treatment identification, and stigma, it can also create a sense of passive inevitability from the patient's perspective: a *chemical imbalance* happens to you, and then you are depressed. Understanding the impact of lifestyle behaviors on neurotransmitters, cells, and circuits as outlined in the previous chapters of this book can give people an appreciation for some of the environmental and epigenetic contributors to their disorder that may be within their control (Fernandes et al. 2017).

If we consider disease from a lifestyle medicine perspective, we might define a disorder called *physical inactivity syndrome* that includes such symptoms as cardiometabolic dysregulation, depression, insomnia, and cognitive decline. As people observe relationships between their health behaviors and symptoms, it creates an opening to consider the interacting directions of causality in their disorder. What level of physical activity is optimal for humans? What happens to you as an individual when your level of activity falls below a certain point? Is exercise a treatment for your depression, or is it restoring balance in your life?

The point of this approach is not to dismiss the advances of neurobiology, psychotherapy, and pharmacology but rather to engage patients in taking perspective on the limitations of a reductionist view of psychiatric distress and avoiding a "fix it" mentality. As people are able to recognize the role of lifestyle in triggering and perpetuating their symptoms, it may help them to view their experience of disease differently. If positive health behaviors are viewed as helping people restore balance and approach a more evolutionarily adaptive state, then it becomes logical to embrace these behaviors as lifetime wellness choices rather than a time-limited treatment for an episode of disease. This change in perspective may help people appreciate their lifestyle choices as a route to optimizing their performance, function, and life satisfaction.

ENGAGEMENT WITH THE ENVIRONMENT

People who are raised in urban environments have higher risk for developing severe mental illness (Haddad et al. 2015). In contrast, engagement with nature has demonstrated benefits for mood and anxiety (Bowler et al. 2010). Physical exercise creates opportunities for engagement with the natural environment. Going out for a walk or a run comes with opportunities to see the sunrise or notice the phase of the moon, hear birds singing, glimpse a fox or rabbit slipping into the bushes, or smell the fragrance of lilacs or eucalyptus trees. Going into a green space or natural area increases opportunities for encounters with nature. These experiences are grounding. They remind us that our lives are embedded in a larger world, a simpler place where we are not alone.

Noticing the lives of plants and animals may facilitate mindfulness. Stopping to appreciate a beautiful scene naturally pulls us from our thoughts into the present moment and reminds us that there is life all around us. Animals by their nature live quite mindfully, grounded in their senses and attentive to the present moment. Observing animals can provide inspiration for living mindfully and help people to notice the present more fully. The rhythms of the tide, moon, daylight, weather, and seasons provide connection to the natural world when we attend to them.

Many observers have raised concerns about the impact of today's technology-centered lives on mental health. The most direct lifestyle impact of screen time is on prolonged periods of physical inactivity, which is independently associated with poor health outcomes (Beauchamp et al. 2018). Screen time occurs largely indoors and can absorb long periods of time, threatening to create further disconnection from nature. Helping patients plan time in nature and notice the impact that it has on their well-being may help them find synergy and develop rich, satisfying lifestyle habits.

TAKING RESPONSIBILITY

Cultural expectations of medicine have evolved rapidly in the past century. Placebo response rates have risen dramatically over the decades because we expect pills to treat our health problems. Our advanced health care system may inadvertently reinforce passive engagement with health in which the doctor is viewed as a benevolent authority who diagnoses and recommends treatment and the patient's role is to adhere faithfully. Many people are frustrated by chronic diseases that seem to chain them to a life of trips to the doctor, growing medication lists, and periodic procedures. Many providers are also frustrated with the limited efficacy of our treatments for chronic disease.

Most psychiatric disorders are chronic and relapsing in nature, and most psychotropic medications require continued adherence for efficacy and are associated with side effects. Psychiatrists routinely address patients' concerns about continuing treatment. Lifestyle psychiatry offers providers an opportunity to help people assume increasing responsibility for their mental and physical health as they attempt to reduce their reliance on medications and therapy.

In our lifestyle psychiatry clinic, we advise people about the evidence for lifestyle interventions for managing their disorder, and then we craft a plan for making lifestyle changes. An incremental process of discovering what level of exercise, diet, sleep, mindfulness, and medication leads to best symptom management and optimal functioning helps people internalize responsibility for illness self-management. This often creates a shift from viewing lifestyle changes as a necessary evil that limits one's ability to have fun into a powerful, validating force that gives a person the freedom to live well. Some people will take off into lifestyle optimization as an organizing focus of their life. In a culture of instant gratification and automation, lifestyle psychiatry offers an opportunity to engage people in experiential learning about the power of taking personal responsibility for their health and well-being.

ACHIEVING REWARD FROM HEALTHY BEHAVIORS

Although it may take time and dedication to implement changes in one's lifestyle, the payoff is often well worth the effort. Lifestyle changes are uniquely rewarding. The rewards may vary depending on the issues with which the individual is struggling and also the lifestyle change on which one embarks. An individual pursuing these changes may know intellectually that exercising, eating healthfully, and meditating are all "good for you," but the unexpected transformation that occurs is that many individuals begin to notice the benefits these changes have on their bodies, in their minds, and in their lives overall. Some of these benefits may be noticed immediately, and some may take several months to emerge. The rewards may come in various forms; one might be a reduction in psychiatric symptoms, another could be improvement in physical health, and another might be positive reinforcement from important others in their lives.

For example, a person with major depression and type 2 diabetes may notice feeling more energized and being less isolated after engaging in an exercise class with other individuals. This change and realization are both reinforcing and motivating and may inspire the individual to continue to engage in the exercise routine. The more he or she exercises, the longer these effects will persist and the more rewarding they will become. Sleep, appetite, and confidence may simultaneously improve. After consistently engaging in regular exercise, the person may exhibit lasting improvements in mental and physical health. Perhaps the symptoms of depression will remit, and hemoglobin A1c may improve. Family, friends, and health care providers may also take note and comment to the individual on these changes by complimenting his or her efforts, which, in turn, engenders positive reinforcement and motivates continuation of the exercise routine.

Although medications may be an important component of treatment for many people with psychiatric illnesses, the medication, unfortunately, may also be associated with untoward side effects. Depending on the medication, the side effects may include weight gain and metabolic disorder signs and symptoms along with reduced energy level and altered sleep patterns. Lifestyle changes, however, frequently help prevent and even reverse these harmful side effects of medications. As mentioned in other chapters of this book (e.g., Chapter 3, "Physical Exercise in the Management of Major Depressive Disorders," and Chapter 4, "Physical Exercise in the Management of Anxiety Disorders and Obsessive-Compulsive Disorder"), in many cases, medications may no longer be required for those who engage in intensive lifestyle treatment—thereby mitigating potentially harmful medication side effects. Therefore, yet another reward of implementing healthy lifestyle behaviors is that they may decrease or even obviate the need for often costly medications, thereby reducing or eliminating side effects.

CONFIDENCE AND SELF-EFFICACY

People making lifestyle changes may notice that they not only feel better but also feel more confident about their ability to effect other beneficial changes in their lives. As stated in the previous section, medications may be an important and necessary part of treatment for some people. Unfortunately, however, relying exclusively on taking medications daily to treat a mental illness or physical problem instills in some individuals an unwanted sense of dependency instead of self-efficacy. On the other hand, engaging in lifestyle changes is empowering. Implementing healthy behavioral changes can instill a sense of control over symptoms that previously seemed beyond the person's control. An example is a patient with anxiety who begins to engage in yoga. Following the first yoga session, the individual may notice feeling a bit calmer and may experience enhanced self-esteem for embarking on a new intervention. Over time, the person may become a frequent yoga participant as a result of increased strength, prolonged endurance, and enhanced flexibility. The meditative component of yoga may lead to reduced anxiety, improved confidence, and greater self-esteem. Overall, the individual has a greater sense of control and agency in his or her life.

Self-efficacy is a term developed by psychologist Alberto Bandura (1994, p. 71), who wrote, "Perceived self-efficacy is defined as people's beliefs about their capabilities to produce designated levels of performance that exercise influence over events that affect their lives." He theorized that individuals with a high sense of self-efficacy have chosen to take on new challenges rather than avoiding them. When faced with failure, such people use these situations to learn and grow and thereby become resilient. Bandura goes on to say, "Such an efficacious outlook produces personal accomplishments, reduces stress and lowers vulnerability to depression" (Bandura 1994, p. 71). He suggests that there are four main sources of enhanced self-efficacy: 1) personal successes, 2) witnessing others succeed, 3) encouragement and persuasion from external sources, and 4) altering one's negative perception of one's abilities.

For example, the individual who decides to pursue a lifestyle change through engaging in yoga practice is able to increase self-efficacy through these four factors and, in addition, decreases anxiety and improves physical health. The person is surrounded by others in his or her yoga class who may serve not only as role models but also as motivation to continue to do even better. Additionally, the person receives encouragement from many other sources, including from his or her health care professional and the yoga instructor and by experiencing personal success. Low self-esteem and demeaning self-perceptions are thereby combated and reduced.

Making lifestyle improvements may also help reduce the chances of or even prevent relapse. Consider the patient who has pursued yoga and is now experiencing an unexpected stressful life event that previously might have elicited a return of psychiatric symptoms. With the newfound practice of yoga and meditation, that individual may feel more able to control his or her psychiatric symptoms and have more confidence in addressing the other challenges that may be associated with the event. Embarking on, engaging in, and succeeding in make lasting lifestyle changes can instill in individuals an enhanced sense of confidence, increased agency, and improved self-efficacy that equip and enable them to address, cope with, and possibly even overcome their psychiatric symptoms.

SYNERGY

The authors of Chapter 18, "Physician Lifestyle and Health-Promoting Behavior," identified the role of providers' own lifestyle practices in their health coaching behaviors. Lifestyle psychiatry offers you the opportunity to bring the practices that you rely on to maintain your health, and other practices that you may aspire to, into your care of patients. Consider how you discovered and developed the lifestyle practices that work for you and how they interact to achieve life balance and optimal performance in your professional and personal life. Consider the synergies between your health behaviors that magnify their effects. How does your interest in one domain (e.g., meditation, exercise) motivate your engagement in other domains (e.g., nutrition, sleep)?

Developing and supporting patient-driven interest in health-promoting behaviors with evidence, resources, and behavioral techniques can help individuals achieve their highest level of function and recovery while taking ownership of optimally managing their psychiatric disorder. Aiming for this target, regardless of the disorder being treated, facilitates shared responsibility for achieving the best outcomes. Helping people discover the synergies between their lifestyle practices, traditional treatments, sense of self-efficacy, and brain reward responses can be quite gratifying for patients and providers alike.

DISCUSSION QUESTIONS

1. How can you facilitate a patient's growth beyond behavior change for resolving a specific complaint to internal motivation for achieving wellness?
2. What techniques have you found helpful in facilitating self-efficacy among your patients?

3. Do you help your patients strive for optimal function and performance? What techniques are most successful?

RECOMMENDED READINGS

Lake JA, Spiegel D: Complementary and Alternative Treatments in Mental Health Care. Washington, DC, American Psychiatric Publishing, 2007

McDougall C: Born to Run: A Hidden Tribe, Superathletes and the Greatest Race the World Has Hever Seen. New York, Alfred A. Knopf, 2009

Yudofsky SC: Fatal Pauses: Getting Unstuck Through the Power of No and the Power of Go. Arlington, VA, American Psychiatric Publishing, 2015

REFERENCES

Bandura A: Self-efficacy, in Encyclopedia of Human Behavior, Vol 4. Edited by Ramachaudran VS. New York, Academic Press, 1994, pp 71–81

Beauchamp MR, Puterman E, Lubans DR: Physical inactivity and mental health in late adolescence. JAMA Psychiatry 75(6):543–544, 2018 29710114

Bowler DE, Buyung-Ali LM, Knight TM, et al: A systematic review of evidence for the added benefits to health of exposure to natural environments. BMC Public Health 10:456, 2010 20684754

Fernandes J, Arida RM, Gomez-Pinilla F: Physical exercise as an epigenetic modulator of brain plasticity and cognition. Neurosci Biobehav Rev 80:443–456, 2017 28666827

Haddad L, Schäfer A, Streit F, et al: Brain structure correlates of urban upbringing, an environmental risk factor for schizophrenia. Schizophr Bull 41(1):115–122, 2015 24894884

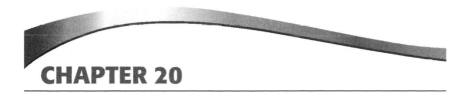

CHAPTER 20

Implications of Lifestyle Medicine and Psychiatry for Health Care Systems and Population Health

Kacy Bonnet, M.D.

Douglas L. Noordsy, M.D.

Keith Humphreys, Ph.D.

KEY POINTS

- Integrated primary lifestyle interventions are effective and could help the health care system become more cost-efficient and satisfying to patients.
- Barriers to lifestyle interventions should be overcome at a systems level.
- A health care system that incentivizes health over treatment and value over volume would drive changes in education and practice priorities.
- Lifestyle interventions can be precisely tailored to subpopulations, are scalable, and have the potential to impact health globally.

COSTS OF OUR CURRENT HEALTH CARE SYSTEM AND THE POTENTIAL IMPACT OF LIFESTYLE INTERVENTIONS

The $3 trillion U.S. health care system has the dubious distinction of being simultaneously unusually expensive yet relatively ineffective at promoting population health and wellness. From 1996 to 2013, inflation-adjusted health care spending increased by nearly a trillion dollars. To put this in perspective, U.S. health care costs now account for 17% of the economy (Dieleman et al. 2016), and expenditures on U.S. health care exceed expenditures on *everything* in France (World Bank Group 2018). This would perhaps be justified if the spending were leading to improvement not only in years lived but also in quality of life. Although life expectancy in the United States has increased over the past several decades, the number of years lived with disability has also increased because of the rising prevalence of chronic health conditions. Cardiovascular disease, diabetes, depression, tobacco use disorder, and anxiety disorders all make the list of diseases that contribute the most to years lived with disability (Murray et al. 2013). Globally, chronic mental health disorders, including substance use disorders, are the leading cause of disability and have increased by 37% from 1900 to 2010 (Whiteford et al. 2013). These conditions lower quality of life, increase psychological distress for individuals and their families, and both initiate and aggravate other chronic conditions.

A system that promotes lifestyle interventions and healthy behavior has the potential to lower health care costs. Many chronic health conditions have a significant behavioral component that lifestyle interventions could modify, thereby improving health and reducing the need for expensive procedures (Sherwood et al. 2016). In addition to advancing a health-promoting public policy environment (e.g., heavily taxing cigarettes, marijuana, and alcohol; including walkability when planning and zoning communities; making health insurance accessible to all), the health care system can play a large part in promoting healthy behavior. The leading modifiable (i.e., not genetic) risk factors for chronic conditions are lifestyle related and include poor dietary patterns; poor stress management; physical inactivity; and use of tobacco, alcohol, and other drugs. According to the Centers for Disease Control and Prevention National Center for Chronic Disease Prevention and Health Promotion report in 2015, chronic disease accounts for 86% of our nation's health care costs, the majority of which can be prevented or cured by lifestyle interventions (Centers for Disease Control and Prevention 2015).

We hope that readers of this chapter will think about what health care could look like if providers used lifestyle interventions as first-line interventions. In the following sections, we touch on how lifestyle-focused care is effective and precise, two pillars that are central to a well-functioning health care system. We then consider the practicalities of a system that focuses on lifestyle and behavior. Last, we discuss some challenges involved in the implementation of a lifestyle-focused system both in the United States and globally.

LIFESTYLE-FOCUSED CARE IS EFFECTIVE CARE

Effective health care is defined as a system that is inclusive of "services that are of proven value and have no significant tradeoffs—that is, the benefits of the services so far outweigh the risks that all patients with specific medical conditions should receive them" (Goodman et al. 2018). This has been shown to be true for lifestyle interventions within cardiovascular medicine: patients who receive supported lifestyle interventions have better outcomes (i.e., fewer cardiac deaths, myocardial infarctions, and bypass surgeries) (Haskell 2003). This is an important concept within health care delivery on the whole because it allows for high-value care to be provided in a sustainable and satisfying way. Physicians are sometimes too quick to turn to expensive and invasive care (e.g., gastric bypass surgery for obesity) rather than prioritizing and sticking with sustained and precise lifestyle care (improved diet and exercise) that is often less expensive. The current health care system tends to focus on pharmaceutical, surgical, and technological interventions while giving less attention to facilitating healthy behaviors, which we know to be effective at preventing chronic disease onset and reducing severity.

Lifestyle interventions are effective because they bring physiological systems back to their nondisease state baseline in ways that are sustainable. Sagner et al. (2014) discussed this concept and explained that if stressors, including unhealthy lifestyle factors, recur and persist, adaptive physiological responses will fail. This leads to dysregulated levels of neurotransmitters, aberrant neural connectivity, and activated cytokines and hormones, which mediate symptoms and pathology. Chronic diseases can thus be understood as conditions in which the body's adaptive capabilities are driven to an imbalanced state, and lifestyle changes can be understood as interventions that prevent or interrupt this dysregulation (McEwen 2012; Sagner et al. 2014). Harnessing the potential of lifestyle interventions and applying them appropriately could thus be very effective for an entire health care system, especially because they are low cost and low risk.

Lifestyle interventions are relatively inexpensive for the health care system because they do not require prescription medications and clinical procedures. They have proven effective in large-scale diabetes management programs (Diabetes Prevention Program Research Group 2012). They are also far less expensive than health care technology, which makes up most of the current health care expenditures (Dieleman et al. 2017). Lifestyle interventions may be necessary to help people establish and maintain healthy behaviors; however, they can be sustained by some individuals without imposing further demands on the health care system. The adage of "give a man a fish, feed him for a day; teach a man to fish, feed him for a lifetime" is apposite here. In the case of lifestyle interventions, teaching a person to fish means inculcating in him or her such practices as daily exercise, balanced nutrition, and mindfulness meditation.

As identified earlier in Part II ("Exercise in the Prevention and Management of Specific Psychiatric Disorders") and Part III ("Healthy Body, Healthy Mind"), diet, exercise, and mind-body interventions most often have moderate effect sizes for psychiatric disorders. Low-cost, low-risk interventions are ideal for first-line treatment when they can effectively treat a substantial proportion of individuals while helping to identify those for whom the risk/benefit ratio of more invasive interventions may be warranted. Lifestyle interventions may also augment the effects of medications and other therapies in individuals with partial response and may be used to replace such treatments for maintenance of remission. When people are successfully restored to balance with a lifestyle intervention, the process often creates recognition of the role of lifestyle decisions in the individual's health and well-being. A lifestyle-focused health care system would track health-related behaviors with an individual throughout his or her lifetime to identify opportunities to fine-tune them for prevention, management of illness, reducing exposure to high-risk procedures, and maintenance of optimal health. A mindset of curating healthy behaviors positions the clinician to monitor lifestyle choices with his or her patients over time, recognizing that people can learn and grow from periods of success and lapses into unhealthy behaviors if approached in a collaborative and motivational fashion. This approach communicates respect for the individual and his or her choices, and as clinicians we find it both gratifying and facilitative of the therapeutic alliance.

LIFESTYLE-FOCUSED CARE: THE ABILITY TO BE PRECISE

Precision medicine is an approach to care that takes "into account individual variability in genes, environment, and lifestyle" and "endeavors to redefine our understanding of disease onset and progression, treatment response, and health outcomes through the more precise measurement of potential contributors" (Gamulin 2016, p. 153). More targeted care can improve outcomes for individuals and populations. It can also encourage appropriate distribution of resources for the most vulnerable, which is ultimately humane and cost-effective for a system of care.

Lifestyle interventions are flexible, and thus, their application can be precisely tailored to an individual or a population. This has been demonstrated by lifestyle interventions within diabetes management, including the National Institutes of Health Diabetes Prevention Program. Of all the intervention arms within the program, lifestyle interventions (specifically, eating less fat and fewer calories and exercising 150 minutes per week) have been translated across diverse populations most successfully and have the most robust effect size, as compared with the use of pharmaceuticals (National Institute of Diabetes and Digestive and Kidney Diseases 2018). Lifestyle interventions can be similarly tailored and equally successful within psychiatry (Firth et al. 2017; Hoffman et al. 2011).

For individual patients within psychiatry, precision care starts when the provider takes a careful and comprehensive history to understand the full range of a patient's health-related behaviors and conceptualization of the patient's choices, as well as barriers to engagement, which might entail a complex interplay between behavior and current environment (Noordsy et al. 2018). This will inform initial recommendations for precision lifestyle interventions. The next step involves getting regular and precise feedback about interventions and outcomes in order to understand what is working and what is not and to reinforce behavior change. Scientists in the field of precision lifestyle medicine refer to this type of practice as using a *small data approach*. Data can be collected, for example, by using activity logs, phone apps, or other recording devices as reviewed in Chapter 17, "Assessment and Behavioral Change Strategies in Clinical Practice."

Large amounts of data (*big data*) can also be aggregated to produce knowledge about the effectiveness of lifestyle interventions for diverse populations and communities. Khoury et al. (2016, p. 400) coined the term *precision public health*, referring to the idea that treatment and prevention strategies can be tailored to specific populations by using public health surveillance, defined as "the systematic, ongoing collection, management, analysis, and interpretation of data to stimulate and guide action." The goal would be to use this knowledge when creating public health policies and campaigns around diet, sleep, weight control, physical activity, and so on, in order to increase reach and effectiveness for the subgroups and populations that are potentially most impacted. If interventions can be precisely tailored to both individuals and groups globally, this would allow for not only optimal engagement but also significantly improved health outcomes.

IMAGINING A NEW SYSTEM

In a health care system that places lifestyle, wellness, and holistic practices at the forefront of care, every practitioner would be versed in the physiological and disease-altering impacts that lifestyle interventions can have, the current evidence for which has been outlined in earlier chapters. According to Sagner et al. (2014, p. 1291), practitioners should "understand lifestyle changes to be the most scientifically valid, clinically effective and achievable treatment possible." Given the need for this change in perspective, education on the role of lifestyle factors in the pathophysiological basis of medical disorders and on lifestyle medicine interventions would likely need to start during medical school and other professional schools and be emphasized throughout residency training and continuing medical education. Some medical schools, including Stanford University, have started to implement this practice by creating courses for their students in lifestyle medicine. Despite not being required, the Stanford Lifestyle Medicine course has been very popular, which speaks to growing interest in this field (Zhou et al. 2017). Studies suggest that education around lifestyle interventions not only is effective for medical trainees but also results in positive impact on patients (see Chapter 18, "Physician Lifestyle and Health-Promoting Behavior," and Malatskey et al. 2017).

Now that we are envisioning a system in which providers are primed to think about diet and exercise as much as pharmaceuticals and interventional technologies, let's imagine what clinical visits might look like. A provider's first goal on evaluation would be to consider all components of a person's life that may contribute to onset and maintenance of his or her disorder and to consider all components of treatment that may be helpful in addressing that condition, including biological, psychological, social, and lifestyle factors. More time would be spent on the assessment of lifetime and current lifestyle practices, including physical activity status, nutrition, stress management, and sleep, than is typically spent in current practice. The encounter would have a consultative, screening, and education focus, with lifestyle behaviors that may be contributing to onset of the disorder identified etiologically and lifestyle interventions being offered on par with other treatment options as supported by evidence.

For example, in evaluating a person with major depressive disorder, the provider might explain the role of inactivity in loss of volume, neuroplasticity, and blood flow in the brain (see Chapter 2, "Physical Exercise and the Brain"). In providing treatment recommendations, the provider might advise that antidepressants and exercise have equal efficacy, and although the effects of antidepressants might be seen sooner, regular exercise may have more sustainable and longer-lasting effects (Chapter 3, "Physical Exercise in the Management of Major Depressive Disorders") Recommendations around lifestyle interventions would be clear and specific—for example, 45 minutes of exercise at least three times a week, a Mediterranean diet with fish oil supplementation, and 8 hours sleep per night—and progress and response that are in line with a patient's goals would be monitored systematically and regularly (Chapter 17). The physician might even consider writing a "prescription" for lifestyle interventions, guidelines for which have already been established in the United Kingdom and in practice in cardiac rehabilitation services there (Seth 2014).

In a system that incentivizes health outcomes, it would be logical to support providers' recommendations for lifestyle change with a multidisciplinary staff and developed infrastructure and by a payment system that reimburses such services. Physicians could be part of a team, including psychologists, social workers, nutritionists, and exercise professionals, who together assume responsibility for providing education and counseling and engaging with patients and families around lifestyle changes. We know that availability of exercise professionals in care settings increases the impact and sustainability of exercise interventions (see Chapter 6, "Physical Exercise in the Management of Schizophrenia Spectrum Disorders"), which would also likely apply to sustained changes in diet with the availability of nutritionists. Clinicians trained in behavior change using the transtheoretical model of change, motivational interviewing techniques, appreciative inquiry, goal-setting theory, acceptance and commitment therapy, cognitive-behavioral therapy for insomnia, and/or the socioecological model (Frates 2017) could enhance outcomes by working with patients on barriers to change. Psychologists or social workers could also be equipped to provide mindfulness training, psychoeducation courses, and group therapy, all of which have evidence for effectiveness in behavior change (Borek and Abraham 2018; Burke and O'Grady 2012).

As you are reading this, you may be thinking, "I have often tried to make lifestyle recommendations, but my patients just do not seem to follow them." Many providers share in this experience and may become discouraged (Abramson et al. 2000). The evidence would suggest, however, that clinician encouragement and prescription of lifestyle intervention does matter. According to several studies, counseling from health care providers can facilitate increased level of physical activity, healthier diet, and general improvement in health outcomes (Lobelo and de Quevedo 2016; Patnode et al. 2017). The discrepancy between providers' perceived inefficacy and the results of several randomized controlled trials suggesting otherwise may be due to limitations in either the provision of counseling or the follow-up by providers regarding behavior changes that patients may have made. Providers' expectations are sometimes too high, and it can be useful to reflect on one's own behavior change efforts (e.g., it took one of the authors of this chapter four attempts over 3 years to completely stop consuming diet soda). Lifestyle change is not a momentary event; it is a process. Tracking and reinforcing adherence to lifestyle interventions, like adherence to other medical interventions, may be important. Although many variables remain untested, one message should be clear: providers can rationally believe in their power to influence lifestyle changes in their patients and need to think seriously about putting this power and privilege to good use.

CHALLENGES TO IMPLEMENTATION AND SUSTAINABILITY OF A LIFESTYLE-FOCUSED SYSTEM IN THE UNITED STATES AND GLOBALLY

So far in this chapter, we have addressed several issues that exist within the current health care system. We also have started to think about a system that emphasizes precise and effective lifestyle interventions. We now discuss some of the challenges of implementation and sustainability of this type of system both in the United States and globally, keeping in mind that challenges evolve over time.

The first and probably the largest barrier to change in the United States is that health care providers and organizations are not incentivized to practice lifestyle medicine. Even now, although providers may wish to counsel their patients on lifestyle interventions, they often avoid doing so because of lack of time and modest reimbursement for personal care (Abramson et al. 2000). The dominant reimbursement model in the current U.S. health care system is fee for service, which incentivizes high-volume, high-cost care rather than optimally effective care. Committed professionals fit lifestyle interventions into their interview and bill for it within the "counseling and coordination" component of their visits.

For lifestyle medicine to be robust, the dominant payment model would need to directly reward value of care—a transformation that would be positive for many other reasons as well. This would mean adopting a system in which providers either are reimbursed with capitated payment for managing a person's health (Porter et al. 2015) or are able to bill more substantially for services that are not procedure based. Similar to Centers for Medicare and Medicaid Services' chronic care management fees, which allow billing for care coordination, billing codes would need to be established for lifestyle interventions, of course based on their impact and clinical outcomes (Chen et al. 2016).

Another model would be to reimburse health care systems on the basis of health outcomes of their patients, specifically incentivizing improved health. The accountable care organization model provides a fixed payment to manage the health care of an individual for a year. To the degree that people remain in an accountable care organization over long periods of time, lifestyle-focused interventions would be cost-effective. The Veterans Health Administration and other health care systems that maintain responsibility for the health care of a population over long periods of time (e.g., Kaiser Permanente) are also settings in which lifestyle interventions could reap long-term health and financial benefits. Specific health outcome–based incentives are yet to be implemented in these settings, however, leading to an emphasis on limiting high-cost care.

There have been efforts to deliver lifestyle-based psychiatric care broadly via the Internet to meet the massive global need (Muñoz and Bunge 2016). Global implementation of a lifestyle-focused system creates challenges, despite the fact that these changes could have significant impact (Katz et al. 2018). Sedentary lifestyle and related diseases are prevalent, and in many places outside the United States, pharmaceuticals and advanced technologies are not readily available, making lifestyle interventions even more important. In 2010, one-third of the world population was characterized as being physically inactive, and 5 million deaths worldwide could be attributed to sedentary behavior (Hallal et al. 2012).

When thinking globally, various cultural and ethical issues merit consideration because they may not have surfaced in trials based primarily in developed countries. In order to translate lifestyle medicine and psychiatry practices into generalizable global practicalities, focus would need to be placed on community-based global participatory research and, as mentioned in the previous section, with data aggregation from large numbers of diverse people. The big data approach brings up many ethical questions around privacy and consent, which is why strong health care partnerships and education of global communities would be essential for developing effective policies and guidelines (Khoury et al. 2016). Health care experts would also need to consider how best to measure the impact of interventions on a global scale. Some options include looking at incidence and prevalence of chronic disease, years lived without disability, subjective reports of health and happiness, and health care costs.

PUTTING IT ALL TOGETHER: A CALL FOR ACTION

For large-scale changes in provision of lifestyle interventions to occur, there would need to be a culture shift among physicians, who are in a unique position to advocate for a health and wellness–oriented system and to influence policymakers. We suggest that current physicians take pause and reflect on whether they would like practicing in this type of system. Do we want to practice in a system that demands more and more of our time without achieving the outcomes that we would wish for our patients? Or is there something different, something better? The system needs to be shaken up (Batalden 2018). What do we define as being within the realm of medical practice? What do our patients expect of health care? Who takes responsibility for health? Consider the possibility of changing diagnostic schemes and starting to think about the problems from a completely different angle. Imagine if obesity and type 2 diabetes were reclassified as *sedentary lifestyle syndrome* or *hypercaloric toxicity*. This etiological approach to defining syndromes can reframe the conceptualization of disease in critically important ways. When defined by relationship to lifestyle behaviors, interventions that focus on exercise, nutrition, sleep, and stress management become inherently logical primary solutions to both patients and providers.

Health care improvement experts W. Edwards Deming and Paul Batalden defined the maxim that "Every system is perfectly designed to get the results it gets" (see www.ihi.org/communities/blogs/origin-of-every-system-is-perfectly-designed-quote). The current U.S. health care system is designed to generate new technology, procedures, and pharmaceuticals at a high volume. This comes at a cost, however, both in a literal and a figurative sense. As we have touched on earlier, the dollar cost is alarming and rising unsustainably. At the same time, people remain impaired by chronic diseases associated with sedentary lifestyle, poor diet, lack of sleep, smoking, alcohol use, and high levels of stress. The rapid rise of Internet-based activities that promote sedentary behavior also raises concern about future trends.

We believe that lifestyle interventions have substantial potential to positively impact the current system. If our health care system were designed with a healthy lifestyle–promoting focus, we imagine that the results it would generate would be much closer to achieving healthier and happier people. As a health care community, we (including *you* after having read this book) have the knowledge and the tools to make changes. The next step is to think broadly and work together to actualize these changes. Please join us in this mission by getting involved in any or all of the following ways:

- *Stay up to date on lifestyle medicine.* The American College of Lifestyle Medicine holds an annual conference and publishes the *American Journal of Lifestyle Medicine,* a peer-reviewed journal for clinicians that provides reviews on lifestyle interventions related to nutrition, cardiovascular disease, obesity, anxiety, depression, insomnia, and more.
- *Engage in continuing medical education (CME).* Courses, webinars, conference dates, and lecture series on lifestyle psychiatry and medicine can now be found at most major CME venues and at www.instituteoflifestyle medicine.org and www.lifestylemedicine.org.
- *Spread the word.* Talk to your colleagues and your patients about lifestyle medicine and test out these principles in your own practice setting.
- *Be an advocate.* Join your local psychiatric or behavioral medicine society's political action committee or make connections with your local legislator and share your ideas about lifestyle medicine and psychiatry with them.

A system that incorporates effective and precise lifestyle interventions and is supported by value-based reimbursement could help address the burden of chronic disease and transform the health of the nation in the twenty-first century. Such a transformation could also improve satisfaction with health care at sustainable cost (Bataldon 2018). This can be accomplished only with the efforts of many. The burgeoning evidence in lifestyle medicine research is promising and compelling. We encourage you to act locally to support your patients in recognizing the full range of contributors to their disease and guide them in achieving a healthful life and to act globally to shape the incentives in the health care systems where you work and beyond.

DISCUSSION QUESTIONS

1. How did your education and training shape your conceptualization of health and disease?
2. How can you shift the education you provide to patients about their disorder to support their understanding of lifestyle factors?
3. Where do you place lifestyle interventions in your sequence of treatment options?
4. Which intervention best fits your definition of precision health for an overweight person with depression: a diet, exercise, and sleep intervention or a selective serotonin reuptake inhibitor and gastric bypass surgery? Which would you want for a family member?
5. What are the overt and covert incentives in your practice setting?
6. How can you shape the health care systems where you work to incentivize positive health outcomes?

RECOMMENDED READINGS

Johnson R, Robertson W, Towey M, et al: Changes over time in mental well-being, fruit and vegetable consumption and physical activity in a community-based lifestyle intervention: a before and after study. Public Health 146:118–125, 2017

Ma J, Rosas LG, Lv N: Precision lifestyle medicine: a new frontier in the science of behavior change and population health. Am J Prev Med 50(3):395–397, 2016

Sagner M, Katz D, Egger G, et al: Lifestyle medicine potential for reversing a world of chronic disease epidemics: from cell to community. Int J Clin Pract 68(11):1289–1292, 2014

REFERENCES

Abramson S, Stein J, Schaufele M, et al: Personal exercise habits and counseling practices of primary care physicians: a national survey. Clin J Sport Med 10(1):40–48, 2000 10695849

Batalden P: Getting more from healthcare: quality improvement must acknowledge patient coproduction. BMJ 362:k3617, 2018 30190297

Borek AJ, Abraham C: How do small groups promote behaviour change? An integrative conceptual review of explanatory mechanisms. Appl Psychol Health Well-Being 10(1):30–61, 2018 29446250

Burke RE, O'Grady ET: Group visits hold great potential for improving diabetes care and outcomes, but best practices must be developed. Health Aff (Millwood) 31(1):103–109, 2012 22232100

Centers for Disease Control and Prevention: At a Glance 2015. Atlanta, GA, National Center for Chronic Disease Prevention and Health Promotion, 2015. Available at: https://stacks.cdc.gov/view/cdc/40074/cdc_40074_DS1.pdf. Accessed November 28, 2018.

Chen CT, Ackerly DC, Gottlieb G: Transforming healthcare delivery: why and how accountable care organizations must evolve. J Hosp Med 11(9):658–661, 2016 27596543

Diabetes Prevention Program Research Group: The 10-year cost-effectiveness of lifestyle intervention or metformin for diabetes prevention: an intent-to-treat analysis of the DPP/DPPOS. Diabetes Care 35(4):723–730, 2012 22442395

Dieleman JL, Baral R, Birger M, et al: US spending on personal health care and public health, 1996–2013. JAMA 316(24):2627–2646, 2016 28027366

Dieleman JL, Squires E, Bui AL, et al: Factors associated with increases in US health care spending, 1996–2013. JAMA 318(17):1668–1678, 2017 29114831

Firth J, Stubbs B, Rosenbaum S, et al: Aerobic exercise improves cognitive functioning in people with schizophrenia: a systematic review and meta-analysis. Schizophr Bull 43(3):546–556, 2017 27521348

Frates B: Lifestyle Medicine Course Syllabus. Woodburn, OR, American College of Lifestyle Medicine, 2017

Gamulin S: The forthcoming era of precision medicine. Acta Med Acad 45(2):152–157, 2016 28000491

Goodman D, Fisher ES, Wennberg JE, et al: The Dartmouth Atlas of Health Care. Lebanon, NH, Trustees of Dartmouth College, 2018. Available at: www.dartmouthatlas.org. Accessed May 5, 2018.

Hallal PC, Andersen LB, Bull FC, et al: Global physical activity levels: surveillance progress, pitfalls, and prospects. Lancet 380(9838):247–257, 2012 22818937

Haskell WL: Cardiovascular disease prevention and lifestyle interventions: effectiveness and efficacy. J Cardiovasc Nurs 18(4):245–255, 2003 14518600

Hoffman BM, Babyak MA, Craighead WE, et al: Exercise and pharmacotherapy in patients with major depression: one-year follow-up of the SMILE study. Psychosom Med 73(2):127–133, 2011 21148807

Katz DL, Frates EP, Bonnet JP, et al: Lifestyle as medicine: the case for a true health initiative. Am J Health Promot 32(6):1452–1458, 2018 28523941

Khoury MJ, Iademarco MF, Riley WT: Precision public health for the era of precision medicine. Am J Prev Med 50(3):398–401, 2016 26547538

Lobelo F, de Quevedo IG: The evidence in support of physicians and health care providers as physical activity role models. Am J Lifestyle Med 10(1):36–52, 2016 26213523

Malatskey L, Bar Zeev Y, Tzuk-Onn A, Polak R: Lifestyle medicine course for family medicine residents: preliminary assessment of the impact on knowledge, attitudes, self-efficacy and personal health. Postgrad Med J 93(1103):549–554, 2017 28289150

McEwen BS: Brain on stress: how the social environment gets under the skin. Proc Natl Acad Sci USA 109(suppl 2):17180–17185, 2012 23045648

Muñoz RF, Bunge EL: Prevention of depression worldwide: a wake-up call. Lancet Psychiatry 3(4):306–307, 2016 26827251

Murray CJ, Atkinson C, Bhalla K, et al: The state of US health, 1990–2010: burden of diseases, injuries, and risk factors. JAMA 310(6):591–608, 2013 23842577

National Institute of Diabetes and Digestive and Kidney Diseases: Diabetes Prevention Program. Bethesda, MD, National Institutes of Health, 2018. Available at: www.niddk.nih.gov/about-niddk/research-areas/diabetes/diabetes-prevention-program-dpp. Accessed on May 29, 2018.

Noordsy DL, Burgess JD, Hardy KV, et al: Therapeutic potential of physical exercise in early psychosis. Am J Psychiatry 175(3):209–214, 2018 29490501

Patnode CD, Evans CV, Senger CA, et al: Behavioral counseling to promote a healthful diet and physical activity for cardiovascular disease prevention in adults without known cardiovascular disease risk factors: updated evidence report and systematic review for the US Preventive Services Task Force. JAMA 318(2):175–193, 2017 28697259

Porter ME, Teisberg EO, Kaplan RS, et al: Curriculum on Value-Based Health Care Delivery. Boston, MA, Harvard Business School, May 2015. Available at: www.isc.hbs.edu/health-care/Documents/2015_05_26_MAH_Curriculum_Overview.pdf. Accessed November 28, 2018.

Sagner M, Katz D, Egger G, et al: Lifestyle medicine potential for reversing a world of chronic disease epidemics: from cell to community. Int J Clin Pract 68(11):1289–1292, 2014 25348380

Seth A: Exercise prescription: what does it mean for primary care? Br J Gen Pract 64(618):12–13, 2014 24567552

Sherwood A, Blumenthal JA, Smith PJ, et al: Effects of exercise and sertraline on measures of coronary heart disease risk in patients with major depression: results from the SMILE-II randomized clinical trial. Psychosom Med 78(5):602–609, 2016 26867076

Whiteford HA, Degenhardt L, Rehm J, et al: Global burden of disease attributable to mental and substance use disorders: findings from the Global Burden of Disease Study 2010. Lancet 382(9904):1575–1586, 2013 23993280

World Bank Group: International Comparison Program Database. Washington, DC, World Bank, 2018. Available at: https://data.worldbank.org/indicator/NY.GNP.MKTP.PP.CD. Accessed on May 28, 2018.

Zhou J, Bortz W, Fredericson M: Moving toward a better balance: Stanford School of Medicine's Lifestyle Medicine course is spearheading the promotion of health and wellness in medicine. Am J Lifestyle Med 11(1):36–38, 2017

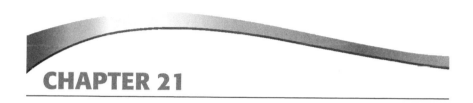

CHAPTER 21

Conclusion

Douglas L. Noordsy, M.D.

IMPLEMENTING LIFESTYLE PSYCHIATRY IN YOUR PRACTICE

This volume was created to prepare psychiatrists and other mental health professionals to deliver lifestyle psychiatry well. As you have seen, the evidence supporting the efficacy of lifestyle interventions in psychiatry is now so robust that clinicians can feel confident recommending them as evidence-based practices for many disorders. Now you have the opportunity to consider how you will incorporate these practices into the care that you deliver. No doubt, you found yourself trying some lifestyle adjustments as you made your way through these chapters. Perhaps you made lifestyle recommendations to your patients or already use some of these interventions in your practice and found support in the current evidence.

Now is the time to consider positioning. How do you decide who might be most likely to benefit from lifestyle interventions? Do you encourage patients to use lifestyle practices as first-line treatment, as part of multimodal therapy, as augmentation for treatment resistance, for maintenance, or to support taper of other treatments? Do you engage patients in shared decision making about their health behaviors? How much attention and detail do you provide to patients about lifestyle interventions relative to other interventions that you employ? How do you track adherence and response to lifestyle interventions over time in subsequent visits?

As academic and political debates grow around the structure and management of our health care system, concepts such as precision health and value-based care are gaining prominence. We are also recognizing the frequency and costs of burnout among health care providers (West et al. 2018). It is perhaps not surprising that lifestyle psychiatry's time has come.

DEFINING THE NEW PSYCHIATRY

As you digest the material in this book, consider the evolution of our field. With decades of biological psychiatry, neuroscience, and advanced imaging techniques, the interface of mind and brain and their contributions to psychiatric disease remains an area of active discovery. This will create ongoing opportunities to optimize the balance between providing expert advice and empowerment of people in their own lifestyle choices as they assume responsibility for their mental health outcomes. The psychiatry of the future must balance advances in genetics, epigenetics, proteomics, and brain biomarkers with strong grounding in lifestyle, health behaviors, and wellness to meet the expectations of consumers and society.

We have an opportunity to provide leadership on health behaviors that can transform public perceptions of mental health and disease. Being a student of lifestyle psychiatry and integrating it skillfully into your practice will prepare you to provide precise, effective, and practical care that will serve you and your patients well, align psychiatry with general medicine, demonstrate integrity, and engender trust. Psychiatry in the twenty-first century can leverage the intersection of neuroscience and behavioral science with technological savvy to approach each individual holistically and engage the power of informed consumers taking ownership of their mental health and wellness. I am confident that having read this volume leaves you better prepared to grasp the opportunities of this exciting time.

REFERENCE

West CP, Dyrbye LN, Shanafelt TD: Physician burnout: contributors, consequences and solutions. J Intern Med 283(6):516–529, 2018 29505159

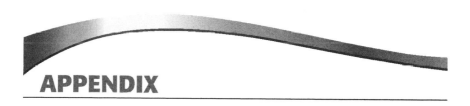

A Guide to Useful Tools for Clinicians

TOOLS INCLUDED IN THE TEXT

Chapter 3

Figure 3–1. Key strategies for counseling patients on exercise as treatment for depression using the 5 As (p. 53). This figure provides a useful mnemonic for guiding progressive behavioral change through the 5 As: ask, advise, assess, assist, and arrange

Chapter 7

Figure 7–1. Borg Rating of Perceived Exertion (p. 122). This rating is a useful guide to use with patients to track the level of exertion during exercise and translate subjective effort into estimated heart rate. The Borg rating × 10 = estimated heart rate.

Chapter 13

Table 13–1. Dietary intake questionnaire (pp. 212–213). This table presents the Mediterranean diet assessment questionnaire used in the Prevención con Dieta Mediterránea (PREDIMED) trials with suggested modifications for use in psychiatric care. This questionnaire is provided in a simple, structured format for assessing quality of diet and tracking improvement over time.

Table 13–2. Dietary recommendations for psychiatric health (pp. 231–232). This table presents evidence-based nutritional guidelines for specific psychiatric disorders that make a quick and easy guide for counseling patients.

Chapter 17

Figure 17–1. Sample template for a personal recovery plan (pp. 311–313). This structured template is designed to help people assess satisfaction with their life in multiple domains, define their vision for recovery, set goals, and track progress toward achieving their goals.

Figure 17–2. Eight ways to practice therapeutic lifestyle changes (p. 315). This practical tool can be used with patients as a therapeutic lifestyle practices diary. It provides a weekly log that patients can use to track their progress in multiple lifestyle domains.

Table 17–1. Guidelines for use of pedometers (p. 319). This table presents a structured guideline for helping people make progressive increases in physical activity using a step tracking device.

RATING SCALES

Simple Physical Activity Questionnaire

The Simple Physical Activity Questionnaire (SIMPAQ) is a structured scale for assessing physical activity specifically designed and validated for people with psychiatric disorders. It was developed by Simon Rosenbaum and Phil Ward at the University of New South Wales in Sydney, Australia. Details can be found at www.simpaq.org. Source: Rosenbaum S, Ward PB: "The Simple Physical Activity Questionnaire." *Lancet Psychiatry* 3:e1, 2016.

Simple Physical Activity Questionnaire (SIMPAQ)

Introduction: I am going to ask you about what you have been doing over the **past seven days**, including time spent in bed, sitting or lying down, walking, exercise, sport and other activities.

1A. What time did you mostly go to bed over the past seven days?
Prompt: between ___ and ___ pm?

Answer: _____ am/pm

1. Average hours in bed per night:

1B. What time did you mostly get out of bed over the past seven days?

Answer: _____ am/pm

2A. That leaves approximately ___ hours a day out of bed. Out of those ___ hours, how long did you spend sitting or lying down, such as when you are eating, reading, watching TV or using electronic devices? *Prompt: e.g. sitting at work, transport, leisure-time or at home.*

Answer: _____ Hours _____ minutes /day

2A. Average hours sedentary per day:

2B. How much of this time is spent napping?

Answer: _____ Hours _____ minutes /day

---

3. That leaves approximately ___ hour a day for other activities. Which days in the past seven days did you walk for exercise or recreation or to get to or from places? How many minutes did you usually spend walking on those days?

Monday	Tuesday	Wednesday	Thursday	Friday	Saturday	Sunday

3. Average hours walking per day:

4A. Now think about any activity that you do for exercise and sport, such as jogging, running, swimming, bike riding, going to the gym, yoga, _____**[e.g. 1]** or _____**[e.g. 2](see manual).** Which days in the past week did you do any of these, or similar activities?

4B What activities did you do and how much time did you spend on each activity on each day?

	Activity and intensity (0-10)	Number of sessions	Minutes	Total
e.g.	Resistance training (5/10); tennis (9/10)	1 ; 1	15; 50	65
Monday				
Tuesday				
Wednesday				
Thursday				
Friday				
Saturday				
Sunday				
	Total			

4. Average hours sport / exercise per day:

---

5 Now think about any other physical activities that you did as part of your work, or activities you did while at home such as gardening or household chores. How many minutes did you spend on these activities on most days? *Prompt: this does not include walking, sport or exercise*

Answer: _____ minutes /day

5. Average hours other activities per day:

Subjective Exercise Experience Scale

The Subjective Exercise Experience Scale (SEES) is an easy-to-use Likert-type rating scale that people can use to record how they feel before and after exercise to track and draw attention to changes in positive well-being (PWB), psychological distress (PD), and fatigue (FAT). It was developed by Edward McAuley and Kerry Courneya at the Exercise Psychology Lab at University of Illinois, Urbana. Details can be found at http://epl.illinois.edu/measures. Source: McAuley E, Courneya, K: "The Subjective Exercise Experiences Scale (SEES): Development and Preliminary Validation." *Journal of Sport and Exercise Psychology* 16:163–177, 1994.

Subjective Exercise Experience Scale

How Do You Feel?

This inventory contains a number of items designed to reflect how you feel at this particular moment in time (i.e., Right Now). Please circle the number on each item that indicates **HOW YOU FEEL RIGHT NOW.**

I FEEL:

1. Great

| 1 | 2 | 3 | 4 | 5 | 6 | 7 |
| not at all | | | moderately | | | very much so |

2. Awful

| 1 | 2 | 3 | 4 | 5 | 6 | 7 |
| not at all | | | moderately | | | very much so |

3. Drained

| 1 | 2 | 3 | 4 | 5 | 6 | 7 |
| not at all | | | moderately | | | very much so |

4. Positive

| 1 | 2 | 3 | 4 | 5 | 6 | 7 |
| not at all | | | moderately | | | very much so |

5. Crummy

| 1 | 2 | 3 | 4 | 5 | 6 | 7 |
| not at all | | | moderately | | | very much so |

6. Exhausted

| 1 | 2 | 3 | 4 | 5 | 6 | 7 |
| not at all | | | moderately | | | very much so |

7. Strong

| 1 | 2 | 3 | 4 | 5 | 6 | 7 |
| not at all | | | moderately | | | very much so |

8. Discouraged

| 1 | 2 | 3 | 4 | 5 | 6 | 7 |
| not at all | | | moderately | | | very much so |

9. Fatigued

| 1 | 2 | 3 | 4 | 5 | 6 | 7 |
| not at all | | | moderately | | | very much so |

10. Terrific

| 1 | 2 | 3 | 4 | 5 | 6 | 7 |
| not at all | | | moderately | | | very much so |

11. Miserable

| 1 | 2 | 3 | 4 | 5 | 6 | 7 |
| not at all | | | moderately | | | very much so |

12. Tired

| 1 | 2 | 3 | 4 | 5 | 6 | 7 |
| not at all | | | moderately | | | very much so |

****

Subjective Exercise Experiences Scale :

PWB $= 1 + 4 + 7 + 10$
PD $= 2 + 5 + 8 + 11$
FAT $= 3 + 6 + 9 + 12$

Noordsy-Dahle Subjective Experience Scale

The Noordsy-Dahle Subjective Experience scale (NDSE) is an easy-to-use rating scale available in both Likert-type and visual analogue formats that people who experience psychosis can use to record how they feel before and after exercise or other lifestyle interventions to track and draw attention to changes in symptoms, energy, and well-being. It was developed by Doug Noordsy and Danielle Dahle at Dartmouth-Hitchcock Medical Center and Stanford University School of Medicine. Source: Ho PA, Dahle DN, Noordsy DL: "Why Do People With Schizophrenia Exercise? A Mixed Methods Analysis Among Community Dwelling Regular Exercisers." *Frontiers in Psychiatry* 9:596, 2018 (open access).

Noordsy-Dahle Subjective Experience scale

How do you feel right now?

Global
how do you feel about your life right now

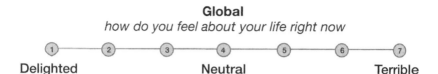

Delighted   Neutral   Terrible

Anxiety
worry, nervousness, fear

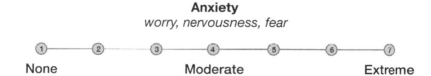

None   Moderate   Extreme

Depression
sadness, hopelessness, worthlessness

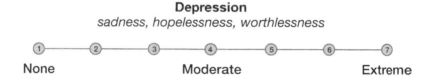

None   Moderate   Extreme

Energy
vigor, strength, power

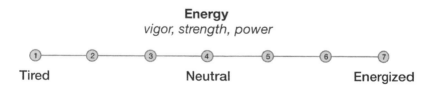

Tired   Neutral   Energized

Hallucinations
voices, direct communications, visions

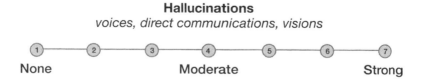

None   Moderate   Strong

Noordsy-Dahle Subjective Experience scale

How do you feel right now?

Delusions
paranoia, suspiciousness

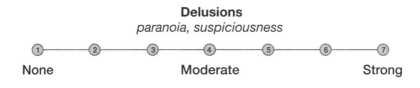

None   Moderate   Strong

Motivation
drive and ambition

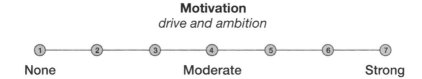

None   Moderate   Strong

Clarity of Thought
clear thinking, not confused

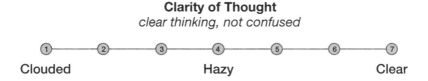

Clouded   Hazy   Clear

Concentration
attention, focus, mental application

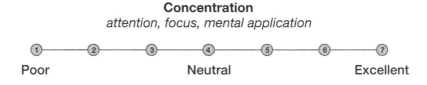

Poor   Neutral   Excellent

Social Interest
prefer to be alone or with others

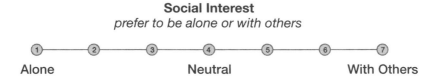

Alone   Neutral   With Others

Index

Page numbers printed in **boldface** type refer to tables and figures.